Bone Marrow Failure Syndromes

Guest Editors

GROVER C. BAGBY, MD
GABRIELLE MEYERS, MD

HEMATOLOGY/ONCOLOGY CLINICS OF NORTH AMERICA

www.hemonc.theclinics.com

April 2009 • Volume 23 • Number 2

SAUNDERS an imprint of ELSEVIER, Inc.

W.B. SAUNDERS COMPANY
A Division of Elsevier Inc.

1600 John F. Kennedy Blvd. • Suite 1800 • Philadelphia, PA 19103-2899

http://www.theclinics.com

HEMATOLOGY/ONCOLOGY CLINICS OF NORTH AMERICA Volume 23, Number 2
April 2009 ISSN 0889-8588, ISBN 13: 978-1-4377-0487-7, ISBN 10: 1-4377-0487-5

Editor: Kerry Holland

Hematology/Oncology Clinics (ISSN 0889-8588) is published bimonthly by Elsevier Inc., 360 Park Avenue South, New York, NY 10010-1710. Months of issue are February, April, June, August, October, and December. Business and Editorial Offices: 1600 John F. Kennedy Blvd., Suite 1800, Philadelphia, PA 19103-2899. Customer Service Office: 11830 Westline Industrial Drive, St. Louis, MO 63146. Periodicals postage paid at New York, NY and additional mailing offices. Subscription prices are $283.00 per year (domestic individuals), $439.00 per year (domestic institutions), $141.00 per year (domestic students/residents), $321.00 per year (Canadian individuals), $537.00 per year (Canadian institutions) $382.00 per year (international individuals), $537.00 per year (international institutions), and $191.00 per year (international and Canadian students/residents). International air speed delivery is included in all *Clinics* subscription prices. All prices are subject to change without notice. **POSTMASTER:** Send address changes to *Hematology/ Oncology Clinics of North America*, 11830 Westline Industrial Drive, St. Louis, MO 63146. Customer Service (orders, claims, online, change of address): Elsevier Periodicals Customer Service, 11830 Westline Industrial Drive, St. Louis, MO 63146. Tel: 1-800-654-2452 (U.S. and Canada). Fax: 314-523-5170. E-mail: journalscustomerservice-usa@ elsevier.com (for print support); journalsonlinesupport-usa@elsevier.com (for online support).

Reprints. For copies of 100 or more, of articles in this publication, please contact the Commercial Reprints Department, Elsevier Inc., 360 Park Avenue South, New York, New York 10010-1710; Tel.: 212-633-3813, Fax: 212-462-1935, E-mail: reprints@elsevier.com.

Hematology/Oncology Clinics of North America is covered in *MEDLINE/PubMed (Index Medicus), EMBASE/ Excerpta Medica, and BIOSIS.*

Printed and bound by CPI Group (UK) Ltd, Croydon, CR0 4YY

Transferred to Digital Print 2011

Contributors

GUEST EDITORS

GROVER C. BAGBY, MD
Professor, Department of Molecular and Medical Genetics; and Department of Medicine, Oregon Health and Sciences University; and Director Emeritus, Knight Cancer Institute at Oregon Health and Sciences University; NW VA Cancer Research Center, VA Medical Center, Portland, Oregon

GABRIELLE MEYERS, MD
Assistant Professor of Medicine, Oregon Health and Sciences University; Hematologic Malignancies Program, Knight Cancer Institute at Oregon Health and Sciences University, Portland, Oregon

AUTHORS

BLANCHE P. ALTER, MD, MPH, FAAP
Clinical Genetics Branch, Division of Cancer Epidemiology and Genetics, National Cancer Institute, National Institutes of Health, Rockville, Maryland

ANDREA BACIGALUPO, MD
Divisione di Ematologia e Trapianto di Midollo Osseo, Ospedale San Martino Largo, Genova, Italy

GROVER C. BAGBY, MD
Professor, Department of Molecular and Medical Genetics; and Department of Medicine, Oregon Health and Sciences University; and Director Emeritus, Knight Cancer Institute at Oregon Health and Sciences University; NW VA Cancer Research Center, VA Medical Center, Portland, Oregon

LAURI BURROUGHS, MD
Clinical Research Division, Fred Hutchinson Cancer Research Center; Acting Professor of Pediatrics, Department of Pediatrics, University of Washington, Seattle, Washington

STEVEN R. ELLIS, PhD
Professor, Department of Biochemistry; and Department of Molecular Biology, University of Louisville, Louisville, Kentucky

NAOHITO FUJISHIMA, MD, PhD
Assistant Professor of Medicine, Division of Hematology, Department of Medicine, Akita University School of Medicine, Akita, Japan

AMY E. GEDDIS, MD, PhD
Assistant Professor, Department of Pediatrics, University of California San Diego, Rady Children's Hospital, San Diego, California

ALLISON M. GREEN, BS
Graduate Student, Section of Pediatric Hematology-Oncology, Department of Pathology, Yale University School of Medicine, New Haven, Connecticut

EVA C. GUINAN, MD
Associate Professor of Pediatrics; and Medical Director, Harvard Catalyst Laboratory of Innovative Translational Technologies; and Director, Harvard Catalyst Linkages Program, Harvard Medical School; Associate Director, Center for Clinical and Translational Research, Dana-Farber Cancer Institute, Boston, Massachusetts

MAKOTO HIROKAWA, MD, PhD
Professor and Chief, Oncology Center, Akita University School of Hospital, Akita, Japan

GARY M. KUPFER, MD
Associate Professor, Section of Pediatric Hematology-Oncology, Department of Pediatrics; and Department of Pathology, Yale University School of Medicine, New Haven, Connecticut

JEFFREY M. LIPTON, MD, PhD
Professor, Elmezzi Graduate School of Molecular Medicine, The Feinstein Institute for Medical Research, Manhasset; Professor, Department of Pediatrics, Albert Einstein College of Medicine, Bronx; Chief, Hematology-Oncology and Stem Cell Transplantation, Schneider Children's Hospital, New Hyde Park, New York

GABRIELLE MEYERS, MD
Assistant Professor of Medicine, Oregon Health and Sciences University; Hematologic Malignancies Program, Knight Cancer Institute at Oregon Health and Sciences University, Portland, Oregon

CHARLES J. PARKER, MD
Professor of Medicine, Division of Hematology and Bone Marrow Transplantation, Department of Medicine, University of Utah School of Medicine, Salt Lake City, Utah

JAKOB PASSWEG, MD
Medicin Chef de Service, Service d'Hematologie, Hopitaux Universitaires de Geneve, Geneva, Switzerland

RAFFAELE RENELLA, MD
Medical Research Council Molecular Haematology Unit, The Weatherall Institute of Molecular Medicine, University of Oxford, John Radcliffe Hospital, Oxford, United Kingdom

SHARON A. SAVAGE, MD, FAAP
Clinical Genetics Branch, Division of Cancer Epidemiology and Genetics, National Cancer Institute, National Institutes of Health, Rockville, Maryland

KENICHI SAWADA, MD, PhD
Professor of Medicine, Division of Hematology; and Division of Nephrology, Department of Medicine, Akita University School of Medicine, Akita, Japan

AKIKO SHIMAMURA, MD, PhD
Clinical Research Division, Fred Hutchinson Cancer Research Center; Associate
Professor of Pediatrics, Department of Pediatrics, University of Washington, Seattle,
Washington

ELAINE M. SLOAND, MD
Senior Clinical Investigator, Hematology Branch, National Heart Lung and Blood Institute,
Bethesda, Maryland

KARL WELTE, MD
Professor of Pediatrics; and Head, Department of Molecular Hematopoiesis, Kinderklinik,
Medizinische Hochschule Hannover, Hannover, Germany

WILLIAM G. WOOD, PhD
Medical Research Council Molecular Haematology Unit, The Weatherall Institute
of Molecular Medicine, University of Oxford, John Radcliffe Hospital, Oxford,
United Kingdom

ANN WOOLFREY, MD
Clinical Research Division, Fred Hutchinson Cancer Research Center; Associate
Professor of Pediatrics, Department of Pediatrics, University of Washington, Seattle,
Washington

CORNELIA ZEIDLER, MD
Department of Molecular Hematopoiesis; and Head, Severe Chronic Neutropenia
Registry, Kinderklinik, Medizinische Hochschule Hannover, Hannover, Germany

Contents

> Acquired severe aplastic anemia can be treated successfully with either immunosuppressive therapy or bone marrow transplantation. Although immunosuppressive therapy can be readily administered to all patients, it is not a curative approach and is associated with a higher risk of clonal evolution than is transplantation, which yields rapid and long-lasting hematologic remission. This article reviews the key diagnostic and prognostic factors that influence the choice of therapy in patients with acquired aplastic anemia.

> In comparison to past decades, children who have acquired aplastic anemia (AA) enjoy excellent overall survival that reflects improvements in supportive care, more accurate exclusion of children who have alternate diagnoses, and advances in transplantation and immunosuppressive therapy (IST). Matched sibling-donor hematopoietic stem cell transplants (HSCT) routinely provide long-term survival in the range of 90%, and 75% of patients respond to IST. In this latter group, the barriers to overall and complication-free survival include recurrence of AA, clonal evolution with transformation to myelodysplasia/acute myelogenous leukemia, and therapy-related toxicities. Improvements in predicting responses to IST, in alternative-donor HSCT, and in rationalizing therapy by understanding the pathophysiology in individual patients are likely to improve short- and long-term outcomes for these children.

> Fanconi anemia (FA) is an autosomal and X-linked recessive disorder characterized by bone marrow failure, acute myelogenous leukemia, solid tumors, and developmental abnormalities. Recent years have seen a dramatic improvement in FA patient treatment, resulting in a greater survival of children into adulthood. These improvements have been made despite the fact that a definitive cellular function for the proteins in the FA pathway has yet to be elucidated. Delineating the cellular functions of the FA pathway could help further improve the treatment options for FA patients and further reduce the probability of succumbing to the disease. This article

reviews the current clinical aspects of FA including presentation, diagnosis, and treatment followed by a review of the molecular aspects of FA as they are currently understood.

Dyskeratosis Congenita 215

Sharon A. Savage and Blanche P. Alter

Dyskeratosis congenita (DC) is an inherited bone marrow failure syndrome characterized clinically by the triad of abnormal nails, reticular skin pigmentation, and oral leukoplakia, and is associated with high risk of developing aplastic anemia, myelodysplastic syndrome, leukemia, and solid tumors. Patients have very short germline telomeres, and approximately half have mutations in one of six genes encoding proteins that maintain telomere function. Accurate diagnosis of DC is critical to ensure proper clinical management, because patients who have DC and bone marrow failure do not respond to immunosuppressive therapy and may have increased morbidity and mortality associated with hematopoietic stem cell transplantation.

Shwachman-Diamond Syndrome: A Review of the Clinical Presentation, Molecular Pathogenesis, Diagnosis, and Treatment 233

Lauri Burroughs, Ann Woolfrey, and Akiko Shimamura

Shwachman-Diamond syndrome is a rare autosomal-recessive, multisystem disease characterized by exocrine pancreatic insufficiency, impaired hematopoiesis, and leukemia predisposition. Other clinical features include skeletal, immunologic, hepatic, and cardiac disorders. This article focuses on the clinical presentation, diagnostic work-up, clinical management, and treatment of patients with Shwachman-Diamond syndrome.

Lineage Restricted Marrow Failure

Diagnosis and Management of Acquired Pure Red Cell Aplasia 249

Kenichi Sawada, Makoto Hirokawa, and Naohito Fujishima

Pure red cell aplasia is a syndrome characterized by a severe normocytic anemia, reticulocytopenia, and absence of erythroblasts from an otherwise normal bone marrow. Although the causes and natural course of this syndrome are variable and although the anemia in some patients can be managed by treatment of an underlying inflammatory or neoplastic disease, the pathogenesis of a large number of cases is autoimmune, including those associated with thymoma, and are best managed with immunosuppressive therapy.

Diamond-Blackfan Anemia: Diagnosis, Treatment, and Molecular Pathogenesis 261

Jeffrey M. Lipton and Steven R. Ellis

Diamond-Blackfan anemia (DBA) is a genetically and clinically heterogeneous disorder characterized by erythroid failure, congenital anomalies, and a predisposition to cancer. Faulty ribosome biogenesis, resulting in proapoptotic erythropoiesis leading to erythroid failure, is hypothesized to be the underlying defect. The genes identified to date that are mutated in DBA all encode ribosomal proteins associated with either the small or large subunit and in these cases haploinsufficiency gives rise to the disease. Extraordinarily robust laboratory and clinical investigations have recently led to demonstrable improvements in clinical care for patients with DBA.

The congenital dyserythropoietic anemias (CDAs) are a heterogeneous group of hereditary disorders that seem to be restricted to the erythroid lineage. They are characterized by morphologic abnormalities of erythroid precursors in the bone marrow, resulting in ineffective erythropoiesis and a suboptimal reticulocyte response. As with many rare disorders, cases of CDA are often misdiagnosed, which may lead to inappropriate management. In this review, the authors highlight the relevant clinical data together with recent molecular advances that should aid decision making in diagnosis and patient management.

Congenital neutropenia (CN) is a genetically heterogeneous bone marrow failure syndrome characterized by a maturation arrest of myelopoiesis at the level of the promyelocyte/myelocyte stage with peripheral blood absolute neutrophil counts below 0.5×10^9/L. From early infancy patients who have CN suffer from bacterial infections. Leukemias occur in both the autosomal dominant and recessive subtypes of CN. The individual risk for each genetic subtype needs to be evaluated further, because the number of patients tested for the underlying genetic defect is still limited. Acquired G-CSFR (CSF3R) mutations are detected in approximately 80% of patients who had CN and who developed acute myeloid leukemia, suggesting that these mutations are involved in leukemogenesis.

Thrombocytopenia in the neonate usually is acquired but in rare cases may be caused by a congenital disorder. This article summarizes the diagnosis, pathophysiology, and management of two congenital inherited platelet disorders that present in the newborn period: congenital amegakaryocytic thrombocytopenia and thrombocytopenia with absent radii.

Marrow Failure and Evolution of Neoplastic Clones

This article discusses the etiology of paroxysmal nocturnal hemoglobinuria (PNH) and its relationship to marrow hyperplasia. The author posits that the defining clinical pathology of PNH (ie, complementmediated intra-vascular hemolysis) is an epiphenomenon that is a consequence of an orchestrated response (ie, natural selection of *PIGA*-mutant stem cells) to a specific type of bone marrow injury (ie, immune mediated). Management of PNH is discussed also.

Myelodysplasia must be considered in the differential diagnosis of patients who have bone marrow failure, but bone marrow cellularity per se may not substantially affect either response to therapy or prognosis. It is unclear whether the primary pathophysiologic defect differs between hyper- and hypoplastic patients who have myelodysplasia. Cellularity does not seem to affect response to immunosuppressive therapy significantly and does not seem to be the major factor affecting improvements in response to lenalidomide, stem cell transplantation, or hematopoietic growth factors.

Patients who have acquired and inherited bone marrow failure syndromes are at risk for the development of clonal neoplasms including acute myeloid leukemia, myelodysplastic syndrome, and paroxysmal nocturnal hemoglobinuria. This article reviews the evidence supporting a model of clonal selection, a paradigm that provides a reasonable expectation that these often fatal complications might be prevented in the future.

RELATED INTEREST
Pediatric Clinics of North America, February 2008 (Vol. 55, No. 1)
Pediatric Oncology
Max J. Coppes, MD, PhD, MBA and Jeffrey S. Dome, MD, *Guest Editors*

THE CLINICS ARE NOW AVAILABLE ONLINE!

Access your subscription at:
www.theclinics.com

Preface

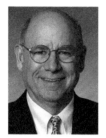 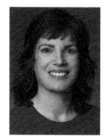

Grover C. Bagby, MD   Gabrielle Meyers, MD
Guest Editors

Before new methodologies allowed such theories to be directly tested, leaders in academic hematology argued about whether marrow injury was a manifestation of external environmental factors or some intrinsic defect in hematopoietic stem cells. As tools that permitted functional studies on stem cells and progenitor cells from mice and humans were developed, it became clear that pathophysiological defects leading to marrow failure can be found either in the stem cells themselves or in the microenvironment in which they reside. Indeed, recent studies on some of these conditions have demonstrated that marrow failure may be the result of interactions of a sick environment with a sick stem cell.

The pathophysiologies and molecular genetics resulting in some of the constitutional marrow failure syndromes are heterogeneous, and, consequently, management strategies differ from subtype to subtype. Therefore, a critical first step in the approach to treating a patient who has bone marrow failure is to establish a proper diagnosis. For this reason, this issue focuses a good deal of attention on this aspect of bone marrow failure syndromes. In the section of global bone marrow failure, there are two articles on acquired aplastic anemia and three on inherited marrow failure syndromes that must be considered in differential diagnosis, particularly in younger patients. While these are rare conditions, failure to rule them out may lead to the use of inappropriate and possibly harmful therapies. For example, treatment of patients who have Fanconi anemia with routine conditioning regimens for stem cell transplantation will result in excessive morbidity and mortality. Therefore, when hematologists meet pancytopenic patients whose bone marrow biopsies show hypocellularity, these inherited disorders must be considered in the interest of the patient and his or her family. In the section on lineage-specific marrow failure, one article on acquired red call aplasia and four articles on inherited diseases are presented. The molecular pathogenesis and treatment of these conditions are distinctly different.

Now that the genes underlying many of these disorders have been identified, there are more questions than answers about pathophysiology. Some dysfunctions are shared, at least ontologically. For example, cells from patients who have dyskeratosis congenita, Diamond-Blackfan anemia, and Shwachman-Diamond syndrome share the common features of disordered ribosome biogenesis. Nonetheless, how these common features lead to a holistic picture of hematopoietic control remains unclear.

Hematol Oncol Clin N Am 23 (2009) xiii–xiv
doi:10.1016/j.hoc.2009.02.001
0889-8588/09/$ – see front matter © 2009 Elsevier Inc. All rights reserved.

There are three reasons that marrow failure syndromes are of interest to hematologists and oncologists. First, understanding hematopoietic control from immunological and molecular genetic points of view standpoints ultimately will lead to better and safer treatments. Second, patients who have these rare syndromes commonly evolve to acute leukemia. Indeed, in some of them (Fanconi anemia and dyskeratosis congenita), the relative risk is nearly 900. Consequently, these tragic disorders provide an important opportunity to identify very early somatic mutations that occur in a leukemic stem cell. As argued in the final article on leukemogenesis, understanding how somatic mutations promote clonal evolution may provide opportunities to intervene and perhaps prevent leukemia in patients at high risk. Finally, epithelial malignancies occur at a high rate in patients who have some of these syndromes, so the considerations on hematopoietic cells also may apply to populations of vulnerable epithelial stem cells in these syndromes. It is increasingly clear that the genes mutated in some of these disorders can be inactivated somatically in neoplastic cells from patients who have sporadic cancers.

The authors assembled for this issue represent an international group of leaders in the field, all of whom deal with the science and human sides of these diseases. We are convinced that readers will find that the advances described herein are exciting and contain lessons of real importance for managing patients. Some of the diseases covered here are categorized as "orphan diseases," but the clinical consequences of ignoring them in one's differential diagnosis can be devastating. The potential impact of science focused on these diseases is enormous, particularly for the fields of mammalian development, hematopoiesis, and carcinogenesis.

Grover C. Bagby, MD
NW VA Cancer Research Center
VA Medical Center Portland
R&D2, Building 103, E221B
3710 SW Veteran's Hospital Road
Portland, OR 97239, USA

Gabrielle Meyers, MD
Center for Hematologic Malignancies
Oregon Health and Sciences University
3181 SW Sam Jackson Park Road
Mail Code UHN73C
Portland, OR 97239, USA

E-mail addresses:
grover@ohsu.edu (G.C. Bagby)
meyersg@ohsu.edu (G. Meyers)

Diagnosis and Treatment of Acquired Aplastic Anemia

Andrea Bacigalupo, MD[a],*, Jakob Passweg, MD[b]

KEYWORDS

- Antithymocyte globulin • Hemopoietic stem cell transplantation
- Bone marrow failure • Cyclosporine • Growth factors

The clinical symptoms of acquired aplastic anemia (AA) depend on the degree of cytopenia and on the time required for it to develop. Severe cytopenia may cause fever, bleeding, and life-threatening infections: often these are young patients, otherwise healthy, sometimes with a preceding history of a recent febrile illness, and occasionally following an episode of elevated serum transaminases with or without cholestasis. These patients require immediate high-intensity care, with appropriate transfusions and antimicrobial therapy and HLA-typing if under the age of 40. An episode of sepsis or a cerebral hemorrhage can be fatal in the first weeks of presentation for these acute patients.

When the cytopenia is less severe, patients are in better clinical condition, and they may also be asymptomatic. Some of these patients are seen by their general practitioner for mild cytopenia, and eventually demonstrate declining peripheral blood counts with time, often over a period of many months. At that point, and especially when their anemia requires red blood cell (RBC) support, they may be referred to the hematologist, who starts a thorough work-up.

DIAGNOSIS

The diagnostic criteria of acquired AA have been defined, and require an empty or hypoplastic marrow, with peripheral blood cytopenia. Severe AA (SAA) is present when patients meet at least two of the following criteria: and absolute neutrophil count less than $0.5 \times 10^9/L$, platelet count less than $20 \times 10^9/L$, or reticulocytes less than $20 \times 10^9/L$.

The diagnosis of acquired AA also requires the exclusion of other conditions associated with pancytopenia, however, among these congenital marrow failure syndromes, such as Fanconi anemia, and myelodysplastic syndromes (MDS) or

[a] Divisione di Ematologia e Trapianto di Midollo Osseo, Ospedale San Martino Largo, Rosanna Benzi 10, Genova 16132, Italy
[b] Service d'Hematologie, Hopitaux Universitaires de Geneve, Geneva, Switzerland
* Corresponding author.
E-mail address: andrea.bacigalupo@hsanmartino.it (A. Bacigalupo).

Hematol Oncol Clin N Am 23 (2009) 159–170
doi:10.1016/j.hoc.2009.01.005
0889-8588/09/$ – see front matter © 2009 Published by Elsevier Inc.

hemonc.theclinics.com

leukemia. Fanconi anemia can be suspected by examining the patient, especially if a child or a teenager, and can be excluded by a chromosomal breakage test using either peripheral blood lymphocytes or dermal fibroblasts exposed to di-epoxibutane or mitomycin C.[1]

Fanconi anemia cells show excessive stress-induced chromosomal breakage. This test is not only of value in children with bone marrow failure, but also young adults can be found to have Fanconi anemia. Some rarer congenital marrow failures, without specific markers, can be more difficult to exclude. These disorders are discussed in detail elsewhere in this issue. MDS can be ruled out by appropriate marrow cytology-histology and cytogenetic analysis, and the same is true for acute leukemia. The distinction between Fanconi anemia, MDS, and AA is important, because treatment is different in these three conditions. Clonal cytogenetic anomalies alone, if the presentation is otherwise typical of AA it is not sufficient to diagnose hypoplastic MDS. Such cases should be treated along the guidelines established for AA (discussed elsewhere in this issue). In the presence of an empty marrow, pancytopenia, and transfusion dependence, the severity of the disease is based on neutrophil (polymorphonuclear [PMN]) count: nonsevere AA (PMN >0.5 × 10^9/L); SAA (PMN 0.2–0.5 × 10^9/L); very SAA (vSAA) (PMN <0.2 × 10^9/L). As will be seen, this may no longer be the case with current treatment strategies.

PAROXYSMAL NOCTURNAL HEMOGLOBINURIA

Paroxysmal nocturnal hemoglobinuria (PNH) in its classic hemolytic form is quite different from AA: patients have a full marrow, with erythroblastic hyperplasia, and white blood cell and platelet counts are normal. In addition, patients complain of episodes of nocturnal hemoglobinuria with dark gray urine in the morning and their ferritin levels are low, because of urinary losses. The expression of glycosyl-phosphatidylinositol on the surface of granulocytes, monocytes, lymphocytes, and erythrocytes is deficient or lacking in classic PNH patients. Some AA patients may have a deficient expression of glycosyl-phosphatidylinositol–liked antigens, however, without hemolysis and without hemoglobinuria: these patients are referred to as "AA-PNH." It is important to recognize these two different clinical settings, because classic PNH and AA-PNH are treated differently: the former may be eligible for eculizumab therapy[2] or allogeneic stem cell transplantation.[3] The latter is treated like any other patients with acquired AA. Several reports have suggested that the presence of a so called "PNH-clone" (a small percentage of cells with defective glycosyl-phosphatidylinositol–associated antigens) is a favorable prognostic predictor for response to immunosuppressive therapy (IS).[4] PNH is reviewed in more detail elsewhere in this issue.

TREATMENT OF ACQUIRED APLASTIC ANEMIA
Supportive Care

Before discussing definitive treatment of acquired AA, one should first consider supportive care. This depends on the severity of cytopenia, and may include RBC transfusions, platelet transfusions, antibiotics, antifungal agents, and antiviral therapy. RBC transfusions should be filtered to decrease the likelihood of alloimmunization and reduce the incidence of viral infection. Whether irradiation of blood products is necessary is not known; many centers do provide irradiated blood products to these patients while undergoing IS treatment and stem cell transplantation. Although it is unlikely that RBC transfusion causes graft-versus-host disease, nevertheless irradiated blood products have been shown to reduce alloimmunization in prospectively transfused animals.[5] Candidates for an allogeneic transplant may benefit from a program of irradiated RBC and platelet transfusions. Antimicrobial therapy depends on the severity of neutropenia and on the presence of symptoms and signs of infection: one should, however, consider the fact that AA patients may present after a history of neutropenia or may face a long period of neutropenia. In these conditions fungal infections, and especially invasive aspergillosis, are known to correlate with the duration of neutropenia, and should warrant the initiation of an early therapy with mold-active drugs. Appropriate transfusion support and antimicrobial treatment may be essential in the early phases of diagnosis and treatment planning. Most centers also provide anti–herpes virus prophylaxis. The use of growth factors is equally controversial; whereas granulocyte colony–stimulating factor (G-CSF) may be of use in neutropenic infections the uncritical use of growth factors may also delay the initiation of appropriate therapy.

Designing a Treatment Strategy

As a general rule treatment is indicated when peripheral blood counts drop to levels that call for RBC or platelets transfusions. Patients with moderate cytopenia not requiring transfusions, also referred to as "hypoplastic anemia," should be followed closely to ascertain whether there is deterioration with time. During this first period they can be offered supportive care or outpatient treatment with anabolic steroids or low-dose steroids or cyclosporin (CsA). Recently, androgens have been shown to increase telomerase activity in human CD34$^+$ cells and this may provide an explanation for their effect, sometimes striking, in patients with AA.[6] This is in keeping with a trial showing increased responses in the group of patients randomized to receive androgens together with IS therapy.[7]

Patients with cytopenia requiring transfusions should be treated as inpatients, with either IS therapy or bone marrow transplantation (BMT), and decision to start treatment should not be delayed, because this may significantly impact on the chance of success.[8] The choice between these two latter treatments is based on severity of the disease and patient age: young patients (<20 years) with vSAA are candidates for first-line transplantation. Older patients with moderate disease are generally offered IS therapy as initial therapy.[9]

IMMUNOSUPPRESSIVE TREATMENT
Combination Therapy

Treatment with antithymocyte globulin (ATG) yields superior survival when compared with supportive care.[6,10] Combinations of ATG with androgens[7] or CsA[11] improves the overall response rates but does not improve survival. The update of the German study comparing ATG + CsA with ATG alone shows a difference in event-free survival, indicating that patients receiving ATG alone required additional courses of IS, as compared with patients receiving ATG + CsA; however, survival at 15 years was comparable.[12] Event-free survival is a relevant outcome, because it indicates survival without transfusions and without additional courses of ATG, and this is relevant for quality of life.[12] The median time to achieve a response is 120 days,[13] and a second treatment should not be planned earlier than 4 months after the initial ATG treatment. Responses can be subdivided into complete and partial: the former requires normal blood counts, although some reports indicate complete response as patients with a hemoglobin greater than 10 G/dL, a PMN count greater than 2×10^9/L, and platelets greater than 100×10^9/L.[13] Partial responses require at least transfusion independence. The probability of becoming transfusion independent varies from 40% to 80% according to the IS regimen and the patient population.

Horse Versus Rabbit Antithymocyte Globulin

Both horse ATG and rabbit ATG have been used successfully in patients with acquired AA.[6] The standard first-line IS treatment is currently horse ATG + CsA and second-line treatment is rabbit ATG + CsA, although the latter has been successfully used also as first-line therapy.[14,15] The infusion of ATG may cause allergic reactions, but with appropriate premedication with steroids or antihistamines, and appropriately slow infusion (up to 24 hours for each dose), almost all patients can complete the prescribed total course of ATG, usually lasting 5 days. ATG does have a first dose effect probably related to cytokine release by lymphocytes and it is a common error to stop treatment for "intolerable" fever and rigors. Infections, hemorrhages, and fever are not an absolute contraindication for treatment with ATG: although these antibodies make cytopenia worse in the first weeks, they should be considered as necessary therapy, just as chemotherapy is required for leukemic patients presenting with cytopenia. In a recent analysis, patients treated beyond the median interval between diagnosis and IS of 23 days have significantly greater risk of failing in multivariate analysis.[8]

Cyclosporin Dependence and Relapse

Current IS regimens including CsA call for full CsA dose (5 mg/kg/d orally) for 6 months; after this time point CsA is tapered, and it is unclear exactly when and how fast this should be done. A recent study of the Italian pediatric group has addressed these two questions. Forty-two children were divided into three groups: (1) very slow tapering (<0.3 mg/kg orally); (2) slow CsA tapering (0.4–0.7 mg/kg orally); and (3) rapid tapering ($\geq$0.8 mg/kg orally). The cumulative incidence of relapse was 8% in the slow–very slow taper group and 60% in the rapid-taper group.[16] Among patients who eventually discontinued CsA, the median duration of CsA treatment at full therapeutic dose (4–6 mg/kg) was 12 months (range, 3–45) and tapering was completed in a median of 19 months (range, 4–64 months). In that study the actuarial probability of discontinuing CsA was 21% at 5 years, 38% at 7 years, and 60% at 10 years, respectively.[17] This study suggests that it is safe to start tapering CsA at 12 months of treatment (rather than 6), and that tapering should be very slow (less than 10% of the dose per month) for at least 1 year to minimize the risk of relapse. Other groups do, however, taper CsA more rapidly and the issue has to be considered as open. Furthermore, little data are available on appropriate drug levels in this disease.

Relapse

Relapse is defined as a patient requiring transfusions of RBCs or platelets after having been independent from transfusion for at least 3 months.[17] The risk of relapse in the pre-CsA era was 35% and was not easily predicted;[17] in a recent Japanese prospective study the risk of relapse was significantly higher in patients receiving ATG + CsA (42%) compared with patients receiving ATG + CsA and G-CSF (15%) ($P = .01$),[18] although 4-year survival was not significantly different (88% versus 94%).[18] This indicates that response can be achieved after hematologic relapse, with an additional course of ATG.[17,19]

Growth Factors

The use of G-CSF has been described in conjunction with ATG and CsA as first-line treatment.[14] The potential advantages of using G-CSF are faster neutrophil recovery,[20] and the opportunity to test for white blood cell increments and to predict early responses and early failures.[14] The authors have recently confirmed that achieving a white blood cell count of $5 \times 10^9/L$ while receiving G-CSF in the first 3 months is predictive of response and survival. Patients who do not achieve a white blood cell count of $5 \times 10^9/L$ have a 72% chance of not responding, a 79% probability of failing primary therapy, and an 84% risk of death.[21] The use of G-CSF allows early identification of nonresponders and early referral for BMT.

The use of daily G-CSF for 4 months, however, has drawbacks. Such treatment is costly and survival was not improved in G-CSF patients in two prospective randomized trials.[18,20] Interestingly, both randomized trials showed no difference in the risk of late clonal disorders in patients receiving or not receiving G-CSF.[18,20] This is in contrast to a retrospective European study showing a borderline increased risk for G-CSF patients,[21] and the Japanese retrospective study also showing increased risk of clonal disorders.[22] A correlation was also found between duration of exposure to G-CSF and clonal disease.[22] The cause-effect relationship is unclear, however, because nonresponders to IS are more likely to develop clonal disorders,[14] and prolonged G-CSF is given precisely to these patients. A third randomized study has been completed by the European Group for Blood and Marrow Transplantation (EBMT) and will be analyzed in the next months. Finally, a further increase of G-CSF to 10 μg/kg/d failed to show any advantage over the conventional 5 μg/kg/d.[23]

Clonal Evolution and Second Malignancies

There are several possible evolutions of the disease that may or may not have to do with its etiology, pathogenesis, and treatment. The appearance or the increase of glycosyl-phosphatidylinositol–negative subpopulations or the evolution toward frank PNH, with increasing levels of L-lactate dehydrogenase, and increasing spleen volume, may be confirming the link between the two disorders.[3] The appearance of cytogenetic clonal abnormalities (eg, trisomy 8) may suggest a pre-existence clone at diagnosis, or the emergence of a +8 clone during stressed hematopoiesis. Some AA cases may proceed to develop frank acute leukemia. The overall risk of developing a clonal cytogenetic abnormality and MDS at 10 years is set between 5% and 20%, and may well depend on the degree of response to IS.[14] An important contribution to this problem was a study by the EBMT published in 1993,[24] comparing second malignancies in patients with AA treated with either IS or BMT. The risk of MDS and acute myelogenous leukemia was significantly higher for IS as compared with BMT patients, suggesting that MDS and acute myelogenous leukemia follows IS treatment, rather than being present at diagnosis: this is because cyclophosphamide (CY), 200 mg/kg, used in transplantation, is unlikely to eradicate a neoplastic clone. Second tumors (especially of the mouth) were frequent in patients receiving radiation before BMT. This is why currently HLA-identical sibling transplants should not receive standard dose radiation. Very low dose (2 Gy) total body radiation (TBI) is being explored in patients undergoing an alternative donor transplant.[25] The factors that may play a pathophysiologic role in clonal evolution in patients with marrow failure states are reviewed elsewhere in this issue.

Factors Predicting Response to Immunosuppressive Therapy

The importance of predicting response is relevant for every disease, but in AA patients, pancytopenia has acute consequences, with daily risk of blood-borne infections or cerebral hemorrhages, and this makes predictive factors very important. In a recent study on almost 1000 patients treated in Europe between 1991 and 2002, the strongest negative predictor was age (>16 years) (RR 1.76, $P = .0009$), followed by an IS protocol other than ATG + CsA (RR 1.29, $P = .02$) and interval between diagnosis and treatment over 23 days (RR 1.32, P = .04).[8] The year of IS treatment (before or after 1997) had a borderline negative effect,[8] suggesting little overall improvement in this last 5 years. Of interest is the fact that severity of the disease, as identified by PMN counts (<0.2, 0.2–0.5, >0.5 × 10^9/L), had no impact on survival, in contrast with results from the original 1988 analysis of the EBMT, showing that PMN count was the strongest predictor of survival.[26] Results have improved dramatically especially in children with vSAA, from 37% in the 1980s to 83% in the 1990s,[8] but this has not been the case for SAA and actually the non-SAA patients showed a trend for worse outcome.[8] Currently, survival can be predicted by age: the 10-year actuarial survival is 73% for patients less than 20 years, 75% for patients aged 21 to 30, 66% for patients aged 31 to 40, and 47% for patients aged over 40 years.

Immunosuppressive Therapy for Older Patients

The author have analyzed the outcome of older patients treated with ATG and cyclosporin:[27] the actuarial 10-year survival was 80% for patients aged 0 to 20 and 21 to 50, it was 45% for patients aged 51 to 70, and it was 25% for patients over the age of 70.[27] Nevertheless, the standardized mortality ratio, indicating the ratio between mortality of patients and of an age-matched population, is 33, 14, and 9, respectively, for the age group less than 50, 50 to 70, and greater than 70.[27] These data suggest that the corrected risk of death is highest in young patients and gets progressively lower with increasing age.

Pregnancies After Immunosuppressive Therapy

Counseling a young woman in remission following IS about the risks of pregnancy is a difficult task. There is only one study of relevance from the EBMT, and it demonstrates that successful pregnancy is possible, but the risk of relapse is approximately 20%. In that study, one of the relapses was fatal.[28] Relapses were more frequent in partial responders as compared with complete responders. If a young woman is in complete remission, off therapy, and is informed about the risk of relapse of the disease, and if she wishes to become pregnant, she can be counseled that a pregnancy is possible.

BONE MARROW TRANSPLANTATION

It is well known that young patients grafted from an HLA-identical sibling have the best outcome, when compared with older patients allografted from alternative donors. A recent study on 1567 patients has confirmed these results: significant predictors of survival were year of transplant greater than 1997, matched sibling donor, age less than 16 years, interval between diagnosis and transplant of less than 83 days, and a conditioning regimen without radiation.[8]

HLA-Identical Siblings

The current survival of children (<16 years) receiving a BMT from an HLA-identical sibling is 91%, and it is 74% for patients older than 16 years.[8] This is true for patients receiving CY, 200 mg/kg, and a BMT. A recent EBMT/IBMTR report suggests that the use of peripheral blood as a stem cell source reduces survival when compared with bone marrow in patients less than 20 years from 85% to 73%, and in patients greater than 20 years from 64% to 52%.[29] The major cause of excess mortality in the peripheral blood arm was chronic graft-versus-host disease. This study would not recommend peripheral blood as a stem cell source in patients with acquired AA, possibly because an increased incidence of chronic graft-versus-host disease does not benefit aplastic patients in the way it might benefit patients with leukemia. A suitable marrow cell dose is recommended, because results of transplantation are highly dependent on the number of nucleated cells infused.[30] CY alone remains the best conditioning regimen for young patients, and ATG seems to reduce the risk of graft failure,[31] although a recent randomized trial has shown some advantage, but no significant difference in survival.[32] The combination of CsA and methotrexate seems to offer a survival advantage over CsA alone (84% versus 75%) used for graft-versus-host disease prophylaxis.[33] Standard CY, 50 mg/kg/d × 4, with 3 days of ATG conditioning, followed by unmanipulated marrow as a stem cell source and CsA and methotrexate as graft-versus-host disease prophylaxis is still standard of care for young patients with acquired AA undergoing an HLA-identical sibling transplant. The use of radiation, peripheral blood, or other conditioning regimens should all be tested in prospective trials, because of their unproved benefit for the patient.

HLA-Identical Bone Marrow Transplantation for Patients Over 30 Years

Notwithstanding the excellent results with a standard BMT in AA, there is still a strong age effect: the actuarial 10-year survival for patients grafted from HLA-identical siblings in the last decade is, respectively, 83%, 73%, 68%, and 51% for ages 1 to 20 (N = 681), 21 to 30 (N = 339), 31 to 40 (N = 146), and 40 and older (N = 111) (R. Oneto, unpublished EBMT data, 2008). Unfortunately, the use of peripheral blood as a stem cell source not only did not solve the problem, but outcome was actually worsened.[29] The authors have explored the use of low-dose CY (30 mg/m^2 × 4) in combination with low-dose fludarabine (FLU) (30 mg/m^2 × 4) and ATG in patients over the age of 30. The initial results are encouraging, with transplant mortality occurring in 30%, but more patients need to be accrued (S. Maury, unpublished EBMT data, 2008). There have been three reports in the literature confirming that the combination FLU-CY produces a high rate of engraftment and very encouraging survival.[34–36] The median age of these patients was actually younger than 30, and the dose of CY higher (60–120 mg/kg), but this new regimen, which derives from the original experience of the Houston group,[37] seems very encouraging.

Unrelated Donor Transplants

The outcome of unrelated donor transplants for patients with AA has improved in the last decade.[38,39] Better selection of HLA matched donors has probably played a major role, but also significant changes in the conditioning regimen have occurred.[25,40,41] The first of these studies tested de-escalating doses of radiation, from 6 Gy down to 2 Gy, and concluded for best results for patients receiving 2 Gy, with 8 of 13 patients surviving.[40] The Japanese study reported 154 SAA patients undergoing an unrelated donor transplant, most receiving 3 Gy TBI:[25] unfavorable factors for survival were older age (>20); conditioning without ATG; and a long (>3 years) interval from diagnosis to transplant. The EBMT study tested a nonradiation-based program:[41] results were overall encouraging with 70% surviving, although rejection was high in young adults over the age of 14. The EBMT is currently testing a conditioning regimen that is very similar to the Japanese regimen: FLU-CY-ATG and low-dose TBI (2 Gy) (A. Bacigalupo, unpublished EBMT data, 2008).

As a consequence of less toxic conditioning regimens and improved donor-recipient matching, survival has almost doubled in the past decade[8,38] from 38% in 1991 to 1996 to 65% in the period 1997 to 2002,[8] and in the latter period survival after unrelated donor transplants in children is 75% versus 63% for adults greater than 16 years of age.[38] Results of unrelated donor transplants have improved to such an extent that treatment strategy may be affected: in children without a matched sibling donor, an unrelated donor search should be started at diagnosis, and transplantation should be seriously considered after one course of IS in the presence of a suitable donor. In young adults between 20 and 30 the same may be true. Adults over the age of 30 should be entered on a prospective trial. Alternative donor transplant is an option for second-line treatment in patients failing one or two courses of IS treatment.

Cord Blood Transplants

A proportion of patients does not have a matched donor in the family, and cannot find a suitable unrelated donor in the world wide network (bone marrow donors world wide). The percentage of these patients who lack a donor varies between 5% and 40%, according to the ethnic origin of the patient. Cord blood transplants is an alternative option that has been successfully explored in patients with hematologic malignancies.[42] Because of the high rate of rejection in AA patients and the low cell numbers of cord blood units, transplants of unrelated cord blood has usually been discouraged in this setting. A recent study from the Japanese group,[43] however, reports 31 cord blood transplants with an overall survival of 42%, but a more encouraging 80% survival for patients receiving the FLU-CY-TBI 2-Gy combination as a conditioning regimen. Cord blood may not be the first option in AA patients lacking a family donor, but some investigators are exploring this stem cell source, and results may be encouraging with appropriate cell dosing, double units, alternative routes of administration, and new conditioning regimens.

FIRST-LINE THERAPY

Table 1 summarizes first- and second-line therapy. First-line therapy is identical in patients up to the age of 40: BMT from identical sibling if available, ATG + CsA if

Table 1 Summary of first- and second-line treatment in patients with severe or very severe acquired aplastic anemia			
	First-Line Treatment	Second-Line Treatment	Other
<20 y, sibling donor	Sibling BMT	—	—
<20 y, no sibling donor	ATG + CsA MUD search	MUD transplant CB transplant Second ATG + CsA	—
20–40 y, sibling donor	Sibling BMT	—	—
20–40 y, no sibling donor	ATG + CsA MUD search	Second course ATG + CsA MUD transplant	Third course ATG MUD transplant
>40 y, sibling donors	ATG + CsA	Sibling BMT	—
>40 y, no sibling donor	ATG + CsA	Second course ATG + CsA MUD search	MUD transplant Third course ATG
Relapse after response to ATG + CsA	ATG + CsA	MUD transplant	—
No response to two courses of ATG + CsA, and no donor	—	—	Supportive care Experimental IS BMT from an alternative donor

Abbreviations: ATG + CsA, Antithymocyte globulin and cyclosporine; BMT, Bone marrow transplantation; CB, Cord blood; IS, Immunosuppression; MUD, Matched unrelated donor.

> **Box 1**
> **Management of acquired aplastic anemia**
>
> 1. Establish correct diagnosis
> 2. Initiate early supportive care
> 3. Perform HLA typing of patient and family members early
> 4. Activate search for an unrelated donor, when a family donor is not available
> 5. Treat early with either BMT or IS
> 6. Do not stop ATG treatment simply because of allergic reactions
> 7. Enter patients in innovative prospective trials

an identical sibling not available. Second-line therapy, however, differs: young patients (<20 years) may proceed to matched unrelated donor BMT, whereas older patients (>20 years) should probably receive a second course of IS, and continue the search for an unrelated donor. An alternative donor transplant can be considered, however, also in patients over the age of 40, if there is heavy transfusion requirement and one believes that further IS may only be delaying a transplant. Over the age of 40 a sibling transplant is usually second line, and matched unrelated donor transplant third line. Patients relapsing after remission from ATG + CsA should receive one course of IS therapy. Patients refractory to two courses of ATG may be entered in prospective protocols testing new agents or experimental transplant procedures.

SUMMARY

Acquired SAA can be treated successfully with either IS therapy or BMT (**Box 1**). Although IS can be readily administered to all patients, it is not a curative approach. In contrast, BMT produces rapid and long-lasting hematologic recovery, without the long-term risk of MDS, but requires a suitable donor and carries the risk of transplant-related mortality.

Survival after BMT from HLA-identical siblings in young patients exceeds 90%, after a conventional CY conditioning, and unmanipulated bone marrow, which is still preferred over peripheral blood as a stem cell source. In some countries patients come to stem cell transplant with a heavy transfusion burden, and highly sensitized. The conditioning regimen may need to be modified in this situation, with the addition of low-dose TBI or low-dose busulfan. Similarly, BMT in patients over the age of 30 may require changes in the conditioning regimen, such as the combination of FLU-CY-ATG. This combination together with low-dose TBI has become the standard regimen for alternative donor transplants in Europe and Japan and is being tested in the United States. The excellent result calls for an unrelated donor search, early in the course of the disease. Age remains a major predictor and requires careful consideration when deciding the treatment strategy.

If one chooses to start with IS therapy, then ATG + CsA remains the preferred first-line combination. For IS patients, age and interval from diagnosis are two major predictors, whereas a low neutrophil count is no longer a negative indicator. This is because of the improved outcome in vSAA patients treated with combined ATG + CsA, but not in patients with less severe AA. The advantage of giving G-CSF, together with ATG + CsA, has been disputed by two randomized trials. In patients responding to IS, CsA should be tapered very slowly over a period of 1 year. Finally, a short interval between diagnosis and treatment is associated with better results so patients should be referred promptly to experienced centers. In addition, AA is a rare disease and patients should participate in well-designed prospective clinical trials.

REFERENCES

1. Bagby GC, Alter BP. Fanconi anemia. Semin Hematol 2006;43(3):147–56, Review.
2. Hillmen P, Young NS, Schubert J, et al. The complement inhibitor eculizumab in paroxysmal nocturnal hemoglobinuria. N Engl J Med 2006;355:1233–43.
3. Luzzatto L, Bessler M, Rotoli B. Somatic mutations in paroxysmal nocturnal hemoglobinuria: a blessing in disguise? Cell 1997;88:1–4.
4. Sugimori C, Chuhjo T, Feng X, et al. Minor population of CD55-CD59- blood cells predicts response to immunosuppressive therapy and prognosis in patients with aplastic anemia. Blood 2006;107:1308–14.
5. Bean MA, Graham T, Appelbaum FR, et al. Gamma-irradiation of pretransplant blood transfusions from unrelated donors prevents sensitization to minor histocompatibility antigens on dog leukocyte antigen-identical canine marrow grafts. Transplantation 1994;57(3):423–6.
6. Young NS, Calado RT, Scheinberg P. Current concepts in the pathophysiology and treatment of aplastic anemia. Blood 2006;108:2509–19.
7. Bacigalupo A, Chaple M, Hows J, et al. Treatment of aplastic anemia (AA) with antilymphocyte globulin (ALG) and methylprednisolone (MPred) with or without androgens: a randomized trial from the EBMT SAA working party. Br J Haematol 1993;83:145–51.
8. Locasciulli A, Oneto R, Bacigalupo A, et al. Severe Aplastic Anemia Working Party of the European Blood and Marrow Transplant Group. Outcome of patients with acquired aplastic anemia given first line bone marrow transplantation or immunosuppressive treatment in the last decade: a report from the European Group for Blood and Marrow Transplantation (EBMT). Haematologica 2007;92:11–8.
9. Bacigalupo A, Brand R, Oneto R, et al. Treatment of acquired severe aplastic anemia: bone marrow transplantation compared with immunosuppressive therapy: the European Group for Blood and Marrow Transplantation experience. Semin Hematol 2000;37:69–80.
10. Camitta B, O'Reilly RJ, Sensenbrenner L, et al. Antithoracic duct lymphocyte globulin therapy of severe aplastic anemia. Blood 1983;62:883–8.
11. Frickhofen N, Heimpel H, Kaltwasser GP, et al. Antithymocyte globulin with or without cyclosporine A: 11-year follow-up of a randomized trial comparing treatments of aplastic anemia. Blood 2003;101:1236–42.
12. Viollier R, Passweg J, Gregor M, et al. Quality-adjusted survival analysis shows differences in outcome after immunosuppression or bone marrow transplantation in aplastic anemia. Ann Hematol 2005;84:47–55.
13. Bacigalupo A, Bruno B, Saracco P, et al. Antilymphocyte globulin, cyclosporine, prednisolone, and granulocyte colony-stimulating factor for severe aplastic anemia: an update of the GITMO/EBMT study on 100 patients. Blood 2000;95:1931–4.
14. Kojima S, Frickhofen N, Deeg HJ, et al. Aplastic anemia. Int J Hematol 2005;82:408–11.
15. Di Bona E, Rodeghiero F, Bruno B, et al. Rabbit antithymocyte globulin (r-ATG) plus cyclosporine and granulocyte colony stimulating factor is an effective treatment for aplastic anaemia patients unresponsive to a first course of intensive immunosuppressive therapy. Br J Haematol 1999;107:330–4.

16. Saracco P, Quarello P, Iori AP, et al. Bone Marrow Failure Study Group of the AIEOP (Italian Association of Paediatric Haematology Oncology). Cyclosporin A response and dependence in children with acquired aplastic anaemia: a multi-centre retrospective study with long-term observation follow-up. Br J Haematol 2008;140:197–205.

17. Schrezenmeier H, Marin P, Ragavachar A, et al. Relapse of aplastic anaemia after immunosuppressive treatment: a report from the European Bone Marrow Trans-plantation Group SAA Working Party. for the EBMT SAA Working Party. Br J Hae-matol 1993;85:371–7.

18. Teramura M, Kimura A, Iwase S, et al. Treatment of severe aplastic anemia with antithymocyte globulin and cyclosporin A with or without G-CSF in adults: a multi-center randomized study in Japan. Blood 2007;110(6):1756–61.

19. Tichelli A, Passweg J, Nissen C, et al. Repeated treatment with horse antil-ymphocyte globulin for severe aplastic anaemia. Br J Haematol 1998;100:393–400.

20. Gluckman E, Rokicka-Milewska R, Hann I, et al. Results and follow-up of a phase III randomized study of recombinant human-granulocyte stimulating factor as support for immunosuppressive therapy in patients with severe aplastic anaemia. Br J Haematol 2002;119:1075–82.

21. Socie G, Mary JY, Schrezenmeier H, et al. Granulocyte-stimulating factor and severe aplastic anemia: a survey by the European Group for Blood and marrow Transplantation (EBMT). Blood 2007;109:2794–6.

22. Ohara A, Kojima S, Hamajima N, et al. Myelodysplastic syndrome and acute myelogenous leukemia as a late clonal complication in children with acquired aplastic anemia. Blood 1997;90:1009–13.

23. Locasciulli A, Bruno B, Rambaldi A, et al. Treatment of severe aplastic anemia with anti-lymphocyte globulin, cyclosporine and two different granulocyte colony stimulating factor regimens: a GITMO prospective randomized study. Haemato-logica 2004;89:1054–61.

24. Sociè G, Henry-Amar M, Bacigalupo A, et al. Malignant tumors occurring after treatment of aplastic anemia. N Engl J Med 1993;329:1152–7.

25. Kojima S, Matsuyama T, Kato S, et al. Outcome of 154 patients with severe aplas-tic anemia who received transplants from unrelated donors: the Japan Marrow Donor Program. Blood 2002;100:799–803.

26. Bacigalupo A, Hows J, Gluckman E, et al. Bone marrow transplantation (BMT) versus immunosuppression (IS) for the treatment of severe aplastic anemia (SAA): a report of the EBMT SAA working party. Br J Haematol 1988;70:177–81.

27. Tichelli A, Socié G, Henry-Amar M, et al. Effectiveness of immunosuppressive therapy in older patients with aplastic anemia. European Group for Blood and Marrow Transplantation Severe Aplastic Anaemia Working Party. Ann Intern Med 1999;130:193–201.

28. Tichelli A, Socié G, Marsh J, et al. for the European Group for Blood and Marrow Transplantation Severe Aplastic Anaemia Working Party. Outcome of pregnancy and disease course among women with aplastic anemia treated with immunosup-pression. Ann Intern Med 2002;137:164–72.

29. Schrezenmeier H, Passweg JR, Marsh JC, et al. Worse outcome and more chronic GVHD with peripheral blood progenitor cells than bone marrow in HLA-matched sibling donor transplants for young patients with severe acquired aplastic anemia: a report from the European Group for blood and marrow trans-plantation and the Center for International blood and marrow transplant research. Blood 2007;110(4):1397–400.

30. Niederwieser D, Pepe M, Storb R, et al. Improvement in rejection, engraftment rate and survival without increase in graft-versus-host disease by high marrow cell dose in patients transplanted for aplastic anaemia. Br J Haematol 1988;69: 23–8.

31. Storb R, Leisenring W, Anasetti C, et al. Long-term follow-up of allogeneic marrow transplants in patients with aplastic anemia conditioned by cyclophosphamide combined with antitymocyte globulin. Blood 1997;89:3890–1.

32. Champlin RE, Perez WS, Passweg JR, et al. Bone marrow transplantation for severe aplastic anemia: a randomized controlled study of conditioning regimens. Blood 2007;109:4582–5.

33. Locatelli F, Bruno B, Zecca M, et al. Cyclosporin A and short-term methotrexate versus cyclosporin A as graft versus host disease prophylaxis in patients with severe aplastic anemia given allogeneic bone marrow transplantation from an HLA-identical sibling: results of a GITMO/EBMT randomized trial. Blood 2000; 96:1690–7.

34. George B, Methews V, Viswabandya A, et al. Fludarabine and cyclophosphamide based reduced intensity conditioning (RIC) regimens reduce rejection and improve outcome in Indian patients undergoing allogeneic stem cell transplantation for severe aplastic anemia. Bone Marrow Transplant 2007;40(1): 13–8.

35. Srinivasan R, Takahashi Y, McCoy JP, et al. Overcoming graft rejection in heavily transfused and allo-immunised patients with bone marrow failure syndromes using fludarabine-based haematopoietic cell transplantation. Br J Haematol 2006;133(3):305–9.

36. Resnick IB, Aker M, Shapira MY, et al. Allogeneic stem cell transplantation for severe acquired aplastic anaemia using a fludarabine-based preparative regimen. Br J Haematol 2006;133(6):649–53.

37. Khouri IF, Lee MS, Romaguera J, et al. Allogeneic hematopoietic transplantation for mantle-cell lymphoma: molecular remissions and evidence of graft-versus-malignancy. Ann Oncol 1999;10:1293–9.

38. Maury S, Balere-Appert ML, Chir Z, et al. French Society of Bone Marrow Transplantation and Cellular Therapy (SFGM-TC). Unrelated stem cell transplantation for severe acquired aplastic anemia: improved outcome in the era of high-resolution HLA matching between donor and recipient. Haematologica 2007;92: 589–96.

39. Viollier R, Socié G, Tichelli A, et al. Recent improvement in outcome of unrelated donor transplantation for aplastic anemia. Bone Marrow Transplant 2008;41(1): 45–50.

40. Deeg HJ, Amylon ID, Harris RE, et al. Marrow transplants from unrelated donors for patients with aplastic anemia: minimum effective dose of total body irradiation. Biol Blood Marrow Transplant 2001;7:208–15.

41. Bacigalupo A, Locatelli F, Lanino E, et al. Severe Aplastic Anemia Working Party of the European Group for Blood and Marrow Transplantation. Fludarabine, cyclophosphamide and anti-thymocyte globulin for alternative donor transplants in acquired severe aplastic anemia: a report from the EBMT-SAA Working Party. Bone Marrow Transplant 2005;36:947–50.

42. Gluckman E, Rocha V. History of the clinical use of umbilical cord blood hematopoietic cells. Cytotherapy 2005;7(3):219–27.

43. Yoshimi A, Kojima S, Taniguchi S, et al. Japan Cord Blood Bank Network. Unrelated cord blood transplantation for severe aplastic anemia. Biol Blood Marrow Transplant 2008;14(9):1057–63.

Acquired Aplastic Anemia in Childhood

Eva C. Guinan, MD[a,b,*]

KEYWORDS

- Aplastic anemia • Immunosuppression
- Stem cell transplantation • Marrow failure • Pediatric

Acquired aplastic anemia (AA) is a relatively infrequent, albeit dramatic, disorder. Although the absence of both a single diagnostic test and centralized registries (in most countries) confound this determination somewhat, the reported all-age incidence ranges from 1 to 4 per million with significant geographic heterogeneity. Although fewer pediatric-specific incidence data are available, AA in children seems to demonstrate the same propensity for higher rates in Asia; for example, the rate in children in Germany has been reported at 2 per million annually, in comparison to a rate of 4.6 per million reported from South Korea.[1,2] Although some differences between adult and pediatric patients (eg, HLA-DR2 frequency in affected individuals[1] and the import of certain potential prognostic variables[3]) have been reported, no consistent distinctions of therapeutic relevance have been well delineated. The diagnostic evaluation of children does require greater attention to the recognition of potential inherited syndromes resulting in marrow failure. These inherited syndromes are reviewed in other articles in this issue. Moreover, the substantial survival advantage of younger patients after hematopoietic stem cell transplantation (HSCT) and their projected at-risk time for late side effects of therapy mandate a somewhat different diagnostic and therapeutic approach.

DEFINITION

There is no single diagnostic test for acquired AA. The term, in principle, defines a final common clinical phenotype that probably results from a number of different, and potentially convergent, pathophysiologies. Several conventions, differing slightly in their specifics, have been used to characterize those diagnostic criteria. Nonetheless

[a] Harvard Catalyst Laboratory of Innovative Translational Technologies, Harvard Catalyst Linkages Program, Harvard Medical School, 25 Shattuck Street, Boston, MA 02115, USA
[b] Center for Clinical and Translational Research, Dana-Farber Cancer Institute, 44 Binney Street, Boston, MA 02115, USA
* Center for Clinical and Translational Research, Dana-Farber Cancer Institute, 44 Binney Street, Boston, MA 02115.
E-mail address: eva_guinan@dfci.harvard.edu

Hematol Oncol Clin N Am 23 (2009) 171–191
doi:10.1016/j.hoc.2009.01.011
0889-8588/09/$ – see front matter © 2009 Elsevier Inc. All rights reserved.

hemonc.theclinics.com

the minimal requirement for diagnosis is pancytopenia in the setting of a hypocellular bone marrow (BM) biopsy without infiltration or fibrosis. Perhaps the most broadly applied additional criteria are documentation of at least two of the following: (1) hemoglobin lower than 10 g/dL, (2) platelet count lower than 50×10^9/L, or (3) neutrophil count lower than 1.5×10^9/L. Acquired AA also is classified usefully by its severity (**Table 1**); at least two similar conventions are in common use for this classification.[4,5] The absolute neutrophil count (ANC) is the discriminator most generally used to make the additional classification of severity (**Table 2**). Which ANC (eg, the count at the onset of pancytopenia, the count at the date of diagnosis, or the count at the date of treatment) is used for this determination is variable, however, leading to potential ambiguity in both the classification and its prognostic value. The literature on acquired AA in childhood generally refers to children who have severe or very severe disease; the implications of moderate disease are significantly different, and these differences highlight the need to scrutinize the characteristics of the patient being treated and the population being reported.

PATHOPHYSIOLOGY

Numerous reviews include detailed discussions of the pathophysiology of acquired AA,[6–10] but there has been little success in elucidating the definitive inciting event in most cases.[10] Large epidemiologic studies and smaller case series have implicated exposures to certain drugs (eg, gold),[11] chemicals (eg, benzene),[12,13] and specific infections (eg, Epstein-Barr virus)[14] as either causative or associated with increased risk. Other than altering the use patterns or the monitoring associated with various pharmaceuticals, such results have done little to provide prognostic or managerial assistance to care providers. In contrast, the clinical observation that AA seemed to respond to immunosuppressive therapy (IST) provided the impetus for subsequent investigations of pathophysiology. The demonstration of various immune mechanisms involved in generating an autoimmune physiology has led to significant therapeutic insights.[9,15–28] Both antigen-specific and nonspecific immune mechanisms of marrow suppression or cytotoxicity have been reported. Peripheral blood (PB) T cells, BM T

Table 1 Classification of aplastic anemia according to severity	
Severity	**Criteria**
Severe	Bone marrow cellularity <25%[a] AND at least two of the following: Peripheral blood neutrophil count <0.5 × 10⁹/L Peripheral blood platelet count <20 ×10⁹/L Peripheral blood reticulocyte count <20 × 10⁹/L
Very severe	Same criteria as severe, but peripheral blood neutrophil count <0.2 × 10⁹/L
Nonsevere	Decreased bone marrow cellularity AND Peripheral blood cytopenias do not fulfill the criteria for severe or very severe aplastic anemia

[a] Or 25%–50%, if residual hematopoietic cells are <30%.

Data from Bacigalupo A, Hows J, Gordon-Smith EC, et al. Bone marrow transplantation for severe aplastic anemia from donors other than HLA identical siblings: a report of the BMT Working Party. Bone Marrow Transplant 1988;3:531–5; and Camitta BM, Thomas ED, Nathan DG, et al. Severe aplastic anemia: a prospective study of the effect early marrow transplantation on acute mortality. Blood 1976;48(1):63–9.

Table 2
Criteria for response after immunosuppressive therapy for severe aplastic anemia in children

Response Category	Criteria
No response	Criteria for severe AA remain fulfilled
Partial response	Criteria for severe AA do not remain fulfilled Does not require transfusion support
Complete response	Hemoglobin normal for age and gender Absolute neutrophil count >1.5 × 10^9/L Platelet count >150 × 10^9/L Does not require transfusion support

cells, and stroma from many AA patients secrete increased quantities of interferon-γ that effectively and nonspecifically inhibit hematopoiesis.[28–33] Over-representation of selected polymorphisms in cytokine genes and genomic-wide transcriptional analysis of T-cell subsets further support the involvement of antigen-independent, innate immune mechanisms in AA.[34–36] Recently, a transcription factor, T bet, that binds to the interferon-γ promoter, was found to be up-regulated in T cells from most patients who have AA.[37] Antigen specificity of the T-cell populations in AA (and other marrow failure disorders) has been demonstrated by the use of molecular clonotypic analyses to identify oligoclonal CD4+ and CD8+ T-cell populations whose frequency can, in some cases, be demonstrated to fluctuate in concert with response to immunosuppressive therapy.[25,38–40] HLA class II–restricted cytolysis of autologous hematopoietic cells can be demonstrated in T-cell clones from some patients who have AA.[41] Evidence for an auto-antigen–specific immune diathesis also is suggested by the finding in some patients, including children, of antibodies to various auto-antigens expressed in primitive hematopoietic cells.[42–44] In concert with findings in a growing number of autoimmune diseases, a deficiency of T-regulatory cells has been described in the majority of patients who have AA.[45]

In vitro studies also have demonstrated that individuals who have AA seem to have numerically and functionally deficient hematopoietic progenitors in both PB and BM, as determined by various criteria, and this finding persists in virtually all individuals regardless of treatment response.[46–48] Indeed, it is likely that some individuals who have AA have an underlying genetic predisposition to marrow failure. The best-described such mechanism is excess telomere shortening. Hematopoietic stem cells, which are a highly proliferative tissue compartment, maintain telomere integrity (and thereby avoid apoptosis) via the telomerase ribonucleoprotein complex. Abnormal telomere shortening in hematopoietic cells has been observed in some patients who have acquired AA, suggesting both that excess proliferation of the limited cell pool and defects in any of the many genes now understood to participate in telomerase and telomere maintenance might have a role in the etiology of AA.[49] In fact, such mutations now have been found, albeit infrequently, in adults and children who have idiopathic AA or in their unaffected family members.[50–52] Additional genes active in the protection of telomere length have been identified since these studies were performed, so it is possible that the incidence is slightly higher than so far depicted. Whether such individuals simply represent the failures of the current diagnostic armamentarium for inherited disorders or whether they represent, in part, a spectrum of predisposing genetic phenotypes who have encountered an inciting event with resultant acquired marrow failure is unknown. In a recent report, fully 20% of children who seemed to have inherited BM failure could not be diagnosed with a specific disorder by any available clinical, histopathologic, laboratory, or genetic criteria.[53] In concert with the growing recognition that patients who have clearly defined myelodysplasia (MDS) have the capacity to respond to IST, such results highlight the remaining gaps in the present understanding of the pathophysiology of marrow failure in general and in specific cases.

DIFFERENTIAL DIAGNOSIS

Given the divergent therapeutic paths for children who have marrow failure of different etiologies, it is critical to exclude as completely as is possible other diagnoses in patients fulfilling the diagnostic criteria. There are many excellent compendia of the wide variety of potential causes of pancytopenia in children and in the general population.[10,54,55] In summary, potential nutritional, metabolic, and infectious conditions should be considered, as should toxic (including pharmacologic) exposures. Viral and other infections may account for as many as 10% to 20% of children presenting with pancytopenia; many such cases may go on to demonstrate recovery.[56] Although most such epidemiologic components of the differential diagnosis are seen across the entire age spectrum, there are some exposures for which children may be at increased risk. For example, there is a peak in the diagnosis of seizure disorders in childhood, and several epilepsy drugs have been associated with marrow failure.[57] There is some suggestion that children may be biologically predisposed to such idiosyncratic reactions.[58] Similarly, the disorder anorexia nervosa has a peak incidence in adolescence and can be accompanied by a quite common macrocytic anemia and by pancytopenia and marrow hypoplasia.[59,60] These examples highlight the need to consider the differential in an age-specific fashion.

Another diagnosis to be considered is paroxysmal nocturnal hemoglobinuria (PNH), a disease marked by gene mutations leading to a deficiency of glycosyl-phosphatidy-linositol (GPI)-linked proteins on the cell surface. This disorder is reviewed in detail in the article by Parker in this issue. At present, the flow cytometric evaluation of peripheral blood for the presence or deficiency of GPI-anchored proteins at the cell surface is the best diagnostic test.[61] These findings can be confirmed if necessary by performing an aerolysin assay, in which toxin binds to and kills GPI-expressing cells with sparing of PNH+ (ie, GPI-deficient) cells.[62] Because immature myeloid cells are relatively deficient in some GPI-linked proteins, such confirmation occasionally is indicated.[61] Nonetheless, a positive test result does not indicate a diagnosis of classic PNH. In fact, cells deficient in GPI-linked protein have been detected in normal volunteers.[63] The nature of the relationship between demonstration of GPI-deficient clones and AA remains a topic of active investigation.[64,65] GPI-linked protein–deficient cells have been detected by immunohistochemistry in the BM of approximately 40% of children who have AA,[66] similar to findings in adults. More recently, however, flow cytometry studies of PB indicated a lower rate, approximately 20%, in children, in comparison with a rate of 68% in a largely adult population.[3,67] AA also is not the only BM failure disorder in which PNH clones can be detected. Patients who have hypoplastic, as well as other, more classic, presentations of MDS can have readily detectable populations of GPI-deficient cells.[61,64] In this setting, PNH positivity seems to be associated with a lower histologic grade of MDS and with decreased marrow cellularity (ie, more AA-like disease), although these findings are somewhat controversial and are derived largely from adult-based studies. Certainly a classic clinical presentation of PNH with significant hemolysis and thrombosis is very uncommon in the pediatric age range, although it has been reported that most such children indeed have concomitant marrow failure.[68]

Leukemia and MDS may present with pancytopenia in the setting of a hypoplastic BM, fulfilling the diagnostic criteria for AA. Using significantly different diagnostic tools than those currently available, investigators previously observed that approximately 2% of childhood acute lymphoblastic leukemia, but not acute myelogenous leukemia (AML), cases are characterized by an antecedent period of pancytopenia, often with a hypocellular BM biopsy found on diagnostic evaluation.[69] Overt leukemia generally presented within a few months. Considered from the reverse perspective, again with less sophisticated molecular diagnostic techniques than those currently available, a number of patients (approximately 4%) carrying a diagnosis of AA after adequate BM histologic confirmation were found to have clonal abnormalities on prospective cytogenetic evaluation or on retrospective sample reassessment.[70,71] No currently available test is infallible in resolving the diagnostic dilemma of AA versus hypoplastic MDS. Although unique morphologic or intracellular findings in PB and BM cells have been suggested as potential discriminators between AA and MDS, these findings have not been broadly applied or validated for diagnostic or management purposes, and virtually no exploration has been performed in isolated pediatric populations.[72] Even the demonstration of aneuploidy fails to resolve this question fully, because there is ongoing debate about the implications of both clonality in general and certain cytogenetic abnormalities specifically in regards to both the diagnosis and prognosis of AA.[73–75] Most of this literature is confined to or is largely contributed to by adult AA populations. Hypoplastic MDS and clonal evolution are reviewed in greater detail in elsewhere in this issue.

From a management perspective, one of the most important diagnostic assessments relates to careful evaluation for one of the inherited bone marrow failure syndromes (IBMFS)[76] of which there are many, as described in detail elsewhere in this issue. Their clinical presentation and variable genetic penetrance make family history and clinical examination inadequate for diagnosis. Although some IBMFS present primarily as single-lineage cytopenias (eg, thrombocytopenia absent radii), others present more frequently with obvious involvement of more than one lineage (eg, Fanconi anemia). Many can evolve, over a variable period, to pancytopenia. Even disorders long thought of as involving a single lineage (eg, Diamond Blackfan anemia) now seem to have potential for aplastic evolution.[77] Although a detailed discussion is beyond the scope of this article, a growing battery of tests (both functional and molecular) can be used to confirm such diagnoses. Rarely, however, are such tests exclusionary; that is, for most of the IBMFS there are individuals who fit the clinical criteria but do not have a known mutation for that syndrome. Functional diagnostic testing also can be misleading. For example, both spontaneous reversion and mosaicism can affect the results of chromosomal breakage testing for Fanconi anemia.[78] As noted previously, fully 20% of individuals in whom a diagnosis of IBMFS is thought to be strongly indicated cannot be assigned a specific diagnosis.[53]

MANAGEMENT

There is an extensive literature detailing, and often comparing, the outcomes of various treatment approaches for children who have acquired AA. In contrast, there are virtually no prospective studies of outcome related to most of the clinical strategies used in the day-to-day care of such children. Thus, in the discussion of generally accepted approaches to commonly encountered issues, there frequently is a paucity of peer-reviewed evidence.

Supportive Care

Attention should be directed first to managing the consequences of the anemia, neutropenia, and thrombocytopenia experienced by the child who has AA. Blood products should be used as needed to maintain adequate function and quality of life but with attention to minimizing alloimmunization. The use of family blood products should be avoided, and all products should be leukoreduced. Transfusional support strategies for children should take into account their developmental stage and activity profile. Children who have ongoing need for red cell transfusion should have appropriate monitoring of iron status, and chelation should be initiated according to the most current guidelines to limit complications of iron overload. Recent studies suggest the importance of iron management to overall outcome in both children and adults who have BM failure syndromes, although few of these data are confined to pediatric AA populations.[2,79,80]

The overall benefit of hematopoietic growth factors, either in overall outcome or in prophylaxis of infectious complications, has been difficult to demonstrate. Moreover, prolonged exposure to granulocyte colony-stimulating factor (G-CSF) has been associated, albeit not consistently, with evolution of AA to MDS and AML.[81–84] There are no studies documenting the outcome of any specific approach to infection prophylaxis in children, or even adults, who have AA. Nonetheless, obtaining and maintaining a detailed history of infections/infectious exposure serves both as guide for individualized patient management and as a prompt to integrate potential drug effects (such as hepatic and hematologic toxicity) into the ongoing evaluation of patient status and management.

Patients who have AA and their families generally formulate long lists of questions regarding diverse activities of daily living, including queries regarding school, athletic activities, pet ownership and handling, diet, travel, and other social interactions. There are no validated guidelines that can be disseminated readily; thus, patients may be served best by the medical team instilling an awareness of activities that unnecessarily increase exposure to infectious agents. Similarly, the nature of activities that may increase the opportunities for spontaneous or trauma-induced hemorrhage should be explained clearly. The potential infectious and hemorrhagic complications of sexual behaviors should be addressed in a developmentally and culturally age-appropriate manner. In addition, hormonal suppression of menstruation should be discussed with all pubertal and near-pubertal girls and their families, and there should be consideration of menstrual suppression in menarchal girls. The form of such suppression may depend on the anticipated course of care.

Treatment

With the improvements in supportive care, particularly transfusion support and the availability of increasingly effective anti-infectious treatments, the mortality of AA in children (and adults) has improved radically. Series reported in the 1970s found median survival times of less than 6 months,[85] and with supportive care alone the 1-year mortality was greater than 80%.[86] Currently the improved ability to support and treat children who have AA results in survival rates ranging from 70% to 100% at 2 to 10 years, strongly suggesting that observation is not an appropriate therapeutic approach for children who have severe or very severe AA. Spontaneous remission in children who have severe AA is rare, although both early and late recovery have been reported, as has somewhat more frequent recovery in children who have less severe disease.[87,88] AA presenting or relapsing during pregnancy may improve spontaneously after delivery or termination.[89,90]

Hematopoietic Stem Cell Transplantation

Matched sibling donor

The triage of allogeneic HSCT versus IST is still debatable in adults but is less so in children, given their excellent survival after matched sibling-donor (MSD) HSCT. These results always have been quite robust, with pediatric series showing disease-free survival rates ranging from 64% to 97%.[91-94] Most articles in which MSD HSCT across all ages is described show survival of younger patients in the 75% to 95% range at 3 to 5 years.[95-98] Factors associated with favorable outcomes in such mixed-age populations include young age, less transfusion history, no intervening therapy, and a short interval from diagnosis to transplantation. Before the era of leukodepletion to decrease transfusional allosensitization, transfusion history was associated with increased graft failure in AA HSCT.[99] Recent reports find that a history of frequent transfusion as well as exposure to interim therapy before HSCT remain associated with greater risk for graft failure and overall worse outcome after MSD HSCT.[100]

The good outcome of children undergoing MSD HSCT may reflect in part the minimally toxic conditioning approach used. Most MSD HSCT for AA have been performed with cyclophosphamide (CY) and anti-thymocyte globulin (ATG), occasionally in concert with other agents.[91,92,95,101] The best overall results often have been obtained with the two agents alone. In a recent combined pediatric/adult study of MSD HSCT for AA in which patients had been conditioned with CY and ATG, 96% demonstrated sustained engraftment with an overall survival rate of 88% at a median follow-up of 9 years.[97] Nonetheless, the role of ATG has been thrown into question by a prospective, randomized MSD study in which patients (of all ages) received standard-dose CY with or without ATG. Both arms had equivalent rates of engraftment, late rejection, and graft-versus-host disease (GVHD) as well as the same overall survival rate of 80%.[102] Conversely, a recent study from India described the potential value of additional fludarabine in the pediatric AA MSD setting, citing less rejection, a faster rate of engraftment, and better overall survival.[92] Thus, alternative approaches may benefit specific populations, practice patterns, and/or medical care settings.

BM has been the most frequent stem cell source in this setting, in part because of the practical, ethical, and possible medical risk issues involved in obtaining cells, particularly peripheral blood stem cells (PBSC), from pediatric donors.[103,104] Moreover, a retrospective registry study in AA demonstrated BM recipients had significantly less chronic GVHD and better overall survival.[105] There is little aggregated information about the use of MSD umbilical cord blood stem cells in pediatric AA HSCT. Only 8 children who had AA were among the 113 receiving MSD umbilical cord blood stem cells in a series demonstrating slower neutrophil engraftment and slightly less acute and chronic GVHD but equivalent overall survival in comparison with BM recipients.[106]

GVHD remains perhaps the most serious acute and chronic complication of MSD for children who have AA. The best studied, most frequently used prophylaxis regimen is cyclosporine (CSA) and short-course methotrexate (MTX).[96,107] The excellence of these results is indicated in a recent trial in a combined age population undergoing MSD HSCT for AA in which a CY/ATG conditioning regimen followed by CSA/MTX prophylaxis for GVHD resulted in a 3% rate of severe acute GVHD and a 26% rate of chronic GVHD.[97] Use of alemtuzumab (anti-CD-52 antibody) in the MSD/AA setting also has had a favorable effect on the rates of acute and chronic GVHD.[108]

Alternative-donor hematopoietic stem cell transplantation

Children without an MSD are treated with IST. For those who do not respond to IST, the option of alternative-donor HSCT should be considered. Alternative donors include matched unrelated donors, mismatched unrelated donors, and mismatched related donors. Although some success was achieved early in the use of matched unrelated donors for acquired AA, long-term survival rates hovered in the range of 20% to 40%.[96,109–113] Poor outcomes were attributable to prolonged time to HSCT, high rates of graft rejection, significant rates of GVHD, and increased toxicity resulting from more aggressive conditioning. All risk factors have been addressed to some extent, and more recent results are improved significantly.[93,113] For example, MSD-like conditioning was associated with poor engraftment with alternative-donor HSCT for AA,[114] whereas aggressive regimens were associated with increased toxicity. Exploration of novel approaches (eg, lower-dose total body irradiation) added to ATG and CY in a cohort of children who had AA and who were receiving BM HSCT was markedly more successful, with a survival rate of 73%.[115] Variations of this approach, including the substitution of alemtuzumab for ATG, produced 100% engraftment and minimal toxicity in a small, prospective pediatric series.[116] Fludarabine/low-dose CY/ATG and fludarabine/CY/alemtuzumab have been evaluated in combined pediatric/adult studies in an attempt to avoid total body irradiation altogether, resulting in low rates of graft failure and in survival rates in excess of 70%.[117–121]

Despite the excellent results in some centers, larger registry data still suggest that survival rates after alternative-donor HSCT are lower than survival rates after IST;[94,122–124] however, alternative-donor HSCT may offer some advantages in failure-free survival.[119] Although retrospective registry and multicenter data demonstrate overall improvement over time, the best results are seen when HSCT is performed in younger patients with good performance status (and younger children have demonstrated better outcome than older children).[119,120,125,126] The relevance of the degree of HLA match and the relative merits of matched unrelated donors, mismatched unrelated donors, and mismatched related donors remain debatable, although a full match at high resolution seems more favorable overall in the unrelated-donor setting.[113,120,125–127]

In most of the reported series, BM was the source for hematopoietic stem cells. The use of umbilical cord blood from unrelated donors has been undertaken successfully in AA, although substantial rates of graft failure and HSCT-related mortality have been reported.[128] Children receiving transplantation for hematologic malignancy have been reported to experience more chronic GVHD, treatment-related mortality, treatment failure, and overall mortality with PBSC than with BM-derived stem cells.[129] Similar analyses limited to pediatric AA are not available. Various strategies for cell manipulation have been applied to patients undergoing alternative-donor HSCT for AA. To limit the toxicity of PBSC, alternate-donor CD34+ selected PBSC have been used with some success.[130–132] Others have developed strategies to limit donor T-cell alloreactivity selectively to reduce GVHD without conferring significant global immunosuppression. Several studies have demonstrated the feasibility of these approaches in children who have IBMFS and/or severe idiopathic AA.[133–136]

Complications of hematopoietic stem cell transplantation for aplastic anemia
Transplantation for AA has been characterized, in general, by significant rates of graft failure.[96,100,119,125,126] This problem has diminished somewhat in incidence over time but has not been eliminated completely.[96,113] Nonetheless, long-term outcomes for children and young adults after HSCT for AA have been very acceptable,[129] and it is believed that the common use of the less-intensive regimens in AA HSCT has contributed to this good outcome. Patients treated with regimens that do not involve total body irradiation often achieve normal growth, predicted final heights, and preserved

fertility.[129,137] Nonetheless, they do not escape other, more generalized HSCT toxicities related to acute immune suppression, chronic immunodeficiency, chronic GVHD, and the sequelae of GVHD treatment as well as the regimen-related toxicity that accrues in even the least-intensive regimen. Infectious diseases, dermatologic problems, cataracts, pulmonary insufficiency, and bone and joint problems are among the more serious late problems reported after MSD HSCT for AA.[138] The cumulative incidence of chronic GVHD after MSD HSCT for AA ranges from negligible to as high as 40%, and affected patients experience both impaired quality of life and reduced overall survival.[95,138] In a large, retrospective analysis of alternative-donor HSCT in AA that was weighted toward younger patients, chronic GVHD rates were in the range of 19% to 29%, with no difference detected by donor type.[126] A single-center pediatric study reported no chronic GVHD when alemtuzumab was used, versus 30% when ATG was used, with no differences between the MSD and alternative-donor groups.[93] Another mixed-age registry study found overall outcome improved in association with better HLA typing in matched unrelated-donor HSCT but failed to detect any impact on the rate of chronic GVHD.[125] Interestingly, the use of fludarabine was associated with less chronic GVHD. These latter studies suggest that innovations in HSCT care may improve some parameters of long-term outcome.

Secondary malignancies are a significant cause of death after HSCT for AA.[125,139,140] Lymphoproliferative disorders, often related to Epstein-Barr virus, are reported relatively early in follow-up.[125,140] The later occurrence of various solid tumors also is reported, generally in association with the risk factors of chronic GVHD and prior irradiation, as also reported in other HSCT populations.

Immunosuppressive Therapy

The data briefly reviewed in the earlier section on pathophysiology serve as the foundation for immunosuppressive management of AA, although the agents themselves are not particularly specific in regard to mode of action. ATG is a commercially available, Food and Drug Administration–approved, polyclonal anti-thymocyte antibody–rich serum fraction made by immunizing either horses or rabbits against human thymic tissue or thymocytes retrieved by cannulation. It has protean properties, being lympholytic and immunomodulatory. It may produce a state of immunologic tolerance by preferential destruction of activated T cells.[22] The species of origin also may confer differential properties; rabbit ATG, but not horse ATG, recently has been shown to support expansion of T-regulatory cells.[141] ATG also stimulates the release of hematopoietic growth factor and cytokine from various cell types.[23] The other most commonly used IST agent, CSA, has immunomodulatory activities in excess of the initially described decrease in T-cell proliferation conferred by calcineurin inhibition and downstream transcriptional regulation mediated by nuclear factor-kappaB.[142] Even filgrastim (G-CSF) has immunomodulatory actions in addition to its more generally recognized hematopoietic activities. Normal human T cells express G-CSF receptors. In healthy human donors, G-CSF causes a shift from T-helper cell type 1 to T-helper cell type 2 cytokine responses,[143] offering a potential mechanism by which it may work synergistically or additively with IST.

Although the most relevant synergies are incompletely understood, the use of ATG and CSA, generally in concert with a corticosteroid, has proven a durable standard of care for children who have acquired AA.[83,122,123,144] Responses to IST usually are categorized as complete, partial, or no response. The specifics may vary from study to study but always are determined by both blood counts and transfusion dependence. Randomized studies across all ages demonstrated improved response rates but not improved overall survival when CSA was added to ATG.[145] As shown in **Table 3**, response rates up to 80% have been reported in pediatric studies, making this regimen the current standard of care for children without an MSD.[4,54,124,146,147] The relative contribution of filgrastim to ATG/CSA with or without a corticosteroid is unclear, with most data being comparative rather than randomized.[81,123,144,148] Addition of the immunosuppressive mycophenolate mofetil has not been demonstrated to date to improve any outcome parameter.[149] Alternative approaches to IST, such as the use of CY, have demonstrated efficacy in some patients,[150] but significant toxicity has limited the broad application of CY.[151] More recently, the use of alemtuzumab, an anti-CD52 antibody with activity against multiple cell types, including T cells and B cells, has been evaluated in combination with CSA. The response rate to date is lower than that seen with ATG/CSA, but the preliminary results are of interest.[152]

The median time to response can be prolonged, with trilineage recovery reported at a median of 96 days from treatment (ATG/CSA/steroid/G-CSF) in a recent large, mixed-age study heavily weighted to pediatric patients.[81] Another pediatric trial of ATG/CSA reported overall response rates of 61%, 74%, and 80% at 3, 6, and 12 months.[71] The ratio of complete response to partial response varies among pediatric studies and may reflect in part the rapidity with which inadequate response is assessed and second-line therapy is initiated.[123,124] Among nonresponders to IST, another course of IST at 2 to 6 months is a frequent second-line treatment. Response rates range from 11% to 63% and seem to be lower in studies weighted toward or conducted in children than in largely adult cohorts.[81,83,119,123,153–155] The variable time to re-treatment confounds these results further. A recent prospective, multicenter study demonstrated that use of alternative-donor HSCT as second-line treatment for children who did not respond to IST conferred markedly better survival with hematologic response than did repeated IST (83.9% ± 16.1% versus 9.5% ± 9.0% at 5 years), although the actuarial overall survival of all patients was high (94.5%) at median of 4 years of follow-up and did not differ by second-line treatment used.[119]

There is little information in regard to prediction of response that is limited to children. Although retrospective analyses of IST demonstrated worse survival (37%) in patients who had very severe AA as compared with those who had severe AA,[156] a large, prospective pediatric IST trial reported the reverse observation of better overall 5-year survival in those who had very severe AA (93%) than in those who had severe AA (81%), although the children with more pronounced neutropenia also received G-CSF.[144] Consecutive case series in or weighted toward younger patients failed to find any relationship with severity.[81,124] A large, multivariate single-institution analysis found younger age and higher baseline absolute reticulocyte and lymphocyte counts to predict IST response at 6 months; this response also translated into increased 5-year survival rates.[124]

Findings thought to reflect an immune etiology also have been associated with response to IST, albeit these associations largely have been made in adult populations. Three of these associations—the presence of HLA-DR15, the presence of a PNH clone, and the presence of AA-associated autoantibody—have been examined in a sizable prospective pediatric study.[3] The presence of HLA-DR15 was less than that in earlier (largely adult) reports, as was the presence of GPI-deficient cells, whereas the prevalence of the autoantibody was similar (14.5%) to that in an earlier pediatric population.[3,67] None of these findings was associated with likelihood of response to IST. Another marker of immune perturbation, detectable cytotoxic T cells with increased levels of intracellular interferon-γ, has been associated with response to IST in a largely adult population but has not been studied in children.[30] The presence of cytogenetic abnormalities at diagnosis does not necessarily define

Table 3
Recent large trials of immunosuppressive therapy for severe aplastic anemia in children

Site	Patient Number	Immunosuppressive Therapy	Response at 6 Months	Relapse (F/U)	Survival (F/U)	Reference
Japan	119	ATG CSA Danazol ±GCSF	55%–77% CR + PR	22% (3 years)	88% (3 years)	(Kojima, et al 2000)[a]
Germany	146	ATG CSA G-CSF[a]	61% CR	14% (5 years)	89% (5 years)	(Fuehrer, et al 2005)
China	51	Variable regimens	27%–79%[b]	NA[b]	NE[b]	(Fang, et al 2006)
Italy	42	ATG CSA	71%	16% (10 years)	83% (10 years)	(Saracco, et al 2008)
Unites States	77	ATG CSA ±MMF ±sirolimus	74% CR + PR	33% (10 years)	80% (10 years)	(Scheinberg, et al 2008)

Abbreviations: ATG, antithymocyte globulin; CR, complete response; CSA, cyclosporin A; F/U, follow-up; G-CSF, granulocyte colony-stimulating factor; MMF, mycophenolate mofetil; NA, not available; PR, partial response.
[a] G-CSF if neutrophil count < 0.5 × 10^9/L.
[b] Regimen-specific information in article.

subsequent evolution of frank MDS/AML, nor does it necessarily define response to IST. This information is difficult to dissect from the literature, however, because many groups use abnormal cytogenetics as an exclusion criterion for AA.[73] Perhaps not surprisingly, patients who have acquired AA and evidence of at least one non-immune etiology (in the form of telomerase-associated mutations and/or telomere shortening) have exhibited poor responses to IST.[52]

Among patients responding to IST, the actuarial probability of relapse ranges from 5% to 35% at 3 to 10 years after treatment.[83,123,124,157,158] If it occurs, relapse can be treated with variable success with another course of IST.[119,155,159] In general, rapid CSA taper is a significant risk factor for relapse.[81,83,157,158] In one pediatric study the risk of relapse was 60% in patients who had a rapid CSA taper but was only 7.6% in those who had a slower taper.[83] In this study the probability of CSA discontinuation was 60.5% at 10 years. In another report, with all ages but weighted toward children, the actuarial probability of CSA discontinuation at 5 years was 38%.[81] These data speak to the CSA dependence of a sizable proportion of patients. Little is known about the optimal dosing of CSA in AA, however, nor has the most appropriate monitoring strategy been determined.

Patients treated with IST have a significant rate of clonal evolution and development of MDS and AML. The relative contributions of an injured and abnormal stem cell compartment, an abnormal and perturbed BM microenvironment, the direct effects of IST, and the selective effects of therapeutics such as G-CSF, all acting either independently or additively, are unclear. Response to IST does not necessarily predict either the acquisition or the time to acquisition of clonal abnormalities.[145] In some cases, however, the use of a second round of IST and a partial response to IST have been associated with increased risk.[83,123,124] The most commonly reported cytogenetic abnormality is monosomy 7. Clones, even monosomy 7, can be transient, stable, or progress to leukemia with a highly variable clinical course.[73,74,83,88,119,123,124]

Both the definition and the cumulative incidence of MDS/AML varies widely by report.[74] A recent multi-institutional pediatric study reported a cumulative incidence of 8% at 10 years,[83] whereas in a single-institution report 2 of 42 patients (4.7%) developed MDS/AML.[123] Retrospective pediatric series have reported cumulative incidences ranging from 8.5%.[82,124] Rates in excess of 20% have been reported previously in children.[160] In a large mixed-age population, trisomy 8 was seen most commonly in prior IST responders, whereas monosomy 7 and other complex abnormalities were somewhat more common in patients who had a poor response to IST.[73] Most strikingly, the speed of evolution of frank MDS/AML was significantly different, with much worse outcomes observed in individuals who had chromosome 7 abnormalities or complex cytogenetic alterations.[73,81] Most reports, but not all, seem to indicate that the use of G-CSF increases this risk in young patients.[81,83,119,160]

REFERENCES

1. Fuhrer M, Durner J, Brunnler G, et al. HLA association is different in children and adults with severe acquired aplastic anemia. Pediatr Blood Cancer 2007;48(2):186–91.
2. Lee JW. Iron chelation therapy in the myelodysplastic syndromes and aplastic anemia: a review of experience in South Korea. Int J Hematol 2008;88(1):16–23.
3. Yoshida N, Yagasaki H, Takahashi Y, et al. Clinical impact of HLA-DR15, a minor population of paroxysmal nocturnal haemoglobinuria-type cells, and an aplastic

anaemia-associated autoantibody in children with acquired aplastic anaemia. Br J Haematol 2008;142:427–35.

4. Bacigalupo A, Hows J, Gluckman E, et al. Bone marrow transplantation (BMT) versus immunosuppression for the treatment of severe aplastic anaemia (SAA): a report of the EBMT SAA working party. Br J Haematol 1988;70(2):177–82.

5. Camitta BM, Thomas ED, Nathan DG, et al. Severe aplastic anemia: a prospective study of the effect of early marrow transplantation on acute mortality. Blood 1976;48(1):63–9.

6. Maciejewski JP, Risitano A, Kook H, et al. Immune pathophysiology of aplastic anemia. Int J Hematol 2002;76(Suppl 1):207–14.

7. Marsh JC, Gordon-Smith EC. Insights into the autoimmune nature of aplastic anaemia. Lancet 2004;364(9431):308–9.

8. Young NS. Acquired aplastic anemia. Ann Intern Med 2002;136(7):534–46.

9. Young NS. Pathophysiologic mechanisms in acquired aplastic anemia. Hematology Am Soc Hematol Educ Program 2006;72–7.

10. Young NS, Kaufman DW. The epidemiology of acquired aplastic anemia. Haematologica 2008;93(4):489–92.

11. McCarty D, Brill J, Harrop D. Aplastic anemia secondary to gold-salt therapy: report of fatal case and a review of literature. JAMA 1962;179:655–7.

12. Aksoy M, Koray D, Akgun T, et al. Haematological effects of chronic benzene poisoning in 217 workers. Br J Ind Med 1971;28:296–302.

13. Smith MT. Overview of benzene-induced aplastic anaemia. Eur J Haematol Suppl 1996;60:107–10.

14. Lau YL, Srivastava G, Lee CW, et al. Epstein-Barr virus associated aplastic anaemia and hepatitis. J Paediatr Child Health 1994;30(1):74–6.

15. Mathe G, Schwarzenberg L. Treatment of bone marrow aplasia by bone marrow graft after conditioning with antilymphocyte globulin: long term results. Exp Hematol 1976;4:256–64.

16. Speck B, Gluckman E, Haak HL, et al. Treatment of aplastic anaemia by antilymphocyte globulin with and without allogeneic bone-marrow infusions. Lancet 1977;2(8049):1145–8.

17. Champlin R, Ho W, Gale R. Antithymocyte globulin treatments in patients with aplastic anemia. N Engl J Med 1983;308(3):113–8.

18. Champlin RE, Feig SA, Sparkes RS, et al. Bone marrow transplantation from identical twins in the treatment of aplastic anaemia: implication for the pathogenesis of the disease. Br J Haematol 1984;56(3):455–63.

19. Storb R, Prentice RL, Thomas ED, et al. Factors associated with graft rejection after HLA-identical marrow transplantation for aplastic anaemia. Br J Haematol 1983;55(4):573–85.

20. Storb R, Thomas ED, Buckner CD, et al. Marrow transplantation in thirty "untransfused" patients with severe aplastic anemia. Ann Intern Med 1980;92(1):30–6.

21. Young NS, Barrett AJ. The treatment of severe acquired aplastic anemia. Blood 1995;85(12):3367–77.

22. Young NS, Calado RT, Scheinberg P. Current concepts in the pathophysiology and treatment of aplastic anemia. Blood 2006;108:2509–19.

23. Taniguchi Y, Frickhofen N, Raghavachar A, et al. Antilymphocyte immunoglobulins stimulate peripheral blood lymphocytes to proliferate and release lymphokines. Eur J Haematol 1990;44(4):244–51.

24. Bacigalupo A, Podesta M, Mingari MC, et al. Immune suppression of hematopoiesis in aplastic anemia: activity of T-gamma lymphocytes. J Immunol 1980;125(4):1449–53.

25. Kook H, Risitano AM, Zeng W, et al. Changes in T-cell receptor VB repertoire in aplastic anemia: effects of different immunosuppressive regimens. Blood 2002; 99(10):3668–75.

26. Nakao S, Harada M, Kondo K, et al. Effect of activated lymphocytes on the regulation of hematopoiesis: suppression of in vitro granulopoiesis by OKT8 + Ia + T cells induced by alloantigen stimulation. J Immunol 1984;132(1):160–4.

27. Nakao S, Takami A, Takamatsu H, et al. Isolation of a T-cell clone showing HLA-DRB1*0405-restricted cytotoxicity for hematopoietic cells in a patient with aplastic anemia. Blood 1997;89(10):3691–9.

28. Nakao S, Yamaguchi M, Shiobara S, et al. Interferon-gamma gene expression in unstimulated bone marrow mononuclear cells predicts a good response to cyclosporine therapy in aplastic anemia. Blood 1992;79(10):2532–5.

29. Laver J, Castro-Malaspina H, Kernan NA, et al. In vitro interferon-gamma production by cultured T-cells in severe aplastic anaemia: correlation with granulomonopoietic inhibition in patients who respond to anti-thymocyte globulin. Br J Haematol 1988;69:545–50.

30. Sloand E, Kim S, Maciejewski JP, et al. Intracellular interferon-gamma in circulating and marrow T cells detected by flow cytometry and the response to immunosuppressive therapy in patients with aplastic anemia. Blood 2002;100(4):1185–91.

31. Zoumbos NC, Gascon P, Djeu JY, et al. Circulating activated suppressor T lymphocytes in apalstic anemia. N Engl J Med 1985;312(5):257–65.

32. Zoumbos NC, Gascon P, Djeu JY, et al. Interferon is a mediator of hematopoietic suppression in aplastic anemia in vitro and possibly in vivo. Proc Natl Acad Sci U S A 1985;82(1):188–92.

33. Young NS. Gamma interferon and aplastic anemia. Blood 1987;70(1):337–9.

34. Gidvani V, Ramkissoon S, Sloand EM, et al. Cytokine gene polymorphisms in acquired bone marrow failure. Am J Hematol 2007;82(8):721–4.

35. Sloand E. Genetic polymorphisms and the risk of acquired idiopathic aplastic anemia. Haematologica 2005;90(8):1009B.

36. Zeng W, Kajigaya S, Chen G, et al. Transcript profile of CD4+ and CD8 + T cells from the bone marrow of acquired aplastic anemia patients. Exp Hematol 2004; 32(9):806–14.

37. Solomou EE, Keyvanfar K, Young NS. T-bet, a Th1 transcription factor, is up-regulated in T cells from patients with aplastic anemia. Blood 2006;107(10): 3983–91.

38. Risitano AM, Kook H, Zeng W, et al. Oligoclonal and polyclonal CD4 and CD8 lymphocytes in aplastic anemia and paroxysmal nocturnal hemoglobinuria measured by V beta CDR3 spectratyping and flow cytometry. Blood 2002; 100(1):178–83.

39. Risitano AM, Maciejewski JP, Green S, et al. In-vivo dominant immune responses in aplastic anaemia: molecular tracking of putatively pathogenetic T-cell clones by TCR beta-CDR3 sequencing. Lancet 2004;364(9431):355–64.

40. Wlodarski MW, Gondek LP, Nearman ZP, et al. Molecular strategies for detection and quantitation of clonal cytotoxic T-cell responses in aplastic anemia and myelodysplastic syndrome. Blood 2006;108(8):2632–41.

41. Nakao S, Takamatsu H, Yachie A, et al. Establishment of a CD4 + T cell clone recognizing autologous hematopoietic progenitor cells from a patient with immune-mediated aplastic anemia. Exp Hematol 1995;23(5):433–8.

42. Hirano N, Butler MO, Guinan EC, et al. Presence of anti-kinectin and anti-PMS1 antibodies in Japanese aplastic anaemia patients. Br J Haematol 2005;128(2): 221–3.

43. Hirano N, Butler MO, Von Bergwelt-Baildon MS, et al. Autoantibodies frequently detected in patients with aplastic anemia. Blood 2003;102(13):4567–75.
44. Takamatsu H, Feng X, Chuhjo T, et al. Specific antibodies to moesin, a membrane-cytoskeleton linker protein, are frequently detected in patients with acquired aplastic anemia. Blood 2007;109(6):2514–20.
45. Solomou EE, Rezvani K, Mielke S, et al. Deficient CD4 + CD25 + FOXP3 + T regulatory cells in acquired aplastic anemia. Blood 2007;110(5):1603–6.
46. Bacigalupo A, Podesta M, Raffo MR, et al. Lack of in vitro colony (CFUC) formation and myelosuppressive activity in patients with severe aplastic anemia after autologous hematologic reconstitution. Exp Hematol 1980;8(6):795–801.
47. Maciejewski JP, Selleri C, Sato T, et al. A severe and consistent deficit in marrow and circulating primitive hematopoietic cells (long-term culture-initiating cells) in acquired aplastic anemia. Blood 1996;88(6):1983–91.
48. Podesta M, Piaggio G, Frassoni F, et al. The assessment of the hematopoietic reservoir after immunosuppressive therapy or bone marrow transplantation in severe aplastic anemia. Blood 1998;91(6):1959–65.
49. Ball SE, Gibson FM, Rizzo S, et al. Progressive telomere shortening in aplastic anemia. Blood 1998;91(10):3582–92.
50. Field JJ, Mason PJ, An P, et al. Low frequency of telomerase RNA mutations among children with aplastic anemia or myelodysplastic syndrome. J Pediatr Hematol Oncol 2006;28(7):450–3.
51. Yamaguchi H, Baerlocher GM, Lansdorp PM, et al. Mutations of the human telomerase RNA gene (TERC) in aplastic anemia and myelodysplastic syndrome. Blood 2003;102(3):916–8.
52. Yamaguchi H, Calado RT, Ly H, et al. Mutations in TERT, the gene for telomerase reverse transcriptase, in aplastic anemia. N Engl J Med 2005;352(14):1413–24.
53. Teo JT, Klaassen R, Fernandez CV, et al. Clinical and genetic analysis of unclassifiable inherited bone marrow failure syndromes. Pediatrics 2008;122(1): e139–48.
54. Kurre P, Johnson FL, Deeg HJ. Diagnosis and treatment of children with aplastic anemia. Pediatr Blood Cancer 2005;45(6):770–80.
55. Young N, Alter B. Aplastic anemia: acquired and inherited. Philadelphia: W.B. Saunders Co.; 1994.
56. Bhatnagar SK, Chandra J, Narayan S, et al. Pancytopenia in children: etiological profile. J Trop Pediatr 2005;51(4):236–9.
57. Toledano R, Gil-Nagel A. Adverse effects of antiepileptic drugs. Semin Neurol 2008;28(3):317–27.
58. Zaccara G, Franciotta D, Perucca E. Idiosyncratic adverse reactions to antiepileptic drugs. Epilepsia 2007;48(7):1223–44.
59. Boullu-Ciocca S, Darmon P, Sebahoun G, et al. [Gelatinous bone marrow transformation in anorexia nervosa]. Ann Endocrinol (Paris) 2005;66(1):7–11 [in French].
60. Myers TJ, Perkerson MD, Witter BA, et al. Hematologic findings in anorexia nervosa. Conn Med 1981;45(1):14–7.
61. Wang SA, Pozdnyakova O, Jorgensen JL, et al. Detection of paroxysmal nocturnal hemoglobinuria clones in patients with myelodysplastic syndromes and related bone marrow diseases, with emphasis on diagnostic pitfalls and caveats. Haematologica 2008;94:29–37.
62. Mukhina GL, Buckley JT, Barber JP, et al. Multilineage glycosylphosphatidylinositol anchor-deficient haematopoiesis in untreated aplastic anaemia. Br J Haematol 2001;115(2):476–82.

63. Araten DJ, Nafa K, Pakdeesuwan K, et al. Clonal populations of hematopoietic cells with paroxysmal nocturnal hemoglobinuria genotype and phenotype are present in normal individuals. Proc Natl Acad Sci U S A 1999;96(9):5209–14.

64. Maciejewski JP, Rivera C, Kook H, et al. Relationship between bone marrow failure syndromes and the presence of glycophosphatidyl inositol-anchored protein-deficient clones. Br J Haematol 2001;115(4):1015–22.

65. Young NS. The problem of clonality in aplastic anemia. Dr. Damshek's riddle, re-stated. Blood 1992;79:1385–92.

66. Rizk S, Ibrahim IY, Mansour IM, et al. Screening for paroxysmal nocturnal hemo-globinuria (PNH) clone in Egyptian children with aplastic anemia. J Trop Pediatr 2002;48(3):132–7.

67. Sugimori C, Chuhjo T, Feng X, et al. Minor population of CD55-CD59- blood cells predicts response to immunosuppressive therapy and prognosis in patients with aplastic anemia. Blood 2006;107(4):1308–14.

68. van den Heuvel-Eibrink MM. Paroxysmal nocturnal hemoglobinuria in children. Paediatr Drugs 2007;9(1):11–6.

69. Breatnach F, Chessells JM, Greaves MF. The aplastic presentation of childhood leukaemia: a feature of common-ALL. Br J Haematol 1981;49(3):387–93.

70. Appelbaum FR, Barrall J, Storb R, et al. Clonal cytogenetic abnormalities in patients with otherwise typical aplastic anemia. Exp Hematol 1987;15(11): 1134–9.

71. Fuhrer M, Burdach S, Ebell W, et al. Relapse and clonal disease in children with aplastic anemia (AA) after immunosuppressive therapy (IST): the SAA 94 expe-rience. German/Austrian Pediatric Aplastic Anemia Working Group. Klin Padiatr 1998;210(4):173–9.

72. Iwasaki T, Murakami M, Sugisaki C, et al. Characterization of myelodysplastic syndrome and aplastic anemia by immunostaining of p53 and hemoglobin F and karyotype analysis: differential diagnosis between refractory anemia and aplastic anemia. Pathol Int 2008;58(6):353–60.

73. Maciejewski JP, Risitano A, Sloand EM, et al. Distinct clinical outcomes for cyto-genetic abnormalities evolving from aplastic anemia. Blood 2002;99(9): 3129–35.

74. Maciejewski JP, Selleri C. Evolution of clonal cytogenetic abnormalities in aplas-tic anemia. Leuk Lymphoma 2004;45(3):433–40.

75. Tsuge I, Kojima S, Matsuoka H, et al. Clonal haematopoiesis in children with acquired aplastic anaemia. Br J Haematol 1993;84(1):137–43.

76. Tamary H, Alter BP. Current diagnosis of inherited bone marrow failure syndromes. Pediatr Hematol Oncol 2007;24(2):87–99.

77. Vlachos A, Ball S, Dahl N, et al. Diagnosing and treating Diamond Blackfan anaemia: results of an international clinical consensus conference. Br J Haema-tol 2008;142(6):859–76.

78. Gregory JJ Jr, Wagner JE, Verlander PC, et al. Somatic mosaicism in Fanconi anemia: evidence of genotypic reversion in lymphohematopoietic stem cells. Proc Natl Acad Sci U S A 2001;98(5):2532–7.

79. Bin JH, Yoo YK, Kim SY, et al. The effects of multiple transfusion on the outcomes of bone marrow transplantation from HLA-matched sibling donor in patients with severe aplastic anemia. Korean J Pediatr Hematol-Oncol 2003;10:30–8.

80. Takatoku M, Uchiyama T, Okamoto S, et al. Retrospective nationwide survey of Japanese patients with transfusion-dependent MDS and aplastic anemia high-lights the negative impact of iron overload on morbidity/mortality. Eur J Haematol 2007;78(6):487–94.

81. Bacigalupo A, Bruno B, Saracco P, et al. Antilymphocyte globulin, cyclosporine, prednisolone, and granulocyte colony-stimulating factor for severe aplastic anemia: an update of the GITMO/EBMT study on 100 patients. European Group for Blood and Marrow Transplantation (EBMT) Working Party on Severe Aplastic Anemia and the Gruppo Italiano Trapianti di Midolio Osseo (GITMO). Blood 2000;95(6):1931–4.

82. Kojima S, Ohara A, Tsuchida M, et al. Risk factors for evolution of acquired aplastic anemia into myelodysplastic syndrome and acute myeloid leukemia after immunosuppressive therapy in children. Blood 2002;100(3):786–90.

83. Saracco P, Quarello P, Iori AP, et al. Cyclosporin A response and dependence in children with acquired aplastic anaemia: a multicentre retrospective study with long-term observation follow-up. Br J Haematol 2008;140(2):197–205.

84. Socie G, Mary JY, Schrezenmeier H, et al. Granulocyte-stimulating factor and severe aplastic anemia: a survey by the European Group for Blood and Marrow Transplantation (EBMT). Blood 2007;109(7):2794–6.

85. Li FP, Alter BP, Nathan DG. The mortality of acquired aplastic anemia in children. Blood 1972;40(2):153–62.

86. Williams DM, Lynch RE, Cartwright GE. Prognostic factors in aplastic anaemia. Clin Haematol 1978;7(3):467–74.

87. Howard SC, Naidu PE, Hu XJ, et al. Natural history of moderate aplastic anemia in children. Pediatr Blood Cancer 2004;43(5):545–51.

88. Najean Y, Haguenauer O. Long-term (5 to 20 years) evolution of nongrafted aplastic anemia. Blood 1990;76(11):2222–8.

89. Goldstein IM, Coller BS. Aplastic anemia in pregnancy: recovery after normal spontaneous delivery. Ann Intern Med 1975;82(4):537–9.

90. Tichelli A, Socie G, Marsh J, et al. Outcome of pregnancy and disease course among women with aplastic anemia treated with immunosuppression. Ann Intern Med 2002;137(3):164–72.

91. Bunin N, Leahey A, Kamani N, et al. Bone marrow transplantation in pediatric patients with severe aplastic anemia: cyclophosphamide and anti-thymocyte globulin conditioning followed by recombinant human granulocyte-macrophage colony stimulating factor. J Pediatr Hematol Oncol 1996;18(1):68–71.

92. George B, Mathews V, Viswabandya A, et al. Fludarabine based reduced intensity conditioning regimens in children undergoing allogeneic stem cell transplantation for severe aplastic anemia. Pediatr Transplant 2008;12(1):14–9.

93. Kennedy-Nasser AA, Leung KS, Mahajan A, et al. Comparable outcomes of matched-related and alternative donor stem cell transplantation for pediatric severe aplastic anemia. Biol Blood Marrow Transplant 2006;12(12):1277–84.

94. Kojima S, Horibe K, Inaba J, et al. Long-term outcome of acquired aplastic anaemia in children: comparison between immunosuppressive therapy and bone marrow transplantation. Br J Haematol 2000;111(1):321–8.

95. Ades L, Mary JY, Robin M, et al. Long-term outcome after bone marrow transplantation for severe aplastic anemia. Blood 2004;103(7):2490–7.

96. Horowitz MM. Current status of allogeneic bone marrow transplantation in acquired aplastic anemia. Semin Hematol 2000;37(1):30–42.

97. Kahl C, Leisenring W, Deeg HJ, et al. Cyclophosphamide and antithymocyte globulin as a conditioning regimen for allogeneic marrow transplantation in patients with aplastic anaemia: a long-term follow-up. Br J Haematol 2005; 130(5):747–51.

98. Locasciulli A, Oneto R, Bacigalupo A, et al. Outcome of patients with acquired aplastic anemia given first line bone marrow transplantation or immunosuppressive

treatment in the last decade: a report from the European Group for Blood and Marrow Transplantation (EBMT). Haematologica 2007;92(1):11–8.

99. Storb R, Prentice RL, Thomas ED. Marrow transplantation for treatment of aplastic anemia. An analysis of factors associated with graft rejection. N Engl J Med 1977;296(2):61–6.

100. Kobayashi R, Yabe H, Hara J, et al. Preceding immunosuppressive therapy with antithymocyte globulin and ciclosporin increases the incidence of graft rejection in children with aplastic anaemia who underwent allogeneic bone marrow transplantation from HLA-identical siblings. Br J Haematol 2006;135(5):693–6.

101. Parkman R, Rappeport J, Camitta B, et al. Successful use of multiagent immunosuppression in the bone marrow transplantation of sensitized patients. Blood 1978;52(6):1163–9.

102. Champlin RE, Perez WS, Passweg JR, et al. Bone marrow transplantation for severe aplastic anemia: a randomized controlled study of conditioning regimens. Blood 2007;109(10):4582–5.

103. Bennett CL, Evens AM, Andritsos LA, et al. Haematological malignancies developing in previously healthy individuals who received haematopoietic growth factors: report from the Research on Adverse Drug Events and Reports (RADAR) project. Br J Haematol 2006;135(5):642–50.

104. Wiener LS, Steffen-Smith E, Fry T, et al. Hematopoietic stem cell donation in children: a review of the sibling donor experience. J Psychosoc Oncol 2007;25(1):45–66.

105. Schrezenmeier H, Passweg JR, Marsh JC, et al. Worse outcome and more chronic GVHD with peripheral blood progenitor cells than bone marrow in HLA-matched sibling donor transplants for young patients with severe acquired aplastic anemia: a report from the European Group for Blood and Marrow Transplantation and the Center for International Blood and Marrow Transplant Research. Blood 2007;110:1397–400.

106. Rocha V, Wagner JE Jr, Sobocinski KA, et al. Graft-versus-host disease in children who have received a cord-blood or bone marrow transplant from an HLA-identical sibling. Eurocord and International Bone Marrow Transplant Registry Working Committee on Alternative Donor and Stem Cell Sources. N Engl J Med 2000;342(25):1846–54.

107. Sorror ML, Leisenring W, Deeg HJ, et al. Re: Twenty-year follow-up in patients with aplastic anemia given marrow grafts from HLA-identical siblings and randomized to receive methotrexate/cyclosporine or methotrexate alone for prevention of graft-versus-host disease. Biol Blood Marrow Transplant 2005;11(7):567–8.

108. Gupta V, Ball SE, Yi QL, et al. Favorable effect on acute and chronic graft-versus-host disease with cyclophosphamide and in vivo anti-CD52 monoclonal antibodies for marrow transplantation from HLA-identical sibling donors for acquired aplastic anemia. Biol Blood Marrow Transplant 2004;10(12):867–76.

109. Bacigalupo A, Hows J, Gordon-Smith EC, et al. Bone marrow transplantation for severe aplastic anemia from donors other than HLA identical siblings: a report of the BMT Working Party. Bone Marrow Transplant 1988;3(6):531–5.

110. Davies SM, Wagner JE, Defor T, et al. Unrelated donor bone marrow transplantation for children and adolescents with aplastic anaemia or myelodysplasia. Br J Haematol 1997;96:749–56.

111. Hows JM, Yin JL, Marsh J, et al. Histocompatible unrelated volunteer donors compared with HLA nonidentical family donors in marrow transplantation for aplastic anemia and leukemia. Blood 1986;68(6):1322–8.

112. Margolis D, Camitta B, Pietryga D, et al. Unrelated donor bone marrow transplantation to treat severe aplastic anaemia in children and young adults. Br J Haematol 1996;94(1):65–72.
113. Viollier R, Socie G, Tichelli A, et al. Recent improvement in outcome of unrelated donor transplantation for aplastic anemia. Bone Marrow Transplant 2008;41(1):45–50.
114. Deeg HJ, Anasetti C, Petersdorf E, et al. Cyclophosphamide plus ATG conditioning is insufficient for sustained hematopoietic reconstitution in patients with severe aplastic anemia transplanted with marrow from HLA-A, B, DRB matched unrelated donors. Blood 1994;83(11):3417–8.
115. Deeg HJ, O'Donnell M, Tolar J, et al. Optimization of conditioning for marrow transplantation from unrelated donors for patients with aplastic anemia after failure of immunosuppressive therapy. Blood 2006;108:1485–91.
116. Vassiliou GS, Webb DK, Pamphilon D, et al. Improved outcome of alternative donor bone marrow transplantation in children with severe aplastic anaemia using a conditioning regimen containing low-dose total body irradiation, cyclophosphamide and Campath. Br J Haematol 2001;114(3):701–5.
117. Bacigalupo A, Locatelli F, Lanino E, et al. Fludarabine, cyclophosphamide and anti-thymocyte globulin for alternative donor transplants in acquired severe aplastic anemia: a report from the EBMT-SAA Working Party. Bone Marrow Transplant 2005;36(11):947–50.
118. Gupta V, Ball SE, Sage D, et al. Marrow transplants from matched unrelated donors for aplastic anaemia using alemtuzumab, fludarabine and cyclophosphamide based conditioning. Bone Marrow Transplant 2005;35(5):467–71.
119. Kosaka Y, Yagasaki H, Sano K, et al. Prospective multicenter trial comparing repeated immunosuppressive therapy with stem-cell transplantation from an alternative donor as second-line treatment for children with severe and very severe aplastic anemia. Blood 2008;111(3):1054–9.
120. Perez-Albuerne ED, Eapen M, Klein J, et al. Outcome of unrelated donor stem cell transplantation for children with severe aplastic anemia. Br J Haematol 2008;141(2):216–23.
121. Urban C, Benesch M, Sykora KW, et al. Non-radiotherapy conditioning with stem cell transplantation from alternative donors in children with refractory severe aplastic anemia. Bone Marrow Transplant 2005;35(6):591–4.
122. Fang JP, Xu HG, Huang SL, et al. Immunosuppressive treatment of aplastic anemia in Chinese children with antithymocyte globulin and cyclosporine. Pediatr Hematol Oncol 2006;23(1):45–50.
123. Pongtanakul B, Das PK, Charpentier K, et al. Outcome of children with aplastic anemia treated with immunosuppressive therapy. Pediatr Blood Cancer 2008; 50(1):52–7.
124. Scheinberg P, Wu CO, Nunez O, et al. Long-term outcome of pediatric patients with severe aplastic anemia treated with antithymocyte globulin and cyclosporine. J Pediatr 2008;153(6):814–9.
125. Maury S, Balere-Appert ML, Chir Z, et al. Unrelated stem cell transplantation for severe acquired aplastic anemia: improved outcome in the era of high-resolution HLA matching between donor and recipient. Haematologica 2007;92(5):589–96.
126. Passweg JR, Perez WS, Eapen M, et al. Bone marrow transplants from mismatched related and unrelated donors for severe aplastic anemia. Bone Marrow Transplant 2006;37(7):641–9.
127. Kojima S, Matsuyama T, Kato S, et al. Outcome of 154 patients with severe aplastic anemia who received transplants from unrelated donors: the Japan Marrow Donor Program. Blood 2002;100(3):799–803.

128. Rubinstein P, Carrier C, Scaradavou A, et al. Outcomes among 562 recipients of placental-blood transplants from unrelated donors. N Engl J Med 1998;339: 1565–77.

129. Eapen M, Ramsay NK, Mertens AC, et al. Late outcomes after bone marrow transplant for aplastic anaemia. Br J Haematol 2000;111(3):754–60.

130. Benesch M, Urban C, Sykora KW, et al. Transplantation of highly purified CD34+ progenitor cells from alternative donors in children with refractory severe aplastic anaemia. Br J Haematol 2004;125(1):58–63.

131. de la Rubia J, Cantero S, Sanz GF, et al. Transplantation of CD34+ selected peripheral blood to HLA-identical sibling patients with aplastic anaemia: results from a single institution. Bone Marrow Transplant 2005;36(4):325–9.

132. Schwinger W, Urban C, Lackner H, et al. Unrelated peripheral blood stem cell transplantation with 'megadoses' of purified CD34+ cells in three children with refractory severe aplastic anemia. Bone Marrow Transplant 2000;25(5): 513–7.

133. Amrolia PJ, Muccioli-Casadei G, Huls H, et al. Adoptive immunotherapy with allodepleted donor T-cells improves immune reconstitution after haploidentical stem cell transplant. Blood 2006;108:1797–808.

134. Andre-Schmutz I, Le Deist F, Hacein-Bey-Abina S, et al. Immune reconstitution without graft-versus-host disease after haemopoietic stem-cell transplantation: a phase 1/2 study. Lancet 2002;360(9327):130–7.

135. Bunin N, Aplenc R, Iannone R, et al. Unrelated donor bone marrow transplantation for children with severe aplastic anemia: minimal GVHD and durable engraftment with partial T cell depletion. Bone Marrow Transplant 2005;35(4): 369–73.

136. Guinan EC, Boussiotis VA, Neuberg D, et al. Transplantation of anergic histoincompatible bone marrow allografts. N Engl J Med 1999;340(22):1704–14.

137. Sanders JE. Endocrine complications of high-dose therapy with stem cell transplantation. Pediatr Transplant 2004;8(Suppl 5):39–50.

138. Deeg HJ, Leisenring W, Storb R, et al. Long-term outcome after marrow transplantation for severe aplastic anemia. Blood 1998;91(10):3637–45.

139. Pierga JY, Socie G, Gluckman E, et al. Secondary solid malignant tumors occurring after bone marrow transplantation for severe aplastic anemia given thoracoabdominal irradiation. Radiother Oncol 1994;30:55–8.

140. Deeg HJ, Socie G, Schoch G, et al. Malignancies after marrow transplantation for aplastic anemia and Fanconi anemia: a joint Seattle and Paris analysis of results in 700 patients. Blood 1996;87(1):386–92.

141. Feng X, Kajigaya S, Solomou EE, et al. Rabbit ATG but not horse ATG promotes expansion of functional CD4 + CD25highFOXP3+ regulatory T cells in vitro. Blood 2008;111(7):3675–83.

142. Matsuda S, Koyasu S. Mechanisms of action of cyclosporine. Immunopharmacology 2000;47(2–3):119–25.

143. Franzke A, Piao W, Lauber J, et al. G-CSF as immune regulator in T cells expressing the G-CSF receptor: implications for transplantation and autoimmune diseases. Blood 2003;102(2):734–9.

144. Fuhrer M, Rampf U, Baumann I, et al. Immunosuppressive therapy for aplastic anemia in children: a more severe disease predicts better survival. Blood 2005; 106(6):2102–4.

145. Frickhofen N, Heimpel H, Kaltwasser JP, et al. Antithymocyte globulin with or without cyclosporin A: 11-year follow-up of a randomized trial comparing treatments of aplastic anemia. Blood 2003;101(4):1236–42.

146. Marsh JCW, Ball SE, Darbyshire P, et al. Guidelines for the diagnosis and management of acquired aplastic anaemia. Br J Haematol 2003;123(5): 782–801.
147. Davies JK, Guinan EC. An update on the management of severe idiopathic aplastic anaemia in children. Br J Haematol 2007;136(4):549–64.
148. Kojima S, Hibi S, Kosaka Y, et al. Immunosuppressive therapy using antithymocyte globulin, cyclosporine, and danazol with or without human granulocyte colony-stimulating factor in children with acquired aplastic anemia. Blood 2000;96(6):2049–54.
149. Scheinberg P, Nunez O, Wu C, et al. Treatment of severe aplastic anaemia with combined immunosuppression: anti-thymocyte globulin, ciclosporin and mycophenolate mofetil. Br J Haematol 2006;133(6):606–11.
150. Tisdale JF, Dunn DE, Maciejewski J. Cyclophosphamide and other new agents for the treatment of severe aplastic anemia. Semin Hematol 2000;37(1):102–9.
151. Tisdale JF, Maciejewski JP, Nunez O, et al. Late complications following treatment for severe aplastic anemia (SAA) with high-dose cyclophosphamide (Cy): follow-up of a randomized trial. Blood 2002;100(13):4668–70.
152. Kim H, Min YJ, Baek JH, et al. A pilot dose-escalating study of alemtuzumab plus cyclosporine for patients with bone marrow failure syndrome. Leuk Res 2009;33(2):222–31.
153. Di Bona E, Rodeghiero F, Bruno B, et al. Rabbit antithymocyte globulin (r-ATG) plus cyclosporine and granulocyte colony stimulating factor is an effective treatment for aplastic anaemia patients unresponsive to a first course of intensive immunosuppressive therapy. Gruppo Italiano Trapianto di Midollo Osseo (GITMO). Br J Haematol 1999;107(2):330–4.
154. Matloub YH, Smith C, Bostrom B, et al. One course versus two courses of antithymocyte globulin for the treatment of severe aplastic anemia in children. J Pediatr Hematol Oncol 1997;19(2):110–4.
155. Tichelli A, Passweg J, Nissen C, et al. Repeated treatment with horse antilymphocyte globulin for severe aplastic anemia. Br J Haematol 1998;100:393–400.
156. Locasciulli A, van't Veer L, Bacigalupo A, et al. Treatment with marrow transplantation or immunosuppression of childhood acquired severe aplastic anemia: a report from the EBMT SAA Working Party. Bone Marrow Transplant 1990; 6(3):211–7.
157. Rosenfeld S, Kimball J, Vining D, et al. Intensive immunosuppression with antithymocyte globulin and cyclosporine as treatment for severe acquired aplastic anemia. Blood 1995;85:3058–65.
158. Schrezenmeier H, Marin P, Raghavachar A, et al. Relapse of aplastic anaemia after immunosuppressive treatment: a report from the European Bone Marrow Transplantation Group SAA Working Party. Br J Haematol 1993;85(2):371–7.
159. Scheinberg P, Nunez O, Young NS. Retreatment with rabbit anti-thymocyte globulin and ciclosporin for patients with relapsed or refractory severe aplastic anaemia. Br J Haematol 2006;133(6):622–7.
160. Ohara A, Kojima S, Hamajima N, et al. Myelodysplastic syndrome and acute myelogenous leukemia as a late clonal complication in children with acquired aplastic anemia. Blood 1997;90(3):1009–13.

Fanconi Anemia

Allison M. Green, BS[a], Gary M. Kupfer, MD[a,b,*]

KEYWORDS

- Fanconi anemia • Bone marrow failure • Genomic instability
- DNA damage and repair • Oxidative stress
- Monobiquitylation • Cytokines • BRCA1/2

Fanconi anemia (FA) is an autosomal and X-linked recessive disorder characterized by bone marrow failure, acute myelogenous leukemia (AML), solid tumors, and developmental abnormalities. At the molecular level, cells derived from FA patients display hypersensitivity to DNA cross-linking agents, resulting in increased numbers of chromosomal abnormalities including translocations and radial chromosomes. This hypersensitivity made treating FA patients a challenge in the past because traditional treatments of their symptoms resulted in more harm than good. Recent years have seen a dramatic improvement in FA patient treatment, however, resulting in a greater survival of children into adulthood. These improvements have been made despite the fact that a definitive cellular function for the proteins in the FA pathway has yet to be elucidated. Delineating the cellular functions of the FA pathway could help further improve the treatment options for FA patients and further reduce the probability of succumbing to the disease. This article reviews the current clinical aspects of FA including presentation, diagnosis, and treatment followed by a review of the molecular aspects of FA as they are currently understood (**Figs. 1** and **2**).

CLINICAL ASPECTS OF FANCONI ANEMIA

In earlier times, children with FA had the inevitable outcome of death, because most FA patients present with aplastic anemia and little in the way of supportive care was available. In the first part of the twentieth century, the advent of modern blood banking allowed the clinician to stem the immediacy of anemia and thrombocytopenia that resulted in death. As a result, the next major issue for these children became infection, even with the development of antibiotics. Neutropenic infections are generally not well tolerated and typically not curable with antibiotics alone, and many FA children succumbed to bacterial and fungal infections. Finally, even when a child could be

[a] Section of Pediatric Hematology-Oncology, Department of Pathology, Yale University School of Medicine, 333 Cedar Street LMP 2073, PO Box 208064, New Haven, CT 06520–8064, USA
[b] Section of Pediatric Hematology-Oncology, Department of Pediatrics, Yale University School of Medicine, 333 Cedar Street LMP 2073, PO Box 208064, New Haven, CT 06520–8064, USA
* Corresponding author. Section of Pediatric Hematology-Oncology, Department of Pediatrics, Yale University School of Medicine, 333 Cedar Street LMP 2073, PO Box 208064, New Haven, CT 06520–8064.
E-mail address: gary.kupfer@yale.edu (G.M. Kupfer).

Hematol Oncol Clin N Am 23 (2009) 193–214
doi:10.1016/j.hoc.2009.01.008
0889-8588/09/$ – see front matter © 2009 Elsevier Inc. All rights reserved.

hemonc.theclinics.com

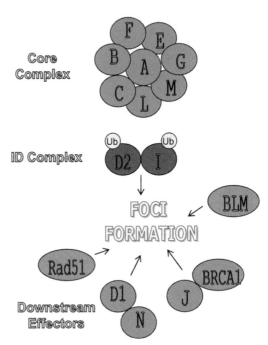

Fig. 1. The FA pathway proteins. The FA pathway is composed of at least 13 genes. Each of these genes, when biallelically mutated, causes FA. The encoded proteins can be subdivided within the FA pathway into three groups: (1) proteins that make up the core complex; (2) the FANCD2 and FANCI proteins, which compose the ID complex; (3) and three downstream effector proteins, FANCD1/BRCA2, FANCJ/BRIP1/BACH1, and FANCN/PALB2. Following treatment with DNA cross-linking agents or during S phase of the cell cycle, FANCD2 and FANCI become monoubiquitylated. An intact core complex is required for these modifications, which result in the translocation of the two proteins to chromatin within cells. Within chromatin, FANCD2 and FANCI colocalize with DNA repair proteins including the downstream effector FA proteins at sites of DNA damage in nuclear foci. FA proteins are in blue.

supported through the huge problem of aplastic anemia, the looming issue of AML nonetheless inevitably and inexorably presented itself. It was the exceptionally rare patient who survived to adulthood.[1–3]

Recent years have revolutionized the care of the FA patient. Although hematopoietic stem cell transplantation (SCT) has been performed on FA patients for almost 30 years, it is only in recent years that such approaches have been done more safely and successfully.[4] Even with the greater survival of children into adulthood as a result of SCT, the specter of potential of solid tumors, such as squamous cell carcinomas of the head, neck, and genitourinary track, remains a serious problem.[5–8]

PRESENTATION

Even though a classic set of features generally characterize these patients, FA children typically present in the first decade of life on recognition of aplastic anemia.[1–3] Nonetheless, classic features of FA consist of thumb and radial absence, malformation, or even less obvious features, such as a deeper cleft between the first two digits. In much the same way as the facial features of children affected by Down's syndrome allow

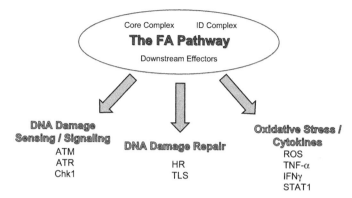

Fig. 2. FA pathway functions. Although an exact mechanism for the FA pathway has yet to be elucidated, it seems to function in sensing DNA damage induced by DNA cross-linking agents, such as mitomycin C, and diepoxybutane likely plays some role in initiating DNA repair. A significant body of work has also pointed to a role for the FA pathway in cell signaling in response to stress stimuli and in apoptosis in the cytoplasm, affecting maintenance of the hematopoietic machinery, so it is likely that at least some of these proteins are multifunctional. ATM, ataxia telangiectasia mutated kinase; ATR, ataxia telangiectasia mutated and Rad3-related kinase; chk1, checkpoint homolog 1; HR, homologous recombination; INF-γ, interferon-γ; ROS, reactive oxygen species; STAT1, signal transducer and activator of transcription; TLS, translesion synthesis; TNF-α, tumor necrosis factor-α.

easy recognition of their affliction, children with FA display a collection of subtle facial features that allow them to be easily recognizable as a group.

A less striking and less specific array of characteristics also may be present and are summarized in **Table 1**. Even more interesting is the fact that a subset of FA patients has no discernible abnormalities at all, in a fraction estimated at up to one third. As a result, the index of suspicion of the clinician must be high to recognize the potential for the diagnosis of FA in the wake of aplastic anemia.

DIAGNOSIS

Once it is recognized that a patient has a production defect resulting in the occurrence of more than one cell line abnormally low, it is incumbent on the clinician to then

Table 1
Physical abnormalities seen in Fanconi anemia patients

Physical Abnormality	Percent of Fanconi Anemia Patients
Skin discolorations	55
Hand, arm, and other skeletal abnormalities	51
Abnormal reproductive organs	35
Small head or eyes	26
Kidney problems	21
Low birth weight	11
Heart defects	6
Gastrointestinal problems (bowel)	5

Data from Alter B. Diagnostic evaluation of FA. In: Owen J, Frohnmayer L, Eiler ME, editors. Fanconi anemia standards for clinical care. 2nd edition. London: The Fanconi Anemia Research Fund; 2003. p. 3–17.

proceed to an examination of the bone marrow. At the time of the bone marrow procedure, it is critical not only to perform aspiration but also a biopsy so that cellularity may be assessed and pathologic examination for evidence of leukemia undertaken. Aspirate samples are sent typically for flow cytometry to rule out further evidence of clonal cell populations and for examination of cell morphology.

The gold standard tests for FA quantify chromosomal breakage in cells exposed to cross-linking agents to which FA cells are hypersensitive. In this test lymphocytes from patients are stimulated and exposed or not to diepoxybutane or mitomycin C (MMC). After inducing mitotic arrest, the cells are then dropped onto slides, and the chromosomes are scored for the number of induced breaks. The hallmark of FA is increased chromosome breakage in a statistically significant way. The chromosomal breakage assay is actually a clue to the basic biology of FA, because the cells themselves that are derived from FA patients display increased cell death when exposed to a whole range of chemical cross-linkers, including diepoxybutane, MMC, and cisplatin.[2-4,9]

On occasion, despite the strong suspicion of FA being present in a patient, the chromosome fragility test can be negative. This phenomenon is associated with somatic reversion in which the hematopoietic lineages (in all or in part) have undergone mutation at a second site within the affected FA gene, resulting in restoration of at least partial function of that FA protein product.[10-13] This phenomenon occurs probably because of a combination of increased genetic instability inherent in the phenotype of FA in combination with selective pressure of the relatively rapidly overturning hematopoietic compartment. Such a phenomenon also has implication for the potential for gene therapy approaches to FA, discussed later. In the face of this possibility, if a negative diepoxybutane or MMC result has been obtained in the setting of strong suspicion of an FA diagnosis, then a skin biopsy should be obtained for culture and subsequent diepoxybutane testing.

ACUTE MYELOGENOUS LEUKEMIA

Even though 90% of FA patients first present with bone marrow failure, a certain percentage nonetheless display AML as the first evidence of FA. These cases of AML are typically M1-M4 FAB subtype and display no characteristic cytogenetic or molecular abnormality, although numerous translocations, deletions, and other aneuploidogenic changes can be found.[14,15] The most ominous part of a diagnosis of AML is the fact that FA patients cannot be treated in a typical fashion as other AML patients, because of their inability to tolerate standard doses of alkylating agents. One might expect that AMLs derived from FA patients would display greater sensitivity to chemotherapy and potentially be more curable, but the morbidity to the patient precludes an aggressive approach. In addition, analysis of cells derived from these AML cases reveals that they are heterogeneous in their cell culture response to agents that normally confer marked toxicity in the patient.

STEM CELL TRANSPLANTATION

The decision to go forward with SCT in an FA patient is one not to be taken lightly. Under the best of circumstances in a patient unafflicted by FA, going forward electively with SCT presents risks and potential for morbidity. Total body irradiation and cyclophosphamide, which are typical parts of conditioning regimens, can result in long-term effects on growth, cognition, and secondary malignancy. In addition, the potential of graft-versus-host disease can result in long-term complications that may result in death. Most clinicians prefer to wait if they have the choice until children are out of the first decade of life, after which such effects are somewhat ameliorated.

It is an even more difficult decision for the FA patient because he or she is so susceptible to toxicity from the regimen. Those caring for the FA patient must realize, however, that an educated guess must be made as to when to transplant the patient so as to pre-empt the onset of leukemia; avoid the long-term effects of blood product provision; and proceed when the patient is in good clinical shape and unaffected by serious infections, such as those from invasive organisms like *Aspergillus*.

An assessment should be made as to the likelihood that proceeding to SCT is necessary. Typically, once the diagnosis of FA has been made, an attempt to identify the complementation group should be made. It has become clear from the experience of FA clinicians that FA-D1 patients are at significant and early risk of progression to AML, often before the presentation of aplastic anemia.[1,16,17] In addition, other genotypes associated with early AML progression include the FA-C Ashkenazi Jewish mutation (deletion of exon 4).[18,19] In general terms, it is thought that such a risk of early AML progression is coincident with a more severely displayed FA phenotype. Finally, a careful watch of patient's cell counts and yearly bone marrow evaluation by the clinician is necessary to identify a decline in numbers that could result in the need for transfusion therapy. Chronic transfusions are generally associated with poorer outcome in the transplant setting, resulting in increased iron burden with the concomitant potential for organ damage, and signaling the potential for neutropenia that can result in infections that can delay or even proscribe the start of SCT.[20-22]

Because the clinical status of FA patients can change rapidly, it is prudent to be prepared for SCT by early identification of a donor well before the need to proceed. Provided the patient has a sibling, that sibling has an approximately 20% chance of being a donor. Because of improved techniques in transplant and the potential for donors in the extended family if ethnically homogeneous, donors can often be found in parents and other family members. If no donor is found in the family then a search is initiated in the unrelated pool, including adults in the National Marrow Donor Registry and cord blood banks. At this time, the typical analysis of HLA loci involves molecular analysis at both alleles, resulting in report on 10 loci. Transplants can proceed with matches of as little as 8 of 10, especially in cord bloods. Several centers are conducting trials with haplo donors from parents.[23-26]

Historically, the challenges of SCT in FA patients have been numerous. The issue of graft failure has been inherent with a prevalence of 10%. Avoiding this outcome necessitates the use of significant conditioning, which is associated with toxicity. In recent years the use of fludaribine has shrunk this number to less than 1%. As a result, efforts at reduction of conditioning have been steady and the use of total body irradiation has been diminished down to doses of 400 to 600 cGy. In addition, the use of cyclophosphamide has also been decreased in recent years. With an allogenic-related transplant, the long-term survival is often greater than 80%.[27-29]

Matched-unrelated transplants have posed a greater challenge with a greater incidence of graft-versus-host disease. Toxicity-associated graft-versus-host disease has proved to occur with greater intensity in the FA patient, perhaps because of the greater degree of toxicity caused by conditioning. Such toxicity is synergistic with the increased graft-versus-host disease risk. With diminished toxicity has come greater graft-versus-host disease control and subsequent increased survival for FA patients undergoing matched-unrelated transplants.[27,30-32]

Secondary effects of SCT predictably have greater consequences for FA patients presumably because of their underlying issues of growth delay, endocrine dysfunction, and risk of malignancy, all of which are associated with long-term effects of undergoing SCT. A markedly increased risk of acquisition of squamous cell carcinoma is seen posttransplantation, out of proportion to that observed anyway in FA patients. These cases are associated with patients having significant toxicity during SCT and are only somewhat linked to human papillomavirus.[7,33,34]

The idea that FA cells are hypersensitive to endogenous and exogenous stimuli suggests that FA stem cells in the bone marrow are susceptible to a sort of "natural selection." This is probably why somatic reversion is observed in some FA patients. As a result, it has been postulated that FA patients are ideal for gene therapy clinical trials. Trials entailing the most common complementation group, FA-A, have been instituted using a lentiviral transduction system of hematopoietic stem cells from FA patients, manipulated ex vivo. In vitro data suggest that hematopoietic stem cells can be transduced with subsequent colony-forming assays suggesting increased growth and reconstitution. Such trails have been disappointing, however, because lack of permanent transduction of progenitors has led to failure to establish long-term hematopoiesis.[35–38]

Traditionally, androgens have proved to be an efficacious treatment in aplastic patients, FA patients included. Androgens generally stimulate more effective hematopoiesis, resulting in an increase in peripheral blood counts. The use of androgens has been marked by their difficulty in use in females, however, given the masculinizing side effects. In addition, their use has been associated with increased risk of liver adenomas.[39,40]

MOLECULAR ASPECTS OF FANCONI ANEMIA

At the molecular level, cells derived from FA patients display hypersensitivity to DNA cross-linking agents, such as MMC and diepoxybutane. Treatment with these agents induces an abnormally prolonged cell cycle arrest in S phase and an accumulation of cells with 4 N DNA.[41] As the result of this response, the FA pathway has been hypothesized to function in sensing DNA damage induced by these agents and in initiating its repair. This hypothesis has been supported by work elucidating the interactions of FA proteins with established DNA repair proteins. A significant body of work has pointed to a role for the FA pathway in cell signaling in response to stress stimuli and in apoptosis in the cytoplasm, however, affecting maintenance of the hematopoietic machinery. Although the exact role of the FA pathway has yet to be discovered, what is known about the FA proteins and their interactions is reviewed.

The FA pathway is composed of at least 13 genes.[42] Each of these genes, when biallelically mutated, causes FA. The encoded proteins (**Table 2**) can be subdivided within the FA pathway into three groups: (1) proteins that make up the core complex; (2) the FANCD2 and FANCI proteins, which compose the ID complex; and (3) three downstream effector proteins, FANCD1/BRCA2, FANCJ/BRIP1/BACH1, and FANCN/PALB2. Many of the FA proteins contain no recognizable motifs, which has made discovering their contributions to the FA pathway and the main function of the FA pathway more challenging. The following section delineates what is known about each of the three FA protein subdivisions and how these groups interact to form an intact FA pathway.

FANCONI ANEMIA CORE COMPLEX PROTEINS

The nuclear "core" complex is composed of 8 of the 13 FA proteins (FANCA, FANCB, FANCC, FANCE, FANCF, FANCG, FANCL, and FANCM). This core complex is required for the monoubiquitylation of FANCD2 and FANCI.[42] Although the reason

Table 2
The 13 Fanconi anemia genes and proteins they encode

Complementation Group	Responsible Gene	Chromosome Location	Protein Molecular Weight (kd)	Known Motifs	Necessary for FANCD2 Monoubiquitylation
A	FANCA	16q24.3	163	2 NLSs, 5 NESs	Yes
B	FANCB	Xp22.31	95	NLS	Yes
C	FANCC	9q22.3	63	None	Yes
D1	FANCD1/BRCA2	13q12.13	380	8 BRC repeats, HD, 3 OBs, TD	No
D2	FANCD2	3p25.3	155, 162	None	Yes
E	FANCE	6p21-22	60	2 NLSs	Yes
F	FANCF	11p15	42	None	Yes
G	FANCG/XRCC9	9p13	68	7 TPRs	Yes
I	FANCI/KIAA1794	15q25-26	146	None	Yes
J	FANCJ/BRIP1/BACH1	17q22-24	130	ATPase, 7 helicase-specific motifs	No
L	FANCL/PHF9	2p16.1	43	3 WD40s, PHD	Yes
M	FANCM	14q21.3	250	7 helicase-specific motifs, degenerate endonuclease domain, ATPase	Yes
N	FANCN/PALB2	16p12	130	2 WD40s	No

for the necessity of an intact FA core complex for these modifications is not well understood, biallelic mutation or deletion of any one of the genes that encode these eight core proteins results in failure to monoubiquitylate FANCD2 and FANCI. The exact mechanism by which the core complex facilitates the monoubiquitylation of FANCD2 and FANCI has yet to be worked out, but a few core complex members contain motifs that allow speculation as to their functions within the complex if not the pathway.

Several of the core complex proteins including FANCA, FANCB, and FANCE contain nuclear localization signals supporting lines of evidence showing that the core complex fully assembles in the nucleus.[43–45] FANCL/PHF9 has been proposed to be the catalytic E3 ubiquitin ligase subunit of the FA core complex required for the monoubiquitylation of FANCD2.[46] FANCL contains three WD40 motifs that are required for interaction with other FA core complex proteins and a plant homeodomain motif that when mutated impairs FANCD2 monoubiquitylation.[47] The FANCL protein has displayed autoubiquitylation activity in vitro;[46] however, in vivo ubiquitin ligase activity has yet to be shown. FANCM has been proposed to act as a scaffolding protein for the FA core complex and is necessary for its localization to chromatin.[48] FANCM possesses seven helicase specific motifs and a degenerate endonuclease domain.[42] Although displaying considerable homology to the archeal Hef (helicase associated endonuclease for fork-structured DNA) protein, which has functional helicase and endonuclease domains and resolves stalled replication forks,[49] the FANCM protein has not displayed any of these activities thus far. The FANCM protein has been shown, however, to display DNA-dependent ATPase activity and promotes the dissociation of DNA triplexes, acting as a DNA translocase.[50] The FANCM protein has been found to require interaction with the FA-associated protein 24 (FAAP24) for functional integrity, because depletion of FAAP24 has been shown to disrupt the chromatin association of FANCM and to destabilize FANCM, leading to failure of the core complex to localize to chromatin.[48] Several of the core complex proteins including FANCA, FANCG, and FANCM are also regulated by phosphorylation and dephosphorylation throughout the cell cycle.[48,51–53] These modifications also seem to be necessary for intact FA pathway function.

Although evidence has shown that an intact core complex is unequivocally necessary for activation of the FA pathway through regulation of the monoubiquitylation of FANCD2, it has been proposed that the core complex proteins may also perform other functions. Consistent with this hypothesis, the eight FA core complex proteins also segregate into several distinct subcomplexes among themselves. FANCB and FANCL directly interact and have been found to interact with FANCA through complex purification experiments. The interaction of these three proteins is disrupted in FA-G and FA-M cells but intact in FA-C, FA-E, and FA-F cells suggesting that two discrete subcomplexes exist, one composed of FANCA, FANCB, FANCG, FANCL, and FANCM, and another composed of FANCC, FANCE, and FANCF.[54] Although the function of these subcomplexes remains elusive, the FANCA protein has been shown directly to interact with a central portion of the BRCA1 protein in a DNA damage-independent manner,[55] the FANCG protein has been shown to interact with XRCC3 and FANCD1/BRCA2,[56] and the FANCM protein has been found to be capable of catalyzing branch migration of Holliday junctions and replication forks in vitro.[50] This suggests that the FANCA, FANCB, FANCG, FANCL, and FANCM subcomplex may participate in the cellular response to DNA cross-links both upstream of FANCD2 and FANCI monoubiquitylation in the core complex and downstream in the aforementioned subcomplex within the FA pathway. The interaction of the two subcomplexes seems to be mediated by FANCG, which interacts with both FANCA and FANCF.[57]

Finally, FANCE seems to mediate the interaction of the core complex with FANCD2 because FANCE has been demonstrated to interact with FANCD2 both in vitro and in vivo.[58]

FANCD2-FANCI

Following treatment with DNA cross-linking agents[59] or during S phase of the cell cycle,[60] FANCD2 and FANCI become monoubiquitylated. These modifications result in the translocation of the two proteins to chromatin within cells where they colocalize with DNA repair proteins including the downstream effector FA proteins at sites of DNA damage.[61–63] An intact core complex is necessary for the monoubiquitylation of FANCD2 on lysine 561[61] and FANCI on lysine 523.[62,63] FANCI is a relatively new member of the FA pathway, identified by a screen for phosphopeptides corresponding to consensus substrates of ataxia telangiectasia mutated kinase (ATM)/ataxia telangiectasia mutated and Rad3-related kinase (ATR).[64] Although the role of the FANCI protein in the FA pathway has yet to be identified, FA-I cells display a lack of FANCD2 monoubiquitylation and a subsequent failure in FANCD2 chromatin-associated foci formation while maintaining a normal intact core complex.[65] Interestingly, FANCI shares sequence homology to FANCD2 and associates with FANCD2 as the FANCI-FANCD2 (ID) complex, which translocates to chromatin following DNA damage.[62] Importantly, monoubiquitylation modifications on FANCD2 and FANCI are important for the preservation of monoubiquitylation on the other protein in the ID complex, respectively.[62] Phosphorylation is also a regulatory mechanism for FANCD2 and FANCI because phosphorylation of key residues on each protein is required for monoubiquitylation and focus formation of both.[66,67] Many of the proteins that colocalize with FANCD2 and FANCI in discrete nuclear foci following treatment with DNA cross-linking agents are proteins that function in DNA damage sensing and repair. These interactions are discussed more in depth later in this article.

THE "DOWNSTREAM" PROTEINS: FANCD1, FANCJ, AND FANCN

The *FANCD1* gene is identical to the familial breast-ovarian cancer susceptibility gene *BRCA2* and as such, biallelic mutation of the *FANCD1/BRCA2* gene results in the FA-D1 subtype of FA, whereas monoallelic mutation results in increased breast and ovarian cancer susceptibility.[68] The main contribution of the FANCD1 protein to the FA pathway is through its ability to recruit Rad51 into the DNA damage-inducible nuclear foci, which FANCD2 translocates into following monoubiquitylation.[69] Rad51 is a recombinase, which like its bacterial homologue RecA binds ssDNA and promotes homologous recombination (HR).[70] The FANCD1/BRCA2 protein consists of eight BRC repeats that have been shown to bind RAD51[71] and five C-terminal domains consisting of a helical domain, three oligonucleotide/oligosaccharide-binding folds, and a tower domain.[72] The oligosaccharide-binding domains participate in ssDNA binding, whereas the tower domain participates in dsDNA binding, allowing the FANCD1/BRCA2 protein to nucleate RAD51 filament formation at ssDNA/dsDNA junctions to promote HR.[72] The protein DSS1 also interacts with FANCD1/BRCA2 and is necessary for the protein's stability.[73]

The *FANCJ* gene is identical to the *BRIP1* (*BRCA1* interacting protein C-terminal helicase 1) and *BACH1* (*BRCA1* associated carboxyl terminal helicase 1) genes.[74–76] As the names of BRIP1 and BACH1 imply, the FANCJ/BRIP1/BACH1 protein directly binds to the BRCT domain of BRCA1.[77] The BRCT domain is a phosphoprotein binding domain, and phosphorylation of FANCJ/BRIP1/BACH1 on serine 990 is required for this interaction.[78] The FANCJ/BRIP1/BACH1 protein is a DNA-dependent ATPase and a 5′ to 3′ DNA helicase, which contains seven helicase-specific motifs.[77] FANCJ has been shown to be a structure-specific helicase, dissociating guanine quadruplex DNA in vitro.[79]

FANCN/PALB2 (partner and localizer of BRCA2) is an interacting protein of FANCD1/BRCA2 on which BRCA2 contributions to DNA double strand break repair and HR are at least partially reliant.[80] The only recognizable motifs in the FANCN/PALB2 protein are two WD40 repeat-like motifs in its carboxyl terminus.[80] Cells deficient in FANCN/PALB2 show cellular phenotypes similar to those seen in cells deficient in FANCD1/BRCA2, such as lack of formation of Rad51 foci after ionizing radiation.[81] FANCN-deficient cells also lack FANCD1/BRCA2 chromatin association, which is necessary for proper double strand break repair and HR.[80]

THE FANCONI ANEMIA PATHWAY AND DNA REPAIR

Cells derived from FA patients display hypersensitivity to DNA cross-linking agents, such as MMC and diepoxybutane.[59] Treatment of cells derived from FA patients with DNA cross-linking drugs has been shown to induce an abnormally prolonged cell cycle arrest in S phase and an accumulation of cells containing 4 N DNA.[41] The mechanism by which the interstrand and intrastrand cross-links induced by these drugs are resolved in mammals is not well understood. Although it is known that nucleotide excision repair, HR, and translesion synthesis (TLS) repair pathways play a role in repairing interstrand and intrastrand cross-links in bacteria and that nucleotide excision repair, Rad6/Rad18-dependent postreplication repair, HR, and cell cycle checkpoint pathways play a role in repairing interstrand and intrastrand cross-links in yeast,[82] lack of a convenient and accurate approach to studying interstrand and intrastrand cross-links in mammals has delayed the field.

In 2005, Nojima and colleagues[83] inferred that multiple pathways are used to resolve interstrand and intrastrand cross-links in chicken DT40 cells and deduced that the FA pathway is epistatic with TLS and HR mediated interstrand and intrastrand cross-links repair. Although a definitive role for the FA proteins in the TLS or HR pathway has yet to be elucidated in vertebrates, many studies have linked the FA pathway to TLS and HR through interactions between FA proteins and proteins that participate in these DNA repair pathways. The following paragraphs briefly describe these known interactions alluding to a role for FA proteins in TLS and HR mediated interstrand and intrastrand cross-links repair.

THE FANCONI ANEMIA PATHWAY AND HOMOLOGOUS RECOMBINATION PROTEINS

One of the most obvious connections between the FA and HR pathways is the interaction between FANCD1/BRCA2 and RAD51. RAD51 is the mammalian homolog of the bacterial RecA protein, which is a ssDNA binding protein necessary for catalyzing the strand invasion step of HR.[84] The interaction between BRCA2 and RAD51 was first discovered through a yeast two-hybrid screen.[85] The importance of this interaction to the FA pathway was not understood until the gene mutated in FA-D1 patients was discovered to be identical to BRCA2.[68] Since then, it has been discovered that the internal BRC repeat motifs within the BRCA2 protein are required for this interaction with RAD51[71] and that this interaction promotes RAD51 nucleoprotein filament formation, which is a necessary early step in the HR pathway.[72] It has also more recently been discovered that the BRCA2 binding protein PALB2 is the protein mutated in the FA-N complementation group.[80] This discovery also then connects FANCN/PALB2 to the HR pathway because FANCN-deficient cells lack FANCD1/BRCA2 chromatin association, which is necessary for proper HR.[80]

The familial breast cancer protein BRCA1 contributes to the HR pathway upstream of BRCA2 and plays a much broader role, participating in multiple cellular processes in response to DNA damage.[86] Although previous studies provided evidence of indirect interactions between BRCA1 and FANCD1/BRCA2,[85,87,88] it was not until 1998 that the two proteins were shown to coimmunoprecipitate and colocalize in nuclear foci during S phase of the cell cycle,[89] foci that were later shown also to contain FANCD2.[59] Interestingly, through the use of yeast two-hybrid analysis, it was discovered that the amino-terminus of the FANCA protein directly interacts with a central section of the BRCA1 protein and this interaction is independent of DNA damage.[55] Finally, perhaps the strongest connection between BRCA1 and the FA pathway lies in the interaction between FANCJ/BRIP1/BACH1 and BRCA1. As its two alternate names suggest, the FANCJ protein was originally identified as a BRCA1 interacting protein because it binds directly to the BRCT domain of BRCA1 and promotes BRCA1s known roles in DNA repair.[77]

The BLM protein is a RecQ family helicase with an ATP-dependent 3'-5' DNA helicase activity. This helicase seems to be highly DNA-structure specific, showing in vivo activity on branched DNA structures, such as Holliday junctions, which can occur during the repair of stalled or collapsed replication forks by HR.[90] Interestingly, purified FANCD2 has also been shown to bind DNA with an increased propensity for dsDNA ends and Holliday junctions.[91] The interaction between the BLM protein and the FA pathway was first elucidated through the purification of a BLM-associated multiprotein complex composed of multiple FA proteins and known BLM-interacting proteins since called the BRAFT complex. Under high salt conditions, BLM and its associated proteins dissociate from the FA proteins leaving the FA core complex.[92] Colocalization in nuclear foci and coimmunoprecipitation of FANCD2 and BLM following DNA damage provide further evidence linking the FA pathway to the HR pathway through interaction with BLM.[93]

In response to forms of DNA damage, such as double strand breaks, the mammalian histone H2A variant H2AX is incorporated into DNA at sites surrounding the damage and is phosphorylated at serine 139 (serine 136 in mice) to generate γH2AX. The γH2AX histone variant serves as a marker of double strand breaks and helps to initiate the accumulation of DNA damage sensing and repairing proteins, such as NBS1 and BRCA1, to these sites of damage to activate DNA damage signaling pathways and ultimately DNA repair through HR or NHEJ.[94] A functional connection between γH2AX and the FA pathway was first discovered in H2AX-/- mouse embryonic fibroblasts. Although UV irradiation in wild-type mouse embryonic fibroblasts prompted the formation of FANCD2 nuclear foci, the formation of FANCD2 foci was abolished in H2AX-/- cells.[95] FANCD2 and H2AX have since been shown to coimmunoprecipitate, an interaction dependent on H2AX phosphorylation. Consistent with the idea that γH2AX is important for FANCD2 recruitment to nuclear foci and for DNA repair, H2AX-/- and phosphorylation-defective H2AX mutant cells have been shown to be hypersensitive to MMC treatment. Interestingly, this sensitivity is not further exacerbated by siRNA-mediated knockdown of FANCD2, suggesting that the two proteins function epistatically in the cellular response to DNA damage induced by MMC treatment.[95]

THE FANCONI ANEMIA PATHWAY AND TRANSLESION SYNTHESIS PROTEINS

To continue replicating through sites of DNA damage, which block replicative polymerases and lead to replication fork stalling, cells use TLS polymerases. Each TLS polymerase is specialized to replicate through a specific type of DNA lesion and keep the replication fork moving regardless of DNA damage.[96] The protein proliferating cell nuclear antigen (PCNA) plays an essential role in this switch from replicative to TLS polymerase. PCNA functions as a polymerase clamp, tethering a polymerase to DNA in need of replication to increase processivity.[97] An interaction between PCNA and FA proteins was first suggested by studies indicating that PCNA colocalizes with FANCD1/BRCA2 and BRCA1 and RAD51 in nuclear foci following treatment with ultraviolet irradiation and hydroxyurea.[89] It was later discovered that PCNA also colocalizes in foci containing FANCD2 in cells treated with hydroxyurea,[98] verifying the observation that DNA damage induces an interaction between PCNA and the FA pathway.

The REV1 protein is a eukaryotic member of the Y family of DNA polymerases, which function as TLS polymerases, replicating through sites of DNA damage. The REV1 protein is an error-prone TLS polymerase that functions as a deoxycytidyl transferase, inserting cytidine nucleotides opposite any template strand nucleotide and abasic sites during TLS-mediated replication.[99] Studies in the DT40 chicken cell line revealed that cells deficient in FANCC, REV1, or another TLS polymerase REV3 showed similar levels of hypersensitivity to cisplatin treatment as measured by cell survival percentage and number of chromosomal aberrations per metaphase, leading to the inference that the proteins function epistatically in response to DNA cross-linking treatment.[100] Further studies in FA-A, FA-G, and FA-D2 patient derived cell lines show that the core complex proteins FANCA and FANCG are required for REV1 nuclear foci formation, whereas FANCD2 is not. Interestingly, mutation of the BRCT domain of REV1, which is necessary for its interaction with PCNA, does not further impair assembly of REV1 into nuclear foci in FANCG-deficient cells, indicating that FANCG may facilitate localization of REV1 in nuclear foci.[101]

The USP1 protein is a ubiquitin specific protease or deubiquitylating enzyme, capable of cleaving ubiquitin moieties off of proteins.[102] The USP1 protein was found to play a role in the FA pathway through a gene family RNAi library screen, which showed that inhibition of USP1 resulted in increased accumulation of ubiquitylated FANCD2. Further experiments showed that USP1 physically interacts with FANCD2 and that the two proteins colocalize in chromatin after DNA damage.[103] This interaction between USP1 and FANCD2 ties the FA pathway to the TLS pathway because USP1 has since been found also to be the deubiquitylating enzyme for PCNA. Similar to results seen with FANCD2, inhibition of USP1 resulted in increased accumulation of monoubiquitylated PCNA.[104] These results have been replicated in a USP1 null chicken DT40 cell line in which eradication of USP1 also resulted in elevated levels of monoubiquitylated FANCD2 and PCNA.[105]

THE FANCONI ANEMIA PATHWAY AND CELL SIGNALING

The FA pathway also interacts with the DNA damage response through the DNA sensing and signaling proteins ataxia telangiectasia and ATM kinase, ATM and ATR kinase, and Chk1 kinase. Cells from patients with ataxia telangiectasia display radiohypersensitivity, cell cycle checkpoint defects, and chromosomal instability. The ATM protein is a serine-threonine kinase and is a member of the phosphatidylinositol-3 kinase–related protein kinase family of kinases. The main function of ATM seems to be recognizing and responding to DNA double strand breaks by initiating a signaling cascade, which results in activation of DNA repair factors and ultimately double strand break repair.[106,107] Taniguchi and colleagues[66] have shown that FANCD2-/- patient-derived cells display a defect in S phase checkpoint response after treatment with IR similar to that seen in ataxia telangiectasia cells. A direct interaction between the

ATM signaling pathway and the FA pathway was made because ATM was shown to phosphorylate FANCD2 on serine 222 in normal cells in response to IR and this phosphorylation event was shown to be necessary for proper cellular response to double strand breaks. Interestingly, the FANCD2-S222A phosphorylation mutant was monoubiquitylated and translocated into discrete nuclear foci following treatment with MMC implying that phosphorylation on serine 222 is not necessary for FANCD2 monoubiquitylation.

Patients with biallelic mutations of the ATR kinase develop Seckel's syndrome, an extremely rare autosomal-recessive disease characterized by microcephaly, growth retardation, and mental retardation. Like ATM, ATR is a serine-threonine kinase and is a member of the phosphatidylinositol-3 kinase–related protein kinase family of kinases. The two proteins also share an overlapping set of protein substrates, which influence DNA repair and cell cycle arrest. Unlike ATM, however, which becomes activated as a result of double strand breaks, ATR becomes activated every S phase of the cell cycle to signal for repair of collapsed replication forks and to prevent early initiation of mitosis.[108] An interaction between ATR and the FA pathway was first hinted at by experiments showing that FANCD2 and ATR colocalized in nuclear foci following treatment with DNA cross-linking agents.[109,110] Further experiments showed that depletion of ATR resulted in inhibition of FANCD2 foci formation and the development of radial chromosomes mimicking those seen in FA patient-derived cells. Interestingly, two major sites of ATR-mediated phosphorylation on FANCD2 are T691 and S717, phosphorylation of which is required for FANCD2 monoubiquitylation and correction of MMC sensitivity in FA-D2 patient-derived cells.[111]

ATR also interacts with other members of the FA pathway. Phosphorylation of FANCG on serine 7 by ATR is necessary for the interaction of FANCG with FANCD1/BRCA2, XRCC2, and FANCD2.[112] ATR has also been shown to phosphorylate FANCI on serines 730 and 1121 and threonine 952.[62] Finally, down-regulation of FANCM or its associated protein FAAP24 dysregulates ATR-meditated checkpoint signaling, further suggesting some interplay between ATR-mediated checkpoint signaling and the FA pathway.[113]

Another of the many substrates of ATR is the effector kinase Chk1. Activation of Chk1 in S phase suspends DNA replication, stabilizes stalled replication forks, and prevents preemptive mitosis initiation.[114] In an examination of the effects of Chk1 on the FA pathway, two highly conserved Chk1 phosphorylation consensus sequences were discovered in the FANCE protein at threonine 346 and serine 374. In vitro and in vivo experiments confirmed these residues as Chk1 phosphorylation sites. Although expression of the FANCE-T346A/S374A double mutant in FA-E cells resulted in a failure to correct MMC sensitivity, FANCD2 monoubiquitylation and foci formation after MMC treatment were left intact. Further experiments showed that FANCE phosphorylated on T346 colocalized with FANCD2 in discrete nuclear foci following UV irradiation, suggesting that phosphorylated FANCE plays a role in DNA damage repair outside of the canonical FA pathway.[115]

THE FANCONI ANEMIA PATHWAY, OXIDATIVE STRESS, CYTOKINE SENSITIVITY

Teleologically, the involvement of very specific developmental abnormalities in FA patients implies that the FA proteins have the potential for other functions aside from those they perform in protecting the genome. Others have argued that the main function of the FA pathway is to regulate oxidative stress, because reactive oxygen species have been documented to be involved in bone marrow failure,[116,117] cancer,[118] endocrinopathies,[119] abnormalities in skin pigmentation,[120] and malformations.[121] This explanation becomes even more plausible when considering the redox-related functions of some FA proteins. Specifically, FANCC has been shown to associate with NADPH cytochrome P-450 reductase and glutathione S-transferase, two proteins with redox functions.[122,123] Microarray studies comparing mRNA expression levels found that nuclear factor-1, heat shock protein 70, and cyclooxygenase 2 were consistently overexpressed in FANCC-deficient cells as compared with their corrected counterparts.[124] The FANCG protein has been shown to interact with cytochrome P-450 2E1, which has been shown to be involved in metabolism of xenobiotics, such as MMC.[125] Finally, both FANCA and FANCG have been shown to be redox-sensitive proteins that multimerize following H_2O_2 treatment, lending plausibility to the hypothesis that the FA pathway may function in oxidative stress management in cells.[126]

Several lines of evidence have shown that excessive apoptosis and consequent malfunction of the hematopoietic stem cell compartment lead to progressive bone marrow failure in FA patients. The FANCC protein functions independently of the FA core complex to suppress apoptosis in hematopoietic cells in response to environmental cues, which induce expression or secretion of certain cytokines.[127] FA patients exhibit altered expression levels of some growth factors and cytokines, including unusually high levels of intracellular tumor necrosis factor-α (TNF-α), a cytokine capable of initiating the apoptotic pathway. Hematopoietic stem cells with inactivating mutations in the FANCC gene are hypersensitive to cytokines, such as interferon-γ and TNF-α.[127] Neoplastic stem cell clones, however, which are resistant to these cytokines, frequently evolve in FA patients and result in leukemia. This phenomenon was more closely examined by Li and colleagues[128] through the use of a murine Fancc-/- model. Recapitulating what likely happens in FA patients, exposure of murine Fancc-/- stem cells to TNF-α results in inhibition of growth in the short term but promotes evolution of clones resistant to TNF-α when treated for longer periods of time. These long-term treated TNF-α–resistant outgrowth cells, when transplanted into wild-type mice, result in AML, mimicking their human counterparts. Importantly, expression of FANCC cDNA in the fancc-/- stem cells prevented the formation of leukemic clonal outgrowths, implying that the FA pathway and the FANCC protein are necessary for an intact cellular response to TNF-α.

The growth inhibition seen in murine fancc-/- stem cells after short-term exposure to TNF-α was further explored by the Pang group and found to correlate with accumulation of reactive oxygen species. Deletion of the TNF-α receptor in fancc-/- mice resulted in a reduction in the amount of reactive oxygen species produced and reduced levels of hematopoietic senescence. Cells from TNF-α–treated fancc-/- mice also showed increased levels of chromosomal aberrations and decreased levels of repair of DNA damage caused by reactive oxygen species, indicating that FANCC may also play a role in the cellular response to oxidative DNA damage.[128]

The FANCC protein has also been found to interact with and be necessary for the proper localization of the STAT1 transcription factor following stimulation with interferon-γ. Loss of functional FANCC results in reduced levels of STAT1 activation and impaired Th1 differentiation, possibly leading to a slight immunologic defect in FA patients.[129] Stimulation with interferon-γ has also been found to activate the RNA-dependent protein kinase PKR, which has been found to be constitutively activated in FANCC-deficient cells. Activated PKR phosphorylates the translation initiation factor eIF2 to arrest protein synthesis. The FANCC protein has been found to interact with the molecular chaperone protein Hsp70, which suppresses PKR activation. The two proteins acting together are able to inactivate PKR and prevent apoptosis caused by interferon-γ stimulation.[130] From these lines of evidence it can be inferred that the

FANCC protein is necessary for the cell to respond properly to interferon-γ stimulation, which is necessary for proper immunologic differentiation and apoptosis avoidance.

SUMMARY

Knowledge about the pathway and the disease seems to grow exponentially with each passing year, because two of the FA proteins (FANCI and FANCN) were discovered and characterized in 2007. The body of work has delineated a pathway with three distinct subdivisions of proteins, but many questions remain to be answered. Some questions involve the function of individual FA proteins: Is FANCL the E3 ubiquitin ligase for FANCD2 and FANCI? Is the helicase activity of FANCM important to the FA pathway or does FANCM solely serve as a DNA translocase? Does the FANCJ helicase interact directly with the FA core complex or downstream partners? Several questions involve the mechanisms of the FA pathway proteins complexes: What are the functions of the subcomplexes composed by core complex proteins? What is the function of the BRAFT complex? What is the function of the FANCD2 and FANCI proteins within nuclear foci? How are the downstream effector FA proteins recruited to these nuclear foci? Other outstanding questions are much broader and involve the pathway itself: Is the FA pathway truly a DNA damage response and repair pathway, an oxidative stress response pathway, or a general stress response pathway for stem cells? Have all of the proteins within the pathway even been discovered? Although the field has come a long way within the past few years, there is still much to learn. Elucidation of the intricacies of the FA pathway will ultimately allow for more individualized and efficacious treatment of FA patients and may provide insights into other cancer susceptibility diseases.

REFERENCES

1. Bagby GC, Alter BP. Fanconi anemia. Semin Hematol 2006;43(3):147–56.
2. D'Andrea AD, Dahl N, Guinan EC, et al. Marrow failure. Hematology Am Soc Hematol Educ Program 2002;58–72.
3. Tischkowitz M, Dokal I. Fanconi anaemia and leukemia: clinical and molecular aspects. Br J Haematol 2004;126(2):176–91.
4. Alter BP. Fanconi's anemia, transplantation, and cancer. Pediatr Transplant 2005; 9(Suppl 7):81–6.
5. Lustig JP, Lugassy G, Neder A, et al. Head and neck carcinoma in Fanconi's anaemia: report of a case and review of the literature. Eur J Cancer B Oral Oncol 1995;31B(1):68–72.
6. Lowy DR, Gillison ML. A new link between Fanconi anemia and human papillomavirus-associated malignancies. J Natl Cancer Inst 2003;95(22):1648–50.
7. Masserot C, Peffault de Latour R, Rocha V, et al. Head and neck squamous cell carcinoma in 13 patients with Fanconi anemia after hematopoietic stem cell transplantation. Cancer 2008;113:3315–22.
8. Socie G, Scieux C, Gluckman E, et al. Squamous cell carcinomas after allogeneic bone marrow transplantation for aplastic anemia: further evidence of a multistep process. Transplantation 1998;66(5):667–70.
9. Auerbach AD. Diagnosis of Fanconi anemia by diepoxybutane analysis. Curr Protoc Hum Genet 2003; Chapter 8: Unit 8.7.
10. Hirschhorn R. In vivo reversion to normal of inherited mutations in humans. J Med Genet 2003;40(10):721–8.

11. Gregory JJ Jr, Wagner JE, Verlander PE, et al. Somatic mosaicism in Fanconi anemia: evidence of genotypic reversion in lymphohematopoietic stem cells. Proc Natl Acad Sci U S A 2001;98(5):2532–7.

12. Soulier J, Leblanc T, Larghero J, et al. Detection of somatic mosaicism and classification of Fanconi anemia patients by analysis of the FA/BRCA pathway. Blood 2005;105(3):1329–36.

13. Lo Ten Foe JR, Kwee ML, Rooimans MA, et al. Somatic mosaicism in Fanconi anemia: molecular basis and clinical significance. Eur J Hum Genet 1997;5(3): 137–48.

14. Xie Y, de Winter JP, Waisfisz Q, et al. Aberrant Fanconi anemia protein profiles in acute myeloid leukemia cells. Br J Haematol 2000;111(4):1057–64.

15. Velez-Ruelas MA, Martinez-Jaramillo G, Arana-Trejo RM, et al. Hematopoietic changes during progression from Fanconi anemia into acute myeloid leukemia: case report and brief review of the literature. Hematology 2006;11(5):331–4.

16. Alter BP, Rosenberg PS, Brody LC, et al. Clinical and molecular features associated with biallelic mutations in FANCD1/BRCA2. J Med Genet 2007;44(1):1–9.

17. Meyer S, Fergusson WD, Whetton AD, et al. Amplification and translocation of 3q26 with overexpression of EVI1 in Fanconi anemia-derived childhood acute myeloid leukemia with biallelic FANCD1/BRCA2 disruption. Genes Chromosomes Cancer 2007;46(4):359–72.

18. Gillio AP, Verlander PC, Batish SD, et al. Phenotypic consequences of mutations in the Fanconi anemia FAC gene: an International Fanconi Anemia Registry study. Blood 1997;90(1):105–10.

19. Auerbach AD. Fanconi anemia: genetic testing in Ashkenazi Jews. Genet Test 1997;1(1):27–33.

20. Farzin A, Davies SM, Smith FO, et al. Matched sibling donor haematopoietic stem cell transplantation in Fanconi anemia: an update of the Cincinnati Children's experience. Br J Haematol 2007;136(4):633–40.

21. Pasquini R, Carreras J, Pasquini MC, et al. HLA-matched sibling hematopoietic stem cell transplantation for Fanconi anemia: comparison of irradiation and non-irradiation containing conditioning regimens. Biol Blood Marrow Transplant 2008;14(10):1141–7.

22. Gluckman E, Wagner JE. Hematopoietic stem cell transplantation in childhood inherited bone marrow failure syndromes. Bone Marrow Transplant 2008;41(2): 127–32.

23. Brown JA, Boussiotis VA. Umbilical cord blood transplantation: basic biology and clinical challenges to immune reconstitution. Clin Immunol 2008;127(3): 286–97.

24. Burt RK, Loh Y, Pearce W, et al. Clinical applications of blood-derived and marrow-derived stem cells for nonmalignant diseases. JAMA 2008;299(8): 925–36.

25. Craddock CF. Full-intensity and reduced-intensity allogeneic stem cell transplantation in AML. Bone Marrow Transplant 2008;41(5):415–23.

26. Brunstein CG, Baker KS, Wagner JE. Umbilical cord blood transplantation for myeloid malignancies. Curr Opin Hematol 2007;14(2):162–9.

27. Chaudhury S, Auerbach AD, Kernan NA, et al. Fludarabine-based cytoreductive regimen and T-cell-depleted grafts from alternative donors for the treatment of high-risk patients with Fanconi anaemia. Br J Haematol 2008;140(6):644–55.

28. Gluckman E, Rocha V, Ionescu I, et al. Results of unrelated cord blood transplant in Fanconi anemia patients: risk factor analysis for engraftment and survival. Biol Blood Marrow Transplant 2007;13(9):1073–82.

29. Bitan M, Or R, Shapira MY, et al. Fludarabine-based reduced intensity conditioning for stem cell transplantation of Fanconi anemia patients from fully matched related and unrelated donors. Biol Blood Marrow Transplant 2006;12(7):712–8.
30. Huck K, Hanenberg H, Nurnberger W, et al. Favourable long-term outcome after matched sibling transplantation for Fanconi-anemia (FA) and in vivo T-cell depletion. Klin Padiatr 2008;220(3):147–52.
31. Balci YI, Akdemir Y, Gumruk F, et al. CD-34 selected hematopoetic stem cell transplantation from HLA identical family members for Fanconi anemia. Pediatr Blood Cancer 2008;50(5):1065–7.
32. Ayas M, Al-Jefri A, Al-Seraihi A, et al. Allogeneic stem cell transplantation in Fanconi anemia patients presenting with myelodysplasia and/or clonal abnormality: update on the Saudi experience. Bone Marrow Transplant. 2008;41(3):261–5.
33. Millen FJ, Rainey MG, Hows JM, et al. Oral squamous cell carcinoma after allogeneic bone marrow transplantation for Fanconi anaemia. Br J Haematol 1997; 99(2):410–4.
34. Rosenberg PS, Alter BP, Socie G, et al. Secular trends in outcomes for Fanconi anemia patients who receive transplants: implications for future studies. Biol Blood Marrow Transplant 2005;11(9):672–9.
35. Croop JM. Gene therapy for Fanconi anemia. Curr Hematol Rep 2003;2(4): 335–40.
36. Yamada K, Ramezani A, Hawley RG, et al. Phenotype correction of Fanconi anemia group a hematopoietic stem cells using lentiviral vector. Mol Ther 2003;8(4):600–10.
37. Kelly PF, Radtke S, von Kalle C, et al. Stem cell collection and gene transfer in Fanconi anemia. Mol Ther 2007;15(1):211–9.
38. Si Y, Ciccone S, Yang FC, et al. Continuous in vivo infusion of interferon-gamma (IFN-gamma) enhances engraftment of syngeneic wild-type cells in Fanca-/- and Fancg-/- mice. Blood 2006;108(13):4283–7.
39. Ozenne V, Paradis V, Vullierme MP, et al. Liver tumours in patients with Fanconi anaemia: a report of three cases. Eur J Gastroenterol Hepatol 2008;20(10):1036–9.
40. Velazquez I, Alter BP. Androgens and liver tumors: Fanconi's anemia and non-Fanconi's conditions. Am J Hematol 2004;77(3):257–67.
41. Akkari YM, Bateman RL, Reifsteck CA, et al. The 4N cell cycle delay in Fanconi anemia reflects growth arrest in late S phase. Mol Genet Metab 2001;74(4): 403–12.
42. Meetei AR, Medhurst AL, Ling C, et al. A human ortholog of archaeal DNA repair protein Hef is defective in Fanconi anemia complementation group M. Nat Genet 2005;37(9):958–63.
43. Lightfoot J, Alon N, Bosnoyan-Collins L, et al. Characterization of regions functional in the nuclear localization of the Fanconi anemia group a protein. Hum Mol Genet 1999;8(6):1007–15.
44. Meetei AR, Levitus M, Xue Y, et al. X-linked inheritance of Fanconi anemia complementation group B. Nat Genet 2004;36(11):1219–24.
45. de Winter JP, Leveille F, van Berkel CGM, et al. Isolation of a cDNA representing the Fanconi anemia complementation group E gene. Am J Hum Genet 2000; 67(5):1306–8.
46. Meetei AR, de Winter JP, Medhurst AL, et al. A novel ubiquitin ligase is deficient in Fanconi anemia. Nat Genet 2003;35(2):165–70.
47. Gurtan AM, Stuckert P, D'Andrea AD. The WD40 repeats of FANCL are required for Fanconi anemia core complex assembly. J Biol Chem 2006;281(16): 10806–905.

48. Kim JM, Kee Y, Gurtan A, et al. Cell cycle dependent chromatin loading of the Fanconi anemia core complex by FANCM/FAAP24. Blood 2008;111(10): 5215–22.
49. Komori K, Fujikane R, Shinagawa H, et al. Novel endonuclease in Archaea cleaving DNA with various branched structure. Genes Genet Syst 2002;77(4): 227–41.
50. Gari K, Decaillet C, Stasiak AZ, et al. The Fanconi anemia protein FANCM can promote branch migration of holliday junctions and replication forks. Mol Cell 2008;29(1):141–8.
51. Yamashita T, Kupfer GM, Naf D, et al. The Fanconi anemia pathway requires FAA phosphorylation and FAA/FAC nuclear accumulation. Proc Natl Acad Sci U S A 1998;95(22):13085–90.
52. Qiao F, Mi J, Wilson JB, et al. Phosphorylation of Fanconi anemia (FA) complementation group G protein, FANCG, at serine 7 is important for function of the FA pathway. J Biol Chem 2004;279(44):46035–45.
53. Mi J, Qiao F, Wilson JB, et al. FANCG is phosphorylated at serines 383 and 387 during mitosis. Mol Cell Biol 2004;24(19):8576–85.
54. Medhurst AL, El Houari L, Steltenpool J, et al. Evidence for subcomplexes in the Fanconi anemia pathway. Blood 2006;108(6):2072–80.
55. Folias A, Matkovic M, Bruun D, et al. BRCA1 interacts directly with the Fanconi anemia protein FANCA. Hum Mol Genet 2002;11(21):2591–7.
56. Hussain S, Witt E, Huber PAJ, et al. Direct interaction of the Fanconi anemia protein FANCG with BRCA2/FANCD1. Hum Mol Genet 2003;12(19):2503–10.
57. Gordon SM, Buchwald M. Fanconi anemia protein complex: mapping protein interactions in the yeast 2- and 3- hybrid systems. Blood 2003;102(1):136–41.
58. Pace P, Johnson M, Tan WM, et al. FANCE: the link between Fanconi anemia complex assembly and activity. EMBO J 2002;21(13):3414–23.
59. Garcia-Higuera I, Taniguchi T, Ganesan S, et al. Interaction of the Fanconi anemia proteins and BRCA1 in a common pathway. Mol Cell 2001;7:249–62.
60. Taniguchi T, Garcia-Higuera I, Andreassen PR, et al. S-phase-specific interaction of the Fanconi anemia protein, FANCD2, with BRCA1 and RAD51. Blood 2002;100:2414–20.
61. Wang X, Andreassen PR, D'Andrea AD. Functional interaction of monoubiquitinated FANCD2 and BRCA2/FANCD1 in chromatin. Mol Cell Biol 2004;24(13):5850–62.
62. Smogorzewska A, Matsuoka S, Vinciguerra P, et al. Identification of the FANCI protein, a monoubiquitinated FANCD2 paralog required for DNA repair. Cell 2007;129(2):289–301.
63. Sims AE, Spiteri E, Sims RJ III, et al. FANCI is a second monoubiquitinated member of the Fanconi anemia pathway. Nat Struct Mol Biol 2007;14(6):564–7.
64. Dorsman JC, Levitus M, Rockx D, et al. Identification of the Fanconi anemia complementation group I gene, FANCI. Cell Oncol 2007;29(3):211–8.
65. Levitus M, Rooimans MA, Steltenpool J, et al. Heterogeneity in Fanconi anemia: evidence for 2 new genetic subtypes. Blood 2004;103(7):2498–503.
66. Taniguchi T, Garcia-Higuera I, Xu B, et al. Convergence of the Fanconi anemia and ataxia telangiectasia signaling pathways. Cell 2002;109(4):459–72.
67. Ishiai M, Kitao H, Smogorzewska A, et al. FANCI phosphorylation functions as a molecular switch to turn on the Fanconi anemia pathway. Nat Struct Mol Biol 2008;15(11):1138–46.
68. Howlett NG, Taniguchi T, Olson S, et al. Biallelic inactivation of BRCA2 in Fanconi anemia. Science 2002;297(5581):606–9.

69. Godthelp BC, Wiegant WW, Waisfisz Q, et al. Inducibility of nuclear Rad51 foci after DNA damage distinguishes all Fanconi anemia complementation groups from D1/BRCA2. Mutat Res 2006;594(1-2):39–48.

70. Shinohara A, Ogawa H, Ogawa T. Rad51 protein involved in repair and recombination in S. cerevisiae is a RecA-like protein. Cell 1992;69(3):457–70.

71. Wong AKC, Pero R, Ormonde PA, et al. RAD51 interacts with the evolutionarily conserved BRC motifs in the human breast cancer susceptibility gene brca2. J Biol Chem 1997;272(51):31941–4.

72. Yang H, Jeffrey PD, Miller J, et al. BRCA2 function in DNA binding and recombination from a BRCA2-DSS1-ssDNA structure. Science 2002;297(5588):1837–48.

73. Li J, Zou C, Bai Y, et al. DSS1 is required for the stability of BRCA2. Oncogene 2006;25(8):1186–94.

74. Levitus M, Waisfisz Q, Godthelp BC, et al. The DNA helicase BRIP1 is defective in Fanconi anemia complementation group J. Nat Genet 2005;37(9):934–5.

75. Levran O, Attwooll C, Henry RT, et al. The BRCA1-interacting helicase BRIP1 is deficient in Fanconi anemia. Nat Genet 2005;37(9):931–3.

76. Litman R, Peng M, Jin Z, et al. BACH1 is critical for homologous recombination and appears to be the Fanconi anemia gene product FANCJ. Cancer Cell 2005;8(3):255–65.

77. Cantor SB, Bell DW, Ganesan S, et al. BACH1, a novel helicase-like protein, interacts directly with BRCA1 and contributes to Its DNA repair function. Cell 2001;105(1):149–60.

78. Yu X, Chini CCS, He M, et al. The BRCT domain is a phospho-protein binding domain. Science 2003;302(5645):639–42.

79. Wu Y, Shin-ya K, Brosh RM Jr. FANCJ helicase defective in Fanconi anemia and breast cancer unwinds G-quadruplex DNA to defend genomic instability. Mol Cell Biol 2008;28(12):4116–28.

80. Xia B, Dorsman JC, Ameziane N, et al. Fanconi anemia is associated with a defect in the BRCA2 partner PALB2. Nat Genet 2007;39(2):159–61.

81. Reid S, Schindler D, Hanenberg H, et al. Biallelic mutations in PALB2 cause Fanconi anemia subtype FA-N and predispose to childhood cancer. Nat Genet 2007;39(2):162–4.

82. Dronkert ML, Kanaar R. Repair of DNA interstrand cross-links. Mutat Res 2001;486(4):217–47.

83. Nojima K, Hochegger H, Saberi A, et al. Multiple repair pathways mediate tolerance to chemotherapeutic cross-linking agents in vertebrate cells. Cancer Res 2005;65(24):11704–11.

84. Shin DS, Chahwan C, Huffman JL, et al. Structure and function of the double strand break repair machinery. DNA Repair (Amst) 2004;4(2):91–8.

85. Sharan SK, Morimatsu M, Albrecht U, et al. Embryonic lethality and radiation hypersensitivity mediated by Rad51in mice lacking Brca2. Nature 1997;386(6627):804–10.

86. Scully R, Xie A, Nagaraju G. Molecular functions of BRCA1 in the DNA damage response. Cancer Biol Ther 2004;3(6):521–7.

87. Rajan JV, Wang ST, Marquis ST, et al. BRCA2 is coordinately regulated with BRCA1 during proliferation and differentiation in mammary epithelial cells. Proc Natl Acad Sci 1996;93(23):13078–83.

88. Scully R, Chen J, Plug A, et al. Association of BRCA1 with Rad51 in mitotic and meiotic cells. Cell 1997;88(2):265–75.

89. Chen J, Silver DP, Walpita D, et al. Stable interaction between the products of the BRCA1 and BRCA2 tumor suppressor genes in mitotic and meiotic cells. Mol Cell 1998;2(3):317–28.

90. Seki M, Tada S, Enomoto T. Function of recQ family helicase in genome stability. Subcell Biochem 2006;40:49–73.

91. Park WH, Margossian S, Horwitz AA, et al. Direct DNA binding activity of the Fanconi anemia D2 protein. J Biol Chem 2005;280(25):23593–8.

92. Meetei AR, Sechi S, Wallisch M, et al. A multiprotein nuclear complex connects Fanconi anemia and Bloom syndrome. Mol Cell Biol 2003;23(10):3417–26.

93. Pichierri P, Franchitto A, Rosselli F. BLM and the FANC proteins collaborate in a common pathway in response to stalled replication forks. EMBO 2004; 23(15):3154–63.

94. Kinner A, Wu W, Staudt C, et al. Gamma-H2AX in recognition and signaling of DNA double strand breaks in the context of chromatin. Nucleic Acids Res 2008;36(17):5678–94.

95. Bogliolo M, Lyakhovich A, Callen E, et al. Histone H2AX and Fanconi anemia FANCD2 function in the same pathway to maintain chromosome stability. EMBO 2007;26(5):1340–51.

96. McCulloch SD, Kunkel TA. The fidelity of DNA synthesis by eukaryotic replicative and translesion synthesis polymerases. Cell Res 2008;18(1):148–61.

97. Andersen PL, Xu F, Xiao W. Eukaryotic DNA damage tolerance and translesion synthesis through covalent modifications of PCNA. Cell Res 2008;18(1):162–73.

98. Hussain S, Wilson JB, Medhurst AL, et al. Direct interaction of FANCD2 with BRCA2 in DNA damage response pathways. Hum Mol Genet 2004;13(12):1241–8.

99. Prakash S, Johnson RE, Prakash L. Eukaryotic translesion synthesis DNA polymerases: specificity of structure and function. Annu Rev Biochem 2005;74: 317–53.

100. Niedzwiedz W, Mosedale G, Johnson M, et al. The Fanconi anemia gene FANCC promotes homologous recombination and error prone DNA repair. Mol Cell 2004;15:607–20.

101. Mirchandani KD, McCaffrey RM, D'Andrea AD. The Fanconi anemia core complex is required for efficient point mutagenesis and Rev1 foci assembly. DNA Repair. 2008;7:902–11.

102. Fujiwara T, Saito A, Suzuki M, et al. Identification and chromosomal assignment of USP1, a novel gene encoding a human ubiquitin-specific protease. Genomics 1998;54(1):155–8.

103. Nijman SM, Huang TT, Dirac AM, et al. The deubiquitinating enzyme USP1 regulates the Fanconi anemia pathway. Mol Cell 2005;17(3):331–9.

104. Huang TT, Nijman SM, Mirchandani KD, et al. Regulation of monoubiquitinated PCNA by DUB autocleavage. Nat Cell Biol 2006;8(4):339–47.

105. Oestergaard VH, Langevin F, Kuiken HJ, et al. Deubiquitination of FANCD2 is required for DNA crosslink repair. Mol Cell 2007;28(5):798–809.

106. Lavin MF. Ataxia-telangiectasia: from a rare disorder to a paradigm for cell signaling and cancer. Mol Cell Biol 2008;9:759–69.

107. Djuzenova C, Flentje M, Plowman PN. Radiation response in vitro of fibroblasts from a Fanconi anemia patient with marked clinical radiosensitivity. Strahlenther Onkol 2004;180(12):789–97.

108. Cimprich KA, Cortez D. ATR: an essential regulator of genome integrity. Mol Cell Biol 2008;9:616–27.

109. Pichierri P, Rosselli F. The DNA crosslink induced S-phase checkpoint depends on ATR-CHK1 and ATR-NBS1-FANCD2 pathways. EMBO 2004;23:1178–87.

110. Andreassen PR, D'Andrea AD, Taniguchi T. ATR couples FANCD2 monoubiqui-tination to the DNA damage response. Genes Dev 2004;18:1958–63.
111. Ho GP, Margossian S, Taniguchi T, et al. Phosphorylation of FANCD2 on two novel sites is required for mitomycin C resistance. Mol Cell Biol 2006;26(18): 7005–15.
112. Wilson JB, Yamamoto K, Marriott AS, et al. FANCG promotes formation of a newly identified protein complex containing BRCA2, FANCD2 and XRCC3. Oncogene 2008;27:3641–52.
113. Collis SJ, Ciccia A, Deans AJ, et al. FANCM and FAAP24 function in ATR medi-ated checkpoint signaling independently of the Fanconi anemia core complex. Mol Cell 32:313–24.
114. Enders GH. Expanded roles for Chk1 in genome maintenance. J Biol Chem 2008;283(26):17749–52.
115. Wang X, Kennedy RD, Ray K, et al. Chk1 mediated phosphorylation of FANCE is required for the Fanconi anemia/BRCA pathway. Mol Cell Biol 2007;27(8): 3098–108.
116. Gordon-Smith EC, Rutherford TR. Fanconi anemia: constitutional, familial aplas-tic anemia. Baillieres Clin Haematol 1989;2:139–52.
117. Bornman L, Baladi S, Richard MJ, et al. Differential regulation and expression of stress proteins and ferritin in human monocytes. J Cell Physiol 1999;178:1–8.
118. Kovacic P, Jacintho JD. Mechanisms of carcinogenesis: focus on oxidative stress and electron transfer. Curr Med Chem 2001;8:773–96.
119. Evans LM, Davies JS, Anderson RA, et al. The effect of GH replacement therapy on endothelial function and oxidative stress in adult growth hormone deficiency. Eur J Endocrinol 2000;142:254–62.
120. Memoli S, Napolitanto A, D'Ischia M, et al. Diffusible melanin-related metabolites are potent inhibitors of lipid peroxidation. Biochim Biophys Acta 1997;1346: 61–8.
121. Wells PG, Kim PM, Laposa RR, et al. Oxidative damage in chemical teratogen-esis. Mutat Res 1997;396:65–78.
122. Kruyt FA, Hoshino T, Liu JM, et al. Abnormal microsomal detoxification impli-cated in Fanconi anemia group C by interaction of the FAC protein with NADPH cytochrome P450 reductase. Blood 1998;92:3050–6.
123. Cumming RC, Lightfoot J, Beard K, et al. Fanconi anemia fropu C protein prevents apoptosis in hematopoietic cells through redox regulation of GSTP1. Nat Med 2001;7:814–20.
124. Zanier R, Briot D, Villard JA, et al. Fanconi anemia C gene product regulates the expression of genes involved in differentiation and inflammation. Oncogene 2004;23:5004–13.
125. Futaki M, Igarashi T, Watanabe S, et al. The FANCG Fanconi anemia protein interacts with CYP2E1: possible role in protection against oxidative DNA damage. Carcinogenesis 2002;23:67–72.
126. Park S, Ciccone SLM, Beck BD, et al. Oxidative stress/damage induces multi-merization and interaction of Fanconi anemia proteins. J Biol Chem 2004; 279(29):30053–9.
127. Fagerlie S, Lensch MW, Pang Q, et al. The Fanconi anemia group C gene product: signaling functions in hematopoietic cells. Exp Hematol 2001;29: 1371–81.
128. Li J, Sejas DP, Zhang X, et al. TNF-α induces leukemic clonal evolution ex vivo in Fanconi anemia group C murine stem cells. J Clin Invest 2007;117(11): 3283–95.

129. Pang Q, Fagerlie S, Christianson TA, et al. The Fanconi anemia protein FANCC binds to and facilitates the activation of STAT1 by gamma interferon and hematopoietic growth factors. Mol Cell Biol 2000;20(13):4724–35.
130. Pang Q, Keeble W, Christianson TA, et al. FANCC interacts with Hsp70 to protect hematopoietic cells from IFNγ/TNF-α mediated cytotoxicity. EMBO 2001;20(16):4478–89.

Dyskeratosis Congenita

Sharon A. Savage, MD, FAAP*, Blanche P. Alter, MD, MPH, FAAP

KEYWORDS

- Dyskeratosis congenita • Telomere • DKC1 • TERC • TERT
- TINF2 • Bone marrow failure

Dyskeratosis congenita (DC) is an inherited bone marrow failure (BMF) and cancer predisposition syndrome caused by defects in telomere biology. The consequences of DC affect all body systems; these may include the diagnostic triad of abnormal nails, reticular skin pigmentation, and oral leukoplakia. BMF, pulmonary fibrosis, liver disease, neurologic and ophthalmic abnormalities, and increased risk for cancer also occur.[1,2] The known clinical complications are listed in **Table 1**.

Patients who have DC have very short germline telomeres compared with those of their healthy relatives, normal controls, and patients who have inherited BMF syndromes (IBMFS).[3,4,5] Mutations in genes important in telomere biology have been identified in approximately half of the patients who have DC.[5] Genotype-phenotype correlations may exist but often are complex to interpret. A broader spectrum of disorders resulting from defects in telomere biology is now appreciated, such as pulmonary fibrosis without other physical or hematologic findings associated with DC. Patients who have DC have a high risk for many medical problems, the most serious of which are BMF, cancer, and pulmonary fibrosis. Accurate diagnosis is critical, because patients who have DC and who develop BMF do not respond to immunosuppression and have a high risk for hematopoietic stem cell transplantation (HSCT)-related complications. This article reviews the clinical features of DC and describes its molecular pathogenesis. The usefulness of telomere length as a diagnostic test and of genetic testing in families is discussed and guidelines for medical management and clinically indicated screening are proposed.

CLINICAL FEATURES

The name, *dyskeratosis congenita*, was derived after the description by Zinsser, in 1910, of two brothers who had nail dystrophy, oral leukoplakia, and skin pigmentation anomalies.[6] Additional reports of patients who had similar features appeared by Engman[7] and by Cole and colleagues,[8] leading to the designation Zinsser-Engman-Cole

This work was supported by the intramural research program of the National Institutes of Health, National Cancer Institute, Division of Cancer Epidemiology and Genetics.

Clinical Genetics Branch, Division of Cancer Epidemiology and Genetics, National Cancer Institute, National Institutes of Health, 6120 Executive Boulevard, Rockville, MD 20852, USA

* Corresponding author.

E-mail address: savagesh@mail.nih.gov (S.A. Savage).

Table 1
Clinical findings in dyskeratosis congenita

System	Findings
Dermatologic	**Lacey, reticular pigmentation,** primarily of the neck and chest; may be subtle or diffuse hyper- or hypopigmentation **Abnormal fingernails and toenails,** may be subtle, with ridging, flaking, or poor growth, or more diffuse with nearly complete loss of nails Early gray hair or hair loss Hyperhidrosis
Growth and development	Short stature Intrauterine growth retardation Developmental delay
Ophthalmic	Epiphora due to stenosis of the lacrimal drainage system Blepharitis Sparse eyelashes, ectropion, entropion, trichiasis Exudative retinopathy (Revesz syndrome)
Dental	Dental caries, may be less frequent now because of improved dental hygiene Periodontal disease Decreased root/crown ratio Taurodontism (enlarged pulp chambers of the teeth)
Ears, nose, throat	**Oral leukoplakia** Deafness (rare) Squamous cell head and neck cancer
Cardiovascular	Rare reported defects include atrial or ventricular septal defects, fibrosis, and dilatated cardiomyopathy
Respiratory	Pulmonary fibrosis
Gastrointestinal	Esophageal stenosis Enteropathy Liver fibrosis
Genitourinary	Urethral stenosis in male patients Epithelial cancers
Musculoskeletal	Osteoporosis Avascular necrosis of the hips and shoulders
Neurologic	Developmental delay Microcephaly Cerebellar hypoplasia (Hoyeraal-Hreidarsson syndrome) Intracranial calcifications (Revesz syndrome)
Psychiatric	Schizophrenia (two case reports)
Endocrine	Hypogonadism
Hematologic	BMF a common presenting sign MDS Leukemia
Immunologic	Immunodeficiency

The diagnostic triad is noted in bold type. Revesz syndrome and Hoyeraal-Hreidarsson syndrome indicate findings specific to those syndromes.

syndrome.[2] Early reports focused on the dermatologic findings. As more cases were described with other medical complications, however, it became clear that DC is a complex, multisystem disorder.[1,2,3]

The clinical diagnosis of classical DC requires at least two features of the triad of dysplastic nails, lacey reticular pigmentation of the upper chest or neck, and oral leukoplakia (**Fig. 1**).[1,9] This diagnostic triad still is important in defining clinically significant disease, but additional features now are appreciated, including BMF, epithelial cancers, myelodysplastic syndrome (MDS), leukemia, epiphora, blepharitis, prematurely gray hair, alopecia, developmental delay, short stature, cerebellar hypoplasia (**Fig. 2**), microcephaly, esophageal stenosis, urethral stenosis, pulmonary fibrosis, liver disease, and avascular necrosis of hips or shoulders (see **Table 1**).[1,9,10] The median age at diagnosis of DC reported by the Dyskeratosis Congenita Registry (DCR) is 15 years (range 0–75 years).[9,11] Thus, many patients may not present until their late teens or adulthood. The DCR required the presence of two of the three features of the triad or one of the triad with at least two minor features.[9,11] The development of the telomere length assay as a diagnostic test for DC coupled with the discovery of more genes as causative of DC, however, has led to modification of the definition of DC.[3,12] The authors accept patients as having DC based on the triad (described previously) or any of the other findings (hematologic or neoplastic complications) consistent with DC and who also have a mutation in a DC gene or very short telomeres. The authors also identify healthy individuals as having DC who have very short telomeres

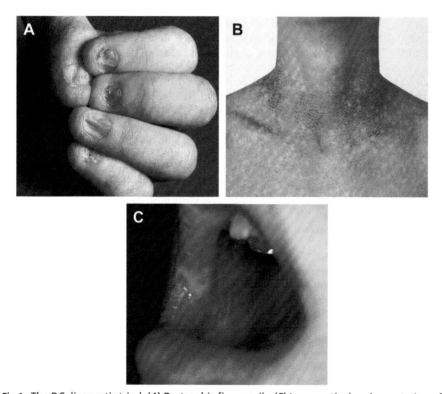

Fig.1. The DC diagnostic triad. (*A*) Dystrophic fingernails. (*B*) Lacey, reticular pigmentation of the neck and upper chest. (*C*) Oral leukoplakia.

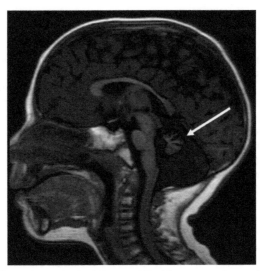

Fig. 2. Brain MRI of a patient who had Hoyeraal-Hreidarsson syndrome. The arrow indicates the characteristic cerebellar hypoplasia.

and are members of a pedigree with bona fide cases in which the gene has not yet been identified.

There are two major severe subsets of DC. The first is Hoyeraal-Hreidarsson syndrome (HH), a severe form of DC characterized by cerebellar hypoplasia, microcephaly, developmental delay, immunodeficiency, intrauterine growth retardation, and BMF. The original descriptions of HH all included cerebellar hypoplasia,[13,14,15] and the authors suggest that documentation of cerebellar hypoplasia (see **Fig. 2**) is required to make the diagnosis of HH. More than 30 such cases have been described, and recent studies showed that patients who have HH have very short telomeres. Several patients who have HH have been found to have mutations in DC genes proved to cause DC, including *DKC1, TINF2*, or *TERT*.[16,17,18]

The second subset is Revesz syndrome (RS), first described in case reports of young children who had BMF and exudative retinopathy.[19,20] These children had bilateral exudative retinopathy (similar to acquired unilateral Coats' retinopathy), intrauterine growth retardation, BMF, sparse fine hair, and central nervous system (CNS) calcifications; some patients also had nail dystrophy and oral leukoplakia. CNS calcification was reported in 15 of the 20 cases in the literature and cerebellar hypoplasia in two cases; two cases had CNS calcifications and cerebellar hypoplasia.[12,17,19] Patients who have RS also have abnormally short telomeres and, so far, mutations have been found in *TINF2*.[12,17]

The authors propose that the appellation HH be restricted to patients who have DC and who have documented cerebellar hypoplasia and that the RS category requires bilateral exudative retinopathy and perhaps also CNS calcifications.

MOLECULAR PATHOGENESIS

The inheritance of DC can be X-linked recessive (XLR), autosomal dominant (AD), or autosomal recessive (AR). There also is a high frequency of sporadic cases, which presumably are due to new mutations in dominant genes. Six genes in the telomere biology pathway have been identified to date as mutated in patients who have DC

(**Table 2**): *DKC1, TERC, TERT, TINF2, NOLA2,* and *NOLA3.*[1,12,18,21,22,23] Approximately half the patients who have DC have a mutation in one of these six genes, whereas the other half await discovery of mutations in additional telomere genes.

Telomeres consist of long nucleotide $(TTAGGG)_n$ repeats and an associated protein complex located at chromosome ends that are essential for the maintenance of chromosomal integrity.[24] Telomeric repeats are lost with each cell division, in part as a result of incomplete replication of the 3' end of the chromosome. Telomere attrition can result in critically short telomeres prompting cellular senescence or cellular crisis, apoptosis, genomic instability, or a reduction in cellular lifespan.[24] Telomerase (*TERT*) is a reverse transcriptase that uses an RNA template (*TERC*) to extend nucleotide repeats at the chromosome end. A protein complex, termed *shelterin*, consists of six proteins that act as a cap at the telomere and regulate telomere length (gene names: *TERF1, TERF2, TINF2, TERF2IP, ACD,* and *POT1*). Additional proteins interact with and regulate the activity of the shelterin complex. Thus, telomere length regulation and telomeric stability require complex interactions of multiple proteins at many different levels.

The locus for the XLR form of DC was mapped in the mid-1980s, and the first DC gene, dyskerin (*DKC1*), was cloned in 1998.[21] Primary fibroblasts and lymphoblasts of men who had *DKC1* mutations had very short telomeres.[4] The dyskerin protein is involved in post-transcriptional pseudouridylation and forms a ribonucleoprotein complex with three other proteins, NOP10, NHP2, and GAR1. AR inheritance of mutations in NOP10 or NHP2 (gene names *NOLA3* and *NOLA2,* respectively) have been identified in three consanguineous families who have DC.[22,23]

TERC, a member of the family of H/ACA small RNAs, serves as the reverse transcription template for the telomerase enzyme.[25] Mutations in the *TERC* gene are present in patients who have DC and occur in an AD manner or de novo.[26] *TERC* mutations also were identified in patients who had aplastic anemia but not other clinical features consistent with DC.[27] These findings prompted subsequent studies that evaluated the telomerase enzyme, *TERT,* in patients who had DC. Mutations in *TERT* were found in patients who had AD and AR DC, in patients who had aplastic anemia and no other signs of DC, and in patients who had pulmonary fibrosis.[18,28,29,30,31,32] The variability in clinical features in patients who had *TERC* or *TERT* mutations suggests the existence of a broad spectrum of telomere biology disorders, often manifested by abnormal levels of telomerase activity and short telomeres.

The authors identified the first component of the shelterin complex as mutated in DC, *TINF2* (protein name: TRF1-interacting nuclear factor 2 [TIN2]).[12] Patients who had *TINF2* mutations can have severe forms of DC, with young age at onset, but the phenotypic spectrum is broad and includes patients who have mild or even no findings.[12,17] *TINF2* is the only gene identified to date as mutated in the RS variant of DC.[12,17] The mechanism by which *TINF2* mutations cause DC has not yet been elucidated, but most patients who have *TINF2* mutations have extremely short telomeres.[12,17]

The primary molecular consequences of mutations in the DC-associated genes are very short telomeres, low levels of telomerase activity, or reduced expression of *TERC*. Genetic anticipation of symptoms and of short telomeres has been suggested in family pedigrees with *TERC* or *TERT* mutations.[26,33] Decreased *TERC* expression and short telomeres were present in patients who had mutations in NOP10 and NHP2.[22,23] It is possible that the *TINF2* mutations may lead to instability of the shelterin complex and telomere dysregulation. Based on these data, DC seems to be a disorder of telomere biology, and the consistent feature in all patients is abnormally short telomeres.[3,5]

Table 2
Dyskeratosis congenita genes

Gene Name	Protein Name	Function	Inheritance	Chromosomal Location[a]	MIM Identifier	Frequency in NCI Cohort[b]	Frequency In DCR[c]
DKC1	DKC1: dyskerin	Component of H/ACA snoRNPs and telomerase RNA (TERC)	XLR	Xq28 NC_000,023.9: 153,644,344–153,659,154	300,126	17%	36%
TERC	TERC: telomerase RNA component	TERC is the RNA component of telomerase. It acts as a template for the addition of telomeric repeat sequences	AD	3q21-q28 NC_000,003.10: 170,965,542–170,965,091	602,322	10%	6%
TERT	TERT: telomerase	A reverse transcriptase that adds the $TTAGGG_n$ repeats to telomeres	AD, AR	5p15.33 NC_000,005.8 1,348,162–1,306,282	187,270	7%	1%
TINF2	TINF2: TRF1-interacting nuclear factor 2	Interacts with telomeric repeat-binding factor-1 and -2 (TRF1 and TRF2) and other shelterin components	AD	14q12 NC_000,014.7: 23,781,720–23,778,689	604,319	24%	11%

| NOLA3 | NOP10: nucleolar protein family A, member 3 | Associates with NHP2, DKC1, and GAR1 in structures corresponding to H/ACA snoRNPs | AR | 15q14-q15 NC_000,015.8: 32,422,654–32,421,209 | 606,471 | 0% | <1% |
| NOLA2 | NHP2: nucleolar protein family A, member 2 | Associates with NOP10, DKC1, and GAR1 in structures corresponding to H/ACA snoRNPs | AR | 5q35.3 NC_000,005.8: 177,513,567–177,509,070 | 606,470 | 0% | <1% |

The genes proved to be mutated in DC and their frequency estimates are shown. Depending on the study, approximately 40% to 50% of patients remained molecularly uncharacterized.

Abbreviations: MIM, Mendelian Inheritance in Man; snoRNP, small nucleolar ribonucleolar proteins.

[a] Based on human genome build 36.3 (National Center for Biotechnology Information), information available on October 7, 2008.

[b] Data from Savage SA, Giri N, Baerlocher GM, et al. TINF2, a component of the shelterin telomere protection complex, is mutated in dyskeratosis congenita. Am J Hum Genet 2008;82(2):501–9; and unpublished data from NCI cohort as a December 1, 2008.

[c] Data from Refs.[11,17,23].

MAKING THE DIAGNOSIS

Patients may develop signs and symptoms of DC at any age, which usually become more severe with increasing age. Accurate diagnosis of DC is critical, especially because therapy for complications, such as BMF or cancer, often is urgent. Telomere length has been evaluated extensively in DC and to some extent in other IBMFS.[5] Multiple methods have been used, including terminal restriction fragment (TRF) measurement on Southern blots, fluorescence in situ hybridization (FISH) with immunostaining, quantitative polymerase chain reaction, single telomere length analysis, and flow cytometry with FISH (flow-FISH).[34,35] Earlier studies used TRF to determine telomere length in DNA isolated from white blood cells or mononuclear cells and reported mean telomere length in patients compared with a small number of age-matched controls or the difference between the average telomere lengths of patients and controls (deltaTEL).[5] Those studies found that patients who had DC had shorter telomeres than controls; the use of telomere length as a diagnostic test was not evaluated at that time.

Flow-FISH, which uses fresh blood samples, has the advantage of providing telomere length data on specific white blood cell subsets.[36] Telomere length in total leukocytes and in leukocyte subsets (granulocytes, total lymphocytes, naïve T cells, memory T cells, B cells, and natural killer cells) was determined by flow-FISH on cells from patients who had DC, their relatives, and patients who had other IBMFS. Data from 400 healthy controls (newborn through 100 years) were used to generate percentiles of normal telomere length, and values below the first percentile for age were considered very short. The diagnostic sensitivity and specificity of very short telomeres was greater than 90% in total lymphocytes, naïve T cells, and B cells for the diagnosis of DC in comparison with healthy relatives of patients who had DC or with non-DC IBMFS patients. Rare healthy relatives who had very short telomeres later were shown to have mutations in the same DC genes as the affected probands. Evaluation of the panel of six leukocyte subsets provided the greatest degrees of sensitivity and specificity; the best statistical performance characteristics were obtained by finding very short telomeres in at least three or four of the subsets.[3]

This study[3] found that many patients who had non-DC IBMFS also had very short telomeres in granulocytes; a similar result was reported in patients who had acquired aplastic anemia.[37] This could be because of increased granulocyte turnover and short lifespan in comparison with other cell types, resulting in more cell divisions of early myeloid progenitor cells (because telomeres shorten with each cell division). In the authors' experience, granulocyte telomere length results are sensitive but not specific for the diagnosis of DC, and the authors rely on the results from lymphocytes and lymphocyte subsets.

In cross-sectional data from normal individuals and those who have non-DC IBMFS, telomere length decreases with age in a nonlinear, S-shaped manner. Telomere length, however, did not seem to decrease with age in the authors' cross-sectional analysis of DC and in some cell types even appeared to increase slightly.[3] If this finding is sustained in longitudinal studies, then deltaTEL also would decrease with age (because the difference between patients who have DC and healthy controls would narrow with age rather than decrease in parallel); thus, deltaTEL should not be used to compare telomere lengths across ages. The lack of age-associated decline in telomere length in DC was not known at the time of the earlier publications using deltaTEL.

Another group recently concluded that telomere length was sensitive but not specific in screening for DC.[38] The flow-FISH method used to determine telomere length differed from previously established methods in several ways.[3,39,40] It used total mononuclear cells and compared patient telomeres to telomeres from a tetraploid acute lymphocytic leukemia cell line, which arbitrarily was assigned as 100%, and then reported patient results as a percentage of the control cell line. The published results did not show the nonlinear, S-shaped distribution of telomere length in healthy individuals, which is well described in the literature.[41,42,43,44] Future studies are required for the interpretation of this method in the context of diagnosis of patients who have DC.

The development of cytopenias often is the first sign in DC; thus, early and accurate diagnosis is essential. Patients who have BMF resulting from DC do not respond to immunosuppressive therapy.[45] They also are at high risk for HSCT-related complications resulting from underlying pulmonary and liver disease.[46,47,48,49,50] In addition, recent studies have shown individuals can be silent carriers of a pathogenic mutation in a DC gene.[12] The authors suggest, therefore, that patients who have BMF in whom Fanconi anemia is ruled out (by a normal chromosome breakage test with crosslinking agents) have telomere length tested by flow-FISH in leukocyte subsets to evaluate for DC. This is the most sensitive and specific screening test for DC at this time. Telomere lengths that are less than the first percentile for age in four of the six leukocyte subsets (described previously), excluding granulocytes, are highly correlated with the diagnosis of DC in the authors' experience.

REASONS TO CONSIDER DYSKERATOSIS CONGENITA IN THE DIFFERENTIAL DIAGNOSIS OF PATIENTS WHO HAVE BONE MARROW FAILURE OR CANCER

The following are standard studies for Fanconi anemia (ie, not consistent with Fanconi anemia).

- Bone marrow failure with normal chromosome breakage responses to diepoxybutane or mitomycin C
- Head/neck cancer in a young person (<50 years of age)
- Anogenital cancer in a young person (<50 years of age)
- Family history of pulmonary fibrosis
- Family history of BMF
- Family history of cancer in young people, especially head and neck cancer

Genetic testing for DC should begin with careful assessment of patient personal and family medical history. Genetic counseling must be provided before and after mutation testing, because testing may identify unsuspected affected or silent carrier diagnoses of DC, which will have effects on individual health care and on family dynamics. Complex issues regarding counseling and testing of children and adolescents need to be considered.[51] Prepregnancy or prenatal genetic counseling is available for families considering the risk to future offspring. Preimplantation genetic diagnosis and prenatal testing also can be considered in families who have a known mutation in a gene for DC.

The physical findings of a patient also should be considered in relation to mutation testing. For example, in male patients who have clinical DC and no affected female relatives, XLR inheritance may be suspected and testing for *DKC1* should be performed. Patients who have *TINF2* mutations may have multiple physical findings and early-onset BMF, although a smaller subset of patients who have mutations in *TINF2* may have mild symptoms.[12,17] There can be variability in the severity of clinical and hematologic findings associated with mutations in *TERC*.[52] Patients who have heterozygous *TERT* mutations may present at slightly older ages with more varied and milder phenotypes than patients who have mutations in other genes.[28,29,30,31,32] AR mutations in *NOLA2* and *NOLA3* have been reported only in consanguineous families.[22,23]

Because mutations have been identified in only approximately half of the known patients who have DC, the absence of a mutation in a known DC gene in patients who have very short telomeres and clinical findings consistent with DC does not rule out the diagnosis. Because of the high rates of complications, including cancer, the authors suggest that patients who have BMF or other clinical signs consistent with DC and who have telomeres below the first percentile for age be considered as having a disorder of telomere biology. The National Cancer Institute's (NCI) cohort study of DC,[53] a part of its IBMFS cohort is evaluating all such patients in a standardized manner to prospectively study the complication rates in these patients and to identify new DC genes.[54,55]

COMPLICATIONS OF DYSKERATOSIS CONGENITA

The clinical features and related medical complications in DC are shown in **Table 1**. Nearly all systems can be affected and the findings may vary greatly between patients. BMF is a common finding in DC and may occur before or after (or even in the absence of) the appearance of the diagnostic triad or other features of DC. The DCR reported an incidence of BMF of 86%,[56] and the NCI cohort study noted a 91% incidence (Blanche P. Alter, MD, MPH and Sharon A. Savage, MD, unpublished data, 2009). Both of these cohorts may be biased, however, because of ascertainment primarily by hematologists or oncologists.

A review of literature reports of cancer in patients who have DC indicates that head and neck squamous cell carcinomas (SCC) were the most common type followed by anorectal SCC, stomach, and lung cancers.[57] MDS and acute myeloid leukemia also are reported in DC. The age at diagnosis of cancer in DC is much younger than the average age of cancer in the NCI's Surveillance, Epidemiology and End Results population-based sporadic cancer registry.[57]

Pulmonary fibrosis is a serious complication in patients who have DC, particularly after HSCT. Studies of patients who have idiopathic pulmonary fibrosis revealed that a subgroup of patients have mutations in *TERT* or *TERC* and shorter telomeres than healthy controls.[28,32,52] The first studies focused on patients who had a family history of idiopathic pulmonary fibrosis; a subsequent study found shorter telomeres and *TERT* or *TERC* mutations in sporadic cases.[58] Although the telomere shortening in these patients was not as dramatic as that seen in patients who had more common features of DC, it suggests that there is a spectrum of disorders of the telomere maintenance pathway caused by mutations in telomere biology genes.

The neurologic consequences of DC are complex. Ataxia may result from cerebellar hypoplasia in the HH variant of DC.[9,11,13,14,15] Patients who present with pancytopenia and ataxia in whom DC is not initially suspected actually may have HH; a mutation in *TINF2* recently was identified in a patient who had these signs.[59] Patients who have DC may have variable degrees of developmental delay or learning disorders and microcephaly; two patients were reported to have had schizophrenia.[60,61]

There are many other clinical complications that significantly affect the quality of life of patients who have DC. There may be gastrointestinal problems of varying severity. Esophageal stenosis requiring dilatation was reported in 17% of patients.[9] Enteropathies and liver fibrosis also have been reported.[9,11] Osteopenia or osteoporosis have occurred at unusually young ages. These bone density complications may be exacerbated by the use of corticosteroids after HSCT for graft versus host disease prophylaxis or treatment. Avascular necrosis of the hips has led to hip replacement surgery in some patients.[30] Ophthalmic problems include obstruction of the lacrimal drainage system leading to constant tearing (epiphora) and abnormal eyelash growth, which can cause corneal erosions or ulcers.[55,62] Bilateral exudative retinopathy is the hallmark of the RS variant of DC and may result in blindness.[12,19,20] Several other ophthalmic complications have been reported, including proliferative retinopathy, retinal or vitreous hemorrhage, glaucoma, and other problems.[62]

The median survival was 44 years of age in cases of DC without HH or RS reported in the medical literature (**Fig. 3**A). The median survival for those who had HH was 5 years; those who had RS had a 75% survival plateau at age 11 (see **Fig. 3**B,C). No patients who had HH or RS, however, have been reported so far who were older than 20 years of age. Thus, survival seems shortened in DC, particularly in those who have the severe subsets. One note of caution is that reports of cases or case series may be biased toward inclusion of those who have severe complications.

MEDICAL MANAGEMENT OF DYSKERATOSIS CONGENITA

The medical management of DC is complex and must be based on patient-specific needs as randomized clinical trials have not been conducted. Patients who have DC and BMF do not respond to immunosuppressive therapy.[45] Failure of response to immunosuppressive therapy in apparently acquired BMF should lead to the consideration of DC as the proper diagnosis. Following the model of the Fanconi anemia consensus guidelines,[63] treatment of BMF is recommended if the hemoglobin is consistently below 8 g/dL, platelets less than 30,000/mm^3, and neutrophils below 1000/mm^3. The first consideration for treatment for hematologic problems, such as BMF or leukemia, should be HSCT, if there is a matched related donor. HSCT from an unrelated donor can be considered, although a trial of androgen therapy (eg, oxymetholone) may be chosen.

In the authors' experience, patients who have DC are more sensitive to androgens than patients who have Fanconi anemia, and the dose must be adjusted to reduce side effects, such as impaired liver function, virilization, or behavioral problems (eg, aggression or mood swings). Starting oxymetholone dosage of 0.5 to 1 mg/kg per day, half the dose used in Fanconi anemia, is used. It may take 2 to 3 months at a constant dose to see a hematologic response. Side effects, including liver enzyme abnormalities, need to monitored carefully. Baseline and follow-up liver ultrasounds should be performed for patients on androgens because of the possibility of liver tumors (adenomas and carcinomas), which have been reported in patients who have Fanconi anemia and in patients whose use of androgens was for other benign hematologic diseases or for nonhematologic reasons.[64]

Hematopoietic growth factors occasionally are considered in patients who have BMF. The authors do not recommend using androgens combined with granulocyte colony-stimulating factor, because splenic rupture occurred in two patients who had DC receiving this combination.[65] Granulocyte colony-stimulating factor with erythropoietin occasionally has been useful but perhaps also should not be used in combination with androgens.[66]

HSCT is the only curative treatment for BMF in patients who have DC. Major indications for HSCT are severe BMF or acute myeloid leukemia. Although there is a high risk for MDS in DC, many of the cases have abnormal cytogenetic clones or morphologic dyspoieses but do not necessarily have severe cytopenias. HSCT clearly is a life-saving measure but has substantial risks from toxicity, radiochemotherapy, or immune-related complications. Reported problems include graft failure, graft versus host disease, sepsis, pulmonary fibrosis, cirrhosis, and veno-occlusive disease,[49,67] resulting in part from underlying pulmonary and liver disease.[46,47,48,49,50] As a result, long-term survival of patients who have DC after HSCT has been poor.[49,67] Studies of

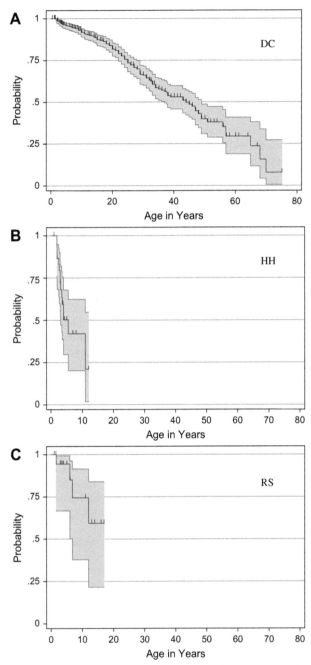

Fig. 3. Survival of patients who had DC based on review of the literature. (*A*) Patients who had DC, not including those who had HH or RS; (*B*) HH, Hoyeraal-Hreidarsson syndrome; (*C*) RS, Revesz syndrome.

reduced-intensity preparative regimens are ongoing in a few institutions and may improve long-term outcomes.[55,68]

The selection of related hematopoietic stem cell donors may be complicated by the variable phenotype seen in DC, including silent carriers. In one family, peripheral blood stem cell mobilization from a matched-sibling HSCT donor yielded suboptimal numbers of CD34+ cells and the HSCT to the proband was complicated by delayed engraftment and sepsis. In a second family, peripheral blood stem cell mobilization was unsuccessful from an apparently healthy matched sibling donor, who subsequently was shown to have a markedly hypocellular bone marrow. The probands and sibling donors later were found to have mutations in TERC.[69]

The authors recently identified a potential donor who was a silent carrier of a TINF2 mutation. The individual was an apparently healthy, HLA-matched sibling of a patient who had DC in need of HSCT. The sibling was found to have very short telomeres before the discovery of the TINF2 gene mutation.[12] The presence of very short telomeres in this potential donor was the basis of a recommendation that he not be used as the donor.[51] Another HLA-matched sibling with normal telomeres was used successfully as the donor and subsequently shown not to have a TINF2 mutation (found in the proband after the transplant). The sibling who had the short telomeres was a silent carrier for the TINF2 mutation.[12] The relatives of patients who have DC who are being considered as HSCT donors should be evaluated carefully for DC. If the causative gene is known in the patient, then it should be tested in the donor. If the gene has not yet been identified, the donors should have telomere length testing done in leukocyte subsets by flow-FISH to rule out silent carriers.

Because patients who have DC are at high risk for SCC of the head and neck or anogenital region and for hematologic malignancies, the authors recommend frequent monitoring of patients for early detection of these complications. Monthly self-examination for oral and head and neck cancer is warranted as is screening annually by a head and neck specialist and semiannually by a dentist, similar to screening recommendations for patients who have Fanconi anemia.[63] Other clinical tests to consider for disease surveillance for patients who have DC include at least twice-yearly complete blood counts; annual bone marrow aspirates, biopsies, and cytogenetics; liver ultrasounds, especially for, but not limited to, those on androgens; annual pulmonary function tests; gynecologic examinations; and skin cancer screening by a dermatologist. These screening measures are being studied prospectively in the NCI DC cohort.[55]

SUMMARY

The identification of large numbers of patients who have DC has led to the recognition of a broad clinical phenotype and an appreciation that these patients have abnormalities in telomere biology. DC is a multisystem disorder that includes a high risk for BMF and cancer. Patients should be monitored closely for these and other complications. Mutations in six telomere biology genes have been identified in DC, representing approximately half of the known patients. Measurement of telomere length in leukocyte subsets determined by flow-FISH is a sensitive and specific screening test for DC in patients who have BMF and normal chromosome breakage tests. If telomeres are less than the first percentile for age, the authors suggest prospective management and screening for DC-related complications and genetic testing for mutations in DC genes. Such studies are required to better understand the clinical consequences of DC, identify the basis for BMF response to androgens, define the best HSCT regimen, and determine the best measures for surveillance and prevention of cancer and other complications.

ACKNOWLEDGMENTS

The authors are grateful to the patients and families for their invaluable contributions to studies of DC. The authors thank Dr. Neelam Giri, National Cancer Institute, for assistance with patient care and data interpretation, and Dr. John Butman, Clinical Center, National Institutes of Health, for assistance with MRI interpretation and images.

REFERENCES

1. Drachtman RA, Alter BP. Dyskeratosis congenita: clinical and genetic heterogeneity. Report of a new case and review of the literature. Am J Pediatr Hematol Oncol 1992;14(4):297–304.
2. Walne AJ, Dokal I. Dyskeratosis congenita: a historical perspective. Mech Ageing Dev 2008;129(1–2):48–59.
3. Alter BP, Baerlocher GM, Savage SA, et al. Very short telomere length by flow fluorescence in situ hybridization identifies patients with dyskeratosis congenita. Blood 2007;110(5):1439–47.
4. Mitchell JR, Wood E, Collins K. A telomerase component is defective in the human disease dyskeratosis congenita. Nature 1999;402(6761):551–5.
5. Savage SA, Alter BP. The role of telomere biology in bone marrow failure and other disorders. Mech Ageing Dev 2008;129(1–2):35–47.
6. Zinsser F. Atrophia Cutis Reticularis cum Pigmentations, Dystrophia Unguium et Leukoplakis oris (Poikioodermia atrophicans vascularis Jacobi). Ikonographia Dermatologica 1910;5:219–23 [in German].
7. Engman MFS. A unique case of reticular pigmentation of the skin with atrophy. Arch Belg Dermatol Syphiligr 1926;13:685–7.
8. Cole HN, Rauschkolb J, Toomey J. Dyskeratosis congenita with pigmentation, dystrophia unguis and leukokeratosis oris. Archives of Dermatology and Syphilology 1930;21:71–95.
9. Dokal I. Dyskeratosis congenita in all its forms. Br J Haematol 2000;110(4): 768–79.
10. Young NS, Alter BP. Aplastic anemia acquired and inherited. Philadelphia: W.B. Saunders Company; 1994.
11. Vulliamy TJ, Marrone A, Knight SW, et al. Mutations in dyskeratosis congenita: their impact on telomere length and the diversity of clinical presentation. Blood 2006;107(7):2680–5.
12. Savage SA, Giri N, Baerlocher GM, et al. TINF2, a component of the shelterin telomere protection complex, is mutated in dyskeratosis congenita. Am J Hum Genet 2008;82(2):501–9.
13. Hoyeraal HM, Lamvik J, Moe PJ. Congenital hypoplastic thrombocytopenia and cerebral malformations in two brothers. Acta Paediatr Scand 1970;59(2):185–91.
14. Hreidarsson S, Kristjansson K, Johannesson G, et al. A syndrome of progressive pancytopenia with microcephaly, cerebellar hypoplasia and growth failure. Acta Paediatr Scand 1988;77(5):773–5.
15. Aalfs CM, van den BH, Barth PG, Hennekam RC. The Hoyeraal-Hreidarsson syndrome: the fourth case of a separate entity with prenatal growth retardation, progressive pancytopenia and cerebellar hypoplasia. Eur J Pediatr 1995; 154(4):304–8.

16. Sznajer Y, Baumann C, David A, et al. Further delineation of the congenital form of X-linked dyskeratosis congenita (Hoyeraal-Hreidarsson syndrome). Eur J Pediatr 2003;162(12):863–7.
17. Walne AJ, Vulliamy T, Beswick R, et al. TINF2 mutations result in very short telomeres: analysis of a large cohort of patients with dyskeratosis congenita and related bone marrow failure syndromes. Blood 2008;112(9):3594–600.
18. Marrone A, Walne A, Tamary H, et al. Telomerase reverse-transcriptase homozygous mutations in autosomal recessive dyskeratosis congenita and Hoyeraal-Hreidarsson syndrome. Blood 2007;110(13):4198–205.
19. Revesz T, Fletcher S, Gazali LI, et al. Bilateral retinopathy, aplastic anaemia, and central nervous system abnormalities: a new syndrome? J Med Genet 1992;29(9):673–5.
20. Kajtar P, Mehes K. Bilateral coats retinopathy associated with aplastic anaemia and mild dyskeratotic signs. Am J Med Genet 1994;49(4):374–7.
21. Heiss NS, Knight SW, Vulliamy TJ, et al. X-linked dyskeratosis congenita is caused by mutations in a highly conserved gene with putative nucleolar functions. Nat Genet 1998;19(1):32–8.
22. Vulliamy T, Beswick R, Kirwan M, et al. Mutations in the telomerase component NHP2 cause the premature ageing syndrome dyskeratosis congenita. Proc Natl Acad Sci U S A 2008;105(23):8073–8.
23. Walne AJ, Vulliamy T, Marrone A, et al. Genetic heterogeneity in autosomal recessive dyskeratosis congenita with one subtype due to mutations in the telomerase-associated protein NOP10. Hum Mol Genet 2007;16(13):1619–29.
24. Aubert G, Lansdorp PM. Telomeres and aging. Physiol Rev 2008;88(2):557–79.
25. Wong JM, Collins K. Telomerase RNA level limits telomere maintenance in X-linked dyskeratosis congenita. Genes Dev 2006;20(20):2848–58.
26. Vulliamy T, Marrone A, Szydlo R, et al. Disease anticipation is associated with progressive telomere shortening in families with dyskeratosis congenita due to mutations in TERC. Nat Genet 2004;36(5):447–9.
27. Yamaguchi H, Baerlocher GM, Lansdorp PM, et al. Mutations of the human telomerase RNA gene (TERC) in aplastic anemia and myelodysplastic syndrome. Blood 2003;102(3):916–8.
28. Armanios MY, Chen JJ, Cogan JD, et al. Telomerase mutations in families with idiopathic pulmonary fibrosis. N Engl J Med 2007;356(13):1317–26.
29. Yamaguchi H, Calado RT, Ly H, et al. Mutations in TERT, the gene for telomerase reverse transcriptase, in aplastic anemia. N Engl J Med 2005;352(14):1413–24.
30. Savage SA, Stewart BJ, Weksler BB, et al. Mutations in the reverse transcriptase component of telomerase (TERT) in patients with bone marrow failure. Blood Cells Mol Dis 2006;37(2):134–6.
31. Vulliamy TJ, Walne A, Baskaradas A, et al. Mutations in the reverse transcriptase component of telomerase (TERT) in patients with bone marrow failure. Blood Cells Mol Dis 2005;34(3):257–63.
32. Tsakiri KD, Cronkhite JT, Kuan PJ, et al. Adult-onset pulmonary fibrosis caused by mutations in telomerase. Proc Natl Acad Sci U S A 2007;104(18):7552–7.
33. Armanios M, Chen JL, Chang YP, et al. Haploinsufficiency of telomerase reverse transcriptase leads to anticipation in autosomal dominant dyskeratosis congenita. Proc Natl Acad Sci U S A 2005;102(44):15960–4.
34. Baird DM. New developments in telomere length analysis. Exp Gerontol 2005;40(5):363–8.
35. Lin KW, Yan J. The telomere length dynamic and methods of its assessment. J Cell Mol Med 2005;9(4):977–89.

36. Baerlocher GM, Lansdorp PM. Telomere length measurements in leukocyte subsets by automated multicolor flow-FISH. Cytometry A 2003;55(1):1–6.

37. Ball SE, Gibson FM, Rizzo S, et al. Progressive telomere shortening in aplastic anemia. Blood 1998;91(10):3582–92.

38. Du HY, Pumbo E, Ivanovich J, et al. TERC and TERT gene mutations in patients with bone marrow failure and the significance of telomere length measurements. Blood 2008.

39. Rufer N, Dragowska W, Thornbury G, et al. Telomere length dynamics in human lymphocyte subpopulations measured by flow cytometry. Nat Biotechnol 1998; 16(8):743–7.

40. Baerlocher GM, Lansdorp PM. Telomere length measurements using fluorescence in situ hybridization and flow cytometry. Methods Cell Biol 2004;75:719–50.

41. Frenck RW Jr, Blackburn EH, Shannon KM. The rate of telomere sequence loss in human leukocytes varies with age. Proc Natl Acad Sci U S A 1998;95(10): 5607–10.

42. Rufer N, Brummendorf TH, Kolvraa S, et al. Telomere fluorescence measurements in granulocytes and T lymphocyte subsets point to a high turnover of hematopoietic stem cells and memory T cells in early childhood. J Exp Med 1999;190(2):157–67.

43. Slagboom PE, Droog S, Boomsma DI. Genetic determination of telomere size in humans: a twin study of three age groups. Am J Hum Genet 1994;55(5):876–82.

44. Zeichner SL, Palumbo P, Feng Y, et al. Rapid telomere shortening in children. Blood 1999;93(9):2824–30.

45. Al Rahawan MM, Giri N, Alter BP. Intensive immunosuppression therapy for aplastic anemia associated with dyskeratosis congenita. Int J Hematol 2006; 83(3):275–6.

46. Yabe M, Yabe H, Hattori K, et al. Fatal interstitial pulmonary disease in a patient with dyskeratosis congenita after allogeneic bone marrow transplantation. Bone Marrow Transplant 1997;19(4):389–92.

47. Ostronoff F, Ostronoff M, Calixto R, et al. Fludarabine, cyclophosphamide, and antithymocyte globulin for a patient with dyskeratosis congenita and severe bone marrow failure. Biol Blood Marrow Transplant 2007;13(3):366–8.

48. Brazzola P, Duval M, Fournet JC, et al. Fatal diffuse capillaritis after hematopoietic stem-cell transplantation for dyskeratosis congenita despite low-intensity conditioning regimen. Bone Marrow Transplant 2005;36(12):1103–5.

49. de la Fuente J, Dokal I. Dyskeratosis congenita: advances in the understanding of the telomerase defect and the role of stem cell transplantation. Pediatr Transplant 2007;11(6):584–94.

50. Dror Y, Freedman MH, Leaker M, et al. Low-intensity hematopoietic stem-cell transplantation across human leucocyte antigen barriers in dyskeratosis congenita. Bone Marrow Transplant 2003;31(10):847–50.

51. Denny CC, Wilfond BS, Peters JA, et al. All in the family: disclosure of "unwanted" information to an adolescent to benefit a relative. Am J Med Genet A 2008; 146A(21):2719–24.

52. Marrone A, Sokhal P, Walne A, et al. Functional characterization of novel telomerase RNA (TERC) mutations in patients with diverse clinical and pathological presentations. Haematologica 2007;92(8):1013–20.

53. National Cancer institute. Inherited bone marrow failure syndromes. Available at: http://marrowfailure.cancer.gov. Accessed March 4, 2009.

54. Rosenberg P, Giri N, Savage SA, et al. Cancer epidemiology in the National Cancer Institute inherited bone marrow failure syndromes cohort: first report. ASH Annual Meeting, San Francisco, CA, December 6–9, 2008.

55. Savage SA, Dokal I, Armanios M, et al. Dyskeratosis congenita: the first NIH clinical research workshop. Pediatr Blood Cancer, manuscript under review.
56. Vulliamy T, Dokal I. Dyskeratosis congenita. Semin Hematol 2006;43(3):157–66.
57. Alter BP. Diagnosis, genetics, and management of inherited bone marrow failure syndromes. Hematology Am Soc Hematol Educ Program 2007;2007:29–39.
58. Alder JK, Chen JJ, Lancaster L, et al. Short telomeres are a risk factor for idiopathic pulmonary fibrosis. Proc Natl Acad Sci U S A 2008;105(35):13051–6.
59. Tsangaris E, Adams SL, Yoon G, et al. Ataxia and pancytopenia caused by a mutation in TINF2. Hum Genet 2008;124(5):507–13.
60. Mahiques L, Febrer I, Vilata JJ, et al. A case of dyskeratosis congenita associated with schizophrenia and two malignancies. J Eur Acad Dermatol Venereol 2006; 20(9):1159–61.
61. Milgrom H, Sroll HL Jr, Crissey JT. Dyskeratosis congenita. A case with new features. Arch Dermatol 1964;89:345–9.
62. Mason III JO, Yunker JJ, Nixon PA, et al. Proliferative retinopathy as a complication of dyskeratosis congenita. Retinal Cases and Brief Reports. in press.
63. Owen J, Frohnmayer L, Eiler ME, editors. Fanconi anemia: standards for clinical care. Eugene (OR): Fanconi Anemia Research Fund, Inc; 2003. p. 184.
64. Velazquez I, Alter BP. Androgens and liver tumors: Fanconi 's anemia and non-Fanconi 's conditions. Am J Hematol 2004;77(3):257–67.
65. Giri N, Pitel PA, Green D, et al. Splenic peliosis and rupture in patients with dyskeratosis congenita on androgens and granulocyte colony-stimulating factor. Br J Haematol 2007;138(6):815–7.
66. Alter BP, Gardner FH, Hall RE. Treatment of dyskeratosis congenita with granulocyte colony-stimulating factor and erythropoietin. Br J Haematol 1997;97(2): 309–11.
67. Berthou C, Devergie A, D'Agay MF, et al. Late vascular complications after bone marrow transplantation for dyskeratosis congenita. Br J Haematol 1991;79(2): 335–6.
68. Tolar J, Orchard PJ, Miller JS, et al. Dyskeratosis congenita: low regimen-related toxicity following hematopoietic cell transplantation (HCT) using a reduced intensity conditioning regimen. ASH Annual Meeting, Atlanta, GA, December 8–11, 2007.
69. Fogarty PF, Yamaguchi H, Wiestner A, et al. Late presentation of dyskeratosis congenita as apparently acquired aplastic anaemia due to mutations in telomerase RNA. Lancet 2003;362(9396):1628–30.

Shwachman-Diamond Syndrome: A Review of the Clinical Presentation, Molecular Pathogenesis, Diagnosis, and Treatment

Lauri Burroughs, MD[a,b,]*, Ann Woolfrey, MD[b,c],
Akiko Shimamura, MD, PhD[b,d]

KEYWORDS

- Shwachman-Diamond syndrome • Aplastic anemia
- Inherited marrow failure • Cancer predisposition
- Hematopoietic cell transplantation • Neutropenia

Shwachman-Diamond syndrome (SDS) is a rare autosomal-recessive, multisystem disease characterized by exocrine pancreatic insufficiency, impaired hematopoiesis, and leukemia predisposition. Other clinical features include skeletal, immunologic, hepatic, and cardiac disorders. Around 90% of patients with clinical features of SDS have biallellic mutations in the evolutionarily conserved Shwachman-Bodian-Diamond Syndrome (*SBDS*) gene located on chromosome 7.[1] The SBDS protein plays a role in ribosome biogenesis and in mitotic spindle stabilization, although its precise

Supported in part by NIH grants P01 HL36444, K23 HL085288, and R01 HL079582.

[a] Clinical Research Division, Fred Hutchinson Cancer Research Center, 1100 Fairview Avenue North, D1-100, PO Box 19024, Seattle, WA 98109–1024, USA

[b] Department of Pediatrics, University of Washington, Seattle, WA, USA

[c] Clinical Research Division, Fred Hutchinson Cancer Research Center, 1100 Fairview Avenue North, D5-380, PO Box 19024, Seattle, WA 98109–1024, USA

[d] Clinical Research Division, Fred Hutchinson Cancer Research Center, 1100 Fairview Avenue North, D2-100, PO Box 19024, Seattle, WA 98109–1024, USA

* Corresponding author. Clinical Research Division, Fred Hutchinson Cancer Research Center, 1100 Fairview Avenue North, D1-100, PO Box 19024, Seattle, WA 98109–1024.

E-mail address: lburroug@fhcrc.org (L. Burroughs).

molecular function remains unclear. This article focuses on the clinical presentation, diagnostic work-up, clinical management, and treatment of patients with SDS.

CLINICAL PRESENTATION
Hematologic Features

Several groups have reported on the hematologic features of patients with SDS.[2–5] The most common hematologic abnormality affecting 88% to 100% of patients with SDS is neutropenia, typically defined as a neutrophil count less than 1500×10^9/L. Roughly one third of patients have chronic neutropenia and the remaining two thirds have intermittent neutropenia. Anemia, either normochromic- normocytic or macrocytic, with reticulocytopenia has also been described in 42% to 82% of patients. Thrombocytopenia (platelet count $<150 \times 10^9$/L) has been reported in 24% to 88% of patients and can lead to fatal bleeding. Similar to patients with other marrow failure syndromes, around 80% of patients with SDS have elevated levels of hemoglobin F, which is likely a sign of stress hematopoiesis. Cytopenias are usually seen at an early age; presentations at later ages have been reported.[6] Roughly 10% to 65% of patients have pancytopenia with some patients developing aplastic anemia.[7] Bone marrow findings are variable and may reveal a hypocellular, normocellular, or hypercellular marrow. Marrow cellularity must be interpreted in the context of the patient's peripheral blood counts because cellularity may be patchy and is subject to sampling variation.

Myelodysplastic Syndrome and Malignancy

Similar to other marrow failure syndromes, patients with SDS have an increased risk for myelodysplasia and malignant transformation, in particular development of acute myelogenous leukemia (AML).[8,9] AML subtypes include AML-M0, AML-M1, AML-M4, AML-M5, and AML-M6. Donadieu and colleagues[10] reported on 55 patients with SDS, median age of 0.5 years (range, birth to 23) from the French Severe Chronic Neutropenia Registry. With a median follow-up of 8 years (range, 0.3–35.6), seven patients developed myelodysplastic syndrome (MDS) or AML, with an estimated risk of 19% at 20 years and 36% at 30 years. Solid tumors have not been described. The mechanisms underlying this tendency toward malignant transformation are unknown. Marrow cytogenetic clonal abnormalities, particularly involving chromosome 7 (monosomy 7, der[7], i[7q]) and del(20q), have commonly been reported.[11] Although certain cytogenetic aberrations, such as monosomy 7, are associated with poor prognosis, the clinical significance of many clonal abnormalities is not clear.[12] Similar cytogenetic abnormalities have been found in patients with MDS or leukemia. A given clonal abnormality may wax and wane over time within a patient and may even become undetectable, further complicating clinical interpretation.[12] To date, there have been no reports of progression to AML among SDS patients presenting with i(7q) abnormalities. In contrast, 42% of patients with other chromosome 7 abnormalities either presented with or progressed to advanced MDS or AML.[11]

Chromosome instability may play a role in MDS or leukemia development.[13] Some have proposed that an increased risk for cancer evolves from accelerated apoptosis, which may lead to replicative stress and increased risk for evolution of malignant clones.[14] This model is developed in detail elsewhere in this issue. Recently, Austin and colleagues[15] demonstrated that SBDS promotes mitotic spindle stability and regulates chromosome segregation. These results suggest that the high frequency of chromosomal abnormalities seen in the bone marrow of patients with SDS may result, at least in part, from a defect in spindle stability.

Infections and Immune Abnormalities

Patients with SDS are susceptible to recurrent bacterial, viral, and fungal infections, in particular, otitis media, sinusitis, mouth sores, bronchopneumonia, septicemia, osteomyelitis, and skin infections.[16] Neutropenia is likely a contributing factor, and possible defects in neutrophil chemotaxis.[2,17,18] Stepanovic and colleagues[19] demonstrated that neutrophils from patients with SDS were unable to orient and migrate toward a chemoattractant gradient, which is essential for normal neutrophil migration to a site of infection or inflammation. Others have suggested that the neutrophil abnormalities may be caused by an abnormal distribution of concanavalin-A receptors on patient's neutrophils or cytoskeletal/microtubular defects.[20] Importantly, despite a deficiency in neutrophil number and function, patients with SDS are able to recruit sufficient neutrophils in response to infections to form abscesses.[16]

Defects in lymphocyte-mediated immunity also have been described.[18,21] Specifically, decreased proportions of circulating B cells, low immunoglobulin (IgG or IgG subclasses) levels, decreased in vitro B-cell proliferation, and lack of specific antibody or isohemaglutinin production have been reported.[11] In addition, decreased percentages of circulating natural killer cells, total circulating T lymphocytes, and decreased proliferative responses and inverse CD4:CD8 ratios have been described.[18]

Gastrointestinal Features

One of the hallmarks of SDS is exocrine pancreatic dysfunction of varying severities caused by absence of acinar cells. Patients classically present in early infancy with malabsorption; steatorrhea; failure to thrive; and low levels of fat-soluble vitamins A, D, E, and K. Importantly, patients with SDS have normal sweat chloride tests, differentiating them from patients with cystic fibrosis, whose pancreatic defect involves the exocrine pancreatic ducts. Low serum pancreatic trypsinogen and low isoamylase are useful markers for pancreatic insufficiency in patients with SDS; however, the age of the patient is important in interpretation. Trypsinogen is generally low in SDS patients younger than 3 years of age but increases to the normal range in older patients where it becomes less useful as a disease marker. Serum isoamylase levels are low in patients with SDS of all ages; however, the use of this test in patients younger than 3 years old is limited because isoamylase levels are also low in healthy children of this age.[22] In addition, fecal elastase levels may be low. Pancreatic enzyme secretion in response to stimulation testing is reduced.

Imaging studies with ultrasound, CT, or MRI often demonstrate a small, structurally abnormal pancreas composed mainly of fat.[23] Pathologic evaluation reveals extensive fatty replacement of the pancreatic acinar tissue and relatively normal pancreatic ducts and islets. For reasons that remain unclear, exocrine pancreatic function spontaneously improves over time in roughly 50% of patients.[3,5] Pancreatic endocrine function generally seems intact as evidenced by normal glucose tolerance tests; however, cases of insulin-dependent diabetes mellitus have been reported (see the other features section for further details).

Hepatomegaly is found in roughly 15% of patients, and 50% to 75% of patients have elevated serum liver enzymes two to three times normal.[3,5,24] Pathologic evaluation of the liver has shown severe panlobular fatty changes with nonspecific periportal and portal inflammatory infiltration, varying degrees of periportal, portal and bridging fibrosis, and microvesicular and macrovesicular steatosis in several patients.[3,4,25–27] These abnormalities typically occur early in life and normalize over time without apparent long-term sequelae. Serious hepatic complications have been reported, however, in patients with SDS following hematopoietic cell transplantation (HCT).[28]

Skeletal Abnormalities

Skeletal abnormalities are commonly reported in patients with SDS. The primary skeletal defects are related to abnormal development of the growth plates, in particular the metaphyses. Metaphyseal dysostosis has been reported in roughly 50% of the patients, is usually asymptomatic, and most commonly involves the femoral head.[4,25] Other sites that may be affected include the knees, humeral heads, wrists, ankles, and vertebrae. Rib cage abnormalities are found in 30% to 50% of patients, including narrow rib cage, shortened ribs with flared anterior ends, and costochondral thickening. Case reports have described respiratory failure in the newborn period as a result of these rib cage abnormalities.[29] Other skeletal abnormalities described in patients with SDS include slipped femoral epiphysis; digit abnormalities (clinodactyly, syndactyly, and supernumerary thumbs); and progressive spinal deformities (kyphosis, scoliosis, and vertebral collapse).[25,30] Low turnover osteopenia and osteoporosis have also been reported independent of vitamin D deficiency.[30,31]

Cardiac Features

Several case reports have described neonatal cardiac manifestations associated with SDS.[32–36] Myocardial necrosis or fibrosis has been primarily seen on histopathology. Savilahti and Rapola[32] reported eight deaths from cardiac failure among 16 patients with SDS. Autopsies demonstrated myocardial necrosis in the left ventricle.[32] Recently, Toiviainen-Salo and colleagues[37] evaluated eight patients with SDS who did not have any cardiac symptoms. All had normal cardiac anatomy and myocardial structure; however, depressed left ventricular contractility during exercise and subtle right ventricular diastolic dysfunctions were seen. Further studies evaluating the clinical importance of these findings are needed.

There also have been several studies describing cardiac complications following HCT in patients with SDS. Specifically, transient congestive heart failure during induction chemotherapy,[38] long-term cardiac hypokinesia after HCT,[39] and fatal pancarditis following HCT[40] have been seen. As a result of these and earlier studies raising concern regarding cardiac complications in patients with SDS, several groups have proposed reduced-intensity conditioning regimens that avoid known cardiotoxic therapies, such as cyclophosphamide (see the section on HCT for further details).

Other Features

Insulin-dependent diabetes,[4] growth hormone deficiency,[21] hypogonadotropic hypogonadism,[41] and hypothyroidism have been described in patients with SDS (Akiko Shimamura, MD, PhD, personal communication, 2009). Failure to thrive is common and is likely multifactorial including pancreatic insufficiency, feeding difficulties, recurrent infections, and metaphyseal dysostosis. Despite pancreatic enzyme replacement, many patients tend to remain below the third percentile for height and weight. Normal height and weight for age, however, does not rule out the diagnosis of SDS. Renal abnormalities including urinary tract anomalies and renal tubular acidosis have also been described.[4,25]

MOLECULAR PATHOGENESIS

SDS is an autosomal-recessive disorder. Approximately 90% of patients meeting the clinical diagnostic criteria for SDS have mutations in the *SBDS* gene. The carrier frequency for this mutation has been estimated at 1 in 110.[42] This highly conserved gene has five exons encompassing 7.9 kb and maps to the 7q11 centromeric region of chromosome 7.[1,42] The SBDS gene encodes a novel 250–amino acid protein lacking homology to known protein functional domains. An adjacent pseudogene, *SBDSP*, shares 97% homology with *SBDS* but contains deletions and nucleotide changes that prevent the generation of a functional protein. Roughly 75% of patients with SDS have *SBDS* mutations resulting from a gene conversion event with this pseudogene.[1] The *SBDS* mRNA and protein are widely expressed throughout human tissues at both the mRNA and protein levels.[1,43,44] The complete absence of *Sbds* expression was lethal in murine models.[45] Although the early truncating *SBDS* mutation 183 TA > CT is common among patients with SDS, patients homozygous for this mutation have not been identified, suggesting that complete loss of the *SBDS* expression is likely lethal in human patients.

CD34[+] hematopoietic cells are quantitatively reduced in the bone marrows of SDS patients compared with healthy control marrows.[46] SDS CD34[+] cells are also qualitatively impaired in progenitor colony formation and long-term colony formation. The ability of marrow stromal cells from SDS patients to support normal CD34[+] cells in long-term colony assays was also diminished.[46] Increased apoptosis[14] and elevated levels of p53 protein[47] have been observed in SDS marrows. Reduction of *Sbds* expression in mouse c-kit+ lineage–hematopoietic cells with lentiviral-mediated RNAi impaired both granulocyte differentiation in vitro and short-term hematopoietic engraftment following transplant in vivo.[48] In a zebrafish model, morpholino-mediated knockdown of sbds resulted in abnormal development of the pancreas and granulocytes.[49]

The crystal structure of the Archael SBDS orthologue revealed a tripartite structure without apparent homology to known protein functional domains.[50,51] Data from SBDS orthologs suggested that SBDS may play a role in ribosome biogenesis, a complex and highly regulated cellular process.[1] The human SBDS protein is present throughout the cell and is particularly concentrated in the nucleolus, the primary site of ribosome biogenesis.[43] In studies of human cells, Ganapathi and colleagues[52] demonstrated that (1) cells from patients with SDS are hypersensitive to low doses of actinomycin D, an inhibitor of rRNA transcription; (2) actinomycin D abolishes nucleolar localization of *SBDS*; (3) SBDS cosediments with the 60S large ribosomal subunit but not with mature ribosomes or polysome in sucrose gradients; (4) *SBDS* coprecipitates with 28S ribosomal RNA (rRNA); and (5) *SBDS* forms a protein complex with nucleophosmin, a multifunctional protein implicated in ribosome biogenesis, leukemogenesis, and centrosomal amplification. An interaction between SBDS and the 60S ribosomal assembly factor Nip7 has also been described.[53] Down-regulation of SBDS in HEK293 cells showed alterations in both the mRNA levels and mRNA polysome loading of genes implicated in nervous system development, bone morphogenesis, and hematopoiesis.[53]

Proteomic analysis of proteins associating with the yeast SBDS orthologue SDO1/YLR022C identified over 20 proteins involved in ribosome biogenesis.[51] Yeast carrying mutations in *SDO1* grow very slowly. Genetic studies demonstrated suppression of the *SDO1*-/- slow-growth phenotype by mutations in *TIF6*.[54] Tif6 is required for pre-60S subunit synthesis and nuclear export.[55] eIF6, the mammalian ortholog of Tif6, associates with the 60S ribosomal subunit and inhibits the joining of the 60S to the 40S ribosomal subunit.[56] The *TIF6* mutations that suppress the *SDO1*-/- slow-growth phenotype were located in a region of Tif6 that reduced the binding of Tif6 to the 60S subunit. *TIF6* mutations also suppress the ribosome biogenesis defects resulting from mutations in *EFL1*, which encodes a cytoplasmic GTPase that promotes dissociation of Tif6 from the 60S subunit in vitro.[57] Genetic analysis revealed an epistatic relationship between *SDO1* and *EFL1*, consistent with data that these two genes function coordinately with *TIF6*.[54] In the absence of *SDO1* expression, 60S ribosomal RNA subunit levels were reduced, and export of the 60S subunit from the nucleus to the cytoplasm was disrupted. These data suggest a model wherein Sdo1 might recruit Efl1 to the pre-60S ribosome, thereby facilitating Tif6 release to allow joining of the 60S and 40S subunits.[54] How disruption in ribosome biogenesis results in specific phenotypic findings in patients with SDS or why the bone marrow seems to be particularly susceptible to ribosome impairment remain to be defined.

SBDS also functions during mitosis to prevent genomic instability.[15] Cultured cells from SDS patients exhibited an increased incidence of mitotic aberrations, characterized by multipolar spindles and centrosomal amplification, compared with controls. Knockdown of SBDS expression with siRNAs in human fibroblasts recapitulated this phenotype, but only after 2 weeks in culture suggesting that the mitotic defects were a downstream result of SBDS loss. Loss of SBDS was associated with increased apoptosis when checkpoint pathways were intact, but resulted in aneuploid cells when p53 was inactivated. Aneuploidy is associated with an increased rate of chromosomal rearrangements, such as breaks and translocations in animal models.[58] SBDS co-localized with the mitotic spindle by immunofluorescence. Recombinant SBDS bound to purified microtubules in vitro resulting in microtubule stabilization both in vitro and in vivo. These data suggest a novel model for a human cancer predisposition syndrome whereby mitotic spindle instability results in chromosomal aberrations. It is intriguing to speculate that the mitotic and ribosomal functions of SBDS might be related because other proteins, such as nucleophosmin[59] and Rrp14,[60] have been shown to function in both ribosome biogenesis and mitosis. Alternatively, it is also possible that these functions might additively contribute to the SDS disease phenotype. Additional mechanistic and biologic studies are required to answer these questions.

DIAGNOSIS, CLINICAL MANAGEMENT, AND TREATMENT
Diagnosis

The diagnosis of SDS is largely based on clinical phenotype, with pancreatic exocrine and bone marrow dysfunction being the central features. There is considerable phenotypic variability between individuals and even within the same individual over time, however, making the diagnosis challenging particularly in older patients where such symptoms as steatorrhea may have resolved or neutropenia may be mild and intermittent. Several disorders must be excluded including cystic fibrosis; Pearson syndrome; Johanson-Blizzard syndrome; severe malnutrition combined with diminished exocrine pancreatic function; and other marrow failure syndromes, such as Fanconi's anemia, dyskeratosis congenita, and severe congenital neutropenia.

Exocrine pancreatic insufficiency may be demonstrated by one of the following: elevated fecal fat excretion following a 72-hour collection in the absence of concomitant intestinal or cholestatic liver disease with imaging studies showing a small or fatty pancreas; and low serum trypsinogen in patients under the age of 3 or low serum iso-amylase testing in patients over the age of 3.[22,61] The use of fecal elastase as a marker for exocrine pancreatic dysfunction in SDS is currently under investigation. Pancreatic stimulation testing with intravenous pancreozymin with or without secretin has been used to evaluate levels of pancreatic enzymes; however, with the advent of serum markers, this invasive procedure has been used less commonly. Signs of marrow failure may include any of the following findings: (1) intermittent or persistent neutropenia (absolute neutrophil count <1500/μL) documented at least three times over a minimum of 3 months without an apparent cause; (2) hypoproductive anemia with a hemoglobin concentration below the age-related adjusted norms; (3) unexplained macrocytosis; (4) platelet count less than 150,000/μL without alternative etiology; or (5) hypocellular bone marrow. Aplastic anemia, MDS, or leukemia may be the presenting hematologic abnormality of a patient with underlying SDS. Additional supportive features include skeletal abnormalities, hepatomegaly with or without elevated serum aminotransferase levels, and immunologic abnormalities. **Box 1** provides a suggested evaluation pathway for SDS. *SBDS* genetic testing provides corroborative data in a patient who has been clinically diagnosed with SDS and allows genetic testing to identify affected family members. Up to 10% of patients with clinical features of SDS lack *SBDS* mutations; the absence (negative test) of the *SBDS* gene mutation does not rule out the diagnosis.[1] It is presently not known whether patients lacking *SBDS* mutations have mutations in an additional as yet unidentified gene for SDS or if they represent a separate distinct disorder. The clinical implications of *SBDS* genetic testing in the diagnosis of patients with SDS has yet to be defined, particularly for those patients who are asymptomatic and lack clinical manifestations of SDS and in those who do not have a positive family history.

Clinical Management

Hematology

All patients with SDS should be monitored by a hematologist. The general recommendation from a clinical consensus conference is to monitor peripheral blood counts for cytopenias every 3 to 4 months.[61] Marrow evaluation with aspirate and biopsy including cytogenetics to assess for marrow cellularity, MDS, acute leukemia, or other clonal disease is recommended on a yearly basis or more often if clinically indicated.[61] Such regular monitoring allows timely institution of therapy before the development of clinical complications. HCT before the development of overt leukemia is associated with better outcomes.

For those neutropenic patients with recurrent or severe infections, granulocyte colony–stimulating factor may be considered. Data regarding malignant myeloid transformation into MDS or AML in SDS patients on granulocyte colony–stimulating factor therapy are inconclusive; however, there is no strong evidence that links granulocyte colony–stimulating factor directly to leukemic conversion.[62] Therefore, granulocyte colony–stimulating factor should not be withheld if clinically indicated to treat infection or to prevent recurrent bacterial or fungal infections.

Gastroenterology

Patients with SDS should also be followed by a gastroenterologist for management of exocrine pancreatic insufficiency. Most patients require oral pancreatic enzyme supplementation. Steatorrhea, however, resolves in roughly 50% of patients; assessment of continued need for pancreatic enzyme supplementation is indicated. Measurement of the fat-soluble vitamins A, D, E, and K should occur with appropriate supplementation as indicated. An abnormal prothrombin time may be a useful marker of vitamin K deficiency.

Skeletal

Data are lacking on the role of bisphosphonates in patients with SDS. Measures to maximize bone density should be implemented including adequate calcium and vitamin D intake, and weight-bearing exercises. In addition, it is important to screen for and correct any underlying endocrine problems that may contribute to osteopenia, such as hypothyroidism or hypoparathyroidism.

Box 1
Recommended work-up for patients with SDS

Diagnostic studies

Marrow function

    Peripheral blood count with smear, mean corpuscular volume

    Reticulocyte count

    Bone marrow aspirate and biopsy: pathologic review and cytogenetics, iron stain

Exocrine pancreatic function

    Trypsinogen (age <3 y) or serum pancreatic isoamylase (age >3 y)

    72-hour fecal fat measurement, fecal elastase

    ± Endoscopic pancreatic stimulation testing

    Vitamin A, D, E, and K levels

Genetic testing

    SBDS mutation analysis

Supportive studies

Liver function

    Alanine transaminase, aspartate transaminase, γ-glutamyltransferase, albumin, prealbumin, prothrombin time

Immune work-up

    Immunoglobulin levels (IgA, IgG, IgM)

    T- and B-lymphocyte subset analysis

    Additional work-up as clinically indicated

Radiologic work-up

    Pancreatic imaging

    Radiographic evaluation for skeletal abnormalities, in particular metaphyseal dysostosis or thoracic dystrophies

    Echocardiogram if clinically indicated

Consultations

Hematology

Gastroenterology

Endocrinology

Genetics

Developmental assessment

Dental evaluation

Treatment: Hematopoietic Cell Transplantation

The primary causes of death in infancy are related to malabsorption, infections, and thoracic dystrophy. In older patients, the main causes of death are hemorrhage and infections caused by associated hematologic abnormalities, such as marrow aplasia, neutropenia, MDS, or acute leukemia. Supportive measures include transfusions, pancreatic enzymes, antibiotics, and granulocyte colony–stimulating factor. The only definitive therapy for marrow failure, MDS, or leukemia is HCT.

Because of the rarity of this disease, the literature on HCT for patients with SDS consists primarily of case reports including various conditioning regimens, donor types, and stem cell sources.[38,40,63–71] Poor outcomes have been reported following HCT because of graft failure or rejection, transplant-related toxicities, and relapsed leukemia. Significant cardiac and other organ toxicities have been described that are believed to be caused by exacerbation of the underlying organ dysfunction by the intensive preparative regimens.

Recently, several groups have published on larger cohorts of patients, which enable more meaningful analysis. Cesaro and colleagues[72] reported 26 patients with SDS from the European Group for Blood and Bone Marrow Transplantation registry given HCT for treatment of severe aplastic anemia (N = 16); MDS-AML (N = 9); or other diagnosis (N = 1; **Table 1**). Various preparative regimens were used; however, most included either busulfan (54%) or total body irradiation (23%) followed by an HLA-matched sibling (N = 6), mismatched family (N = 1), or unrelated graft (N = 19). Most patients were given in vitro (N = 4) or in vivo (N = 17) T-cell depleted marrow grafts. Graft failure occurred in five (19%) patients, and the incidence of grade III to IV acute and chronic graft-versus-host disease were 24% and 29%, respectively. With a median follow-up of 1.1 years, overall survival was 65%. Deaths were primarily caused by infections with or without graft-versus-host disease (N = 5) or major organ toxicities (N = 3). The analysis suggested that presence of MDS-AML or use of total body irradiation–based conditioning regimens were factors associated with poor outcome.

Donadieu and colleagues[39] published French neutropenia registry data that included 10 patients with SDS who received HCT for marrow failure (N = 5) or MDS-leukemia (N = 5). Patients were conditioned with busulfan-cyclophosphamide (N = 6) with or without antithymocyte globulin or total body irradiation plus chemo-therapy (N = 4) followed by HLA-matched sibling (N = 4) or unrelated (N = 6) marrow grafts. With a median follow-up for surviving patients of 6.9 years, the 5-year overall survival was 60%. Marrow engraftment occurred in eight patients. Two patients died before engraftment because of infections in the setting of grade IV graft-versus-host disease and multiorgan dysfunction, and two patients died 10 and 19 months after HCT because of relapse and transplant-related toxicity, respectively. The authors note that although the number of patients was small, mortality among patients with MDS-leukemia seemed to be higher than among those with marrow failure. The authors speculated that older age and associated increased comorbidities might also contribute to higher mortality following HCT for patients with MDS-leukemia.

Recently, two groups reported results of reduced-intensity preparative regimens that spared cyclophosphamide and total body irradiation. Sauer and colleagues[73] reported three patients who received conditioning with fludarabine, treosulfan (a busulfan analog), and melphalan with or without Campath-1H (N = 2) or rabbit an-tithymocyte globulin (N = 1) followed by a HLA-identical sibling (N = 1) and matched-unrelated (N = 1) marrow graft or a 9 of 10 matched cord blood graft (N = 1). Patients received HCT because of pancytopenia (N = 2) or pancytopenia-MDS (N = 1). With a follow-up of 9 and 20 months, two patients are alive. One patient who received a cord blood graft died 98 days after HCT of idiopathic pneumonitis syndrome. Bhatla and colleagues[74] reported seven patients conditioned with Campath-1H, fludarabine, and melphalan followed by HLA-matched related marrow

Table 1
Summary of recent publications for patients who have Shwachman-Diamond syndrome using HCT

Conditioning Regimen (N)	Donor Source (N)	Stem Cell Source (N)	Median Age at HCT (y)	Engraftment (N)	GVHD Prophylaxis (N)	Acute GVHD Grade (N)	cGVHD	TRM	OS	Median f/(y)	Ref
Bu based (14) TBI based (6) Flu (4) Others (2)	Sibling (6) URD (19) Other family (1) T-cell depleted (21)	BM (21) PBSC (3) CB (2)	10.3 (1.2–26.8)	21/26 (81%)	CSP/MTX (14) Other (6) Not specified (6)	I–IV: 15 (71%) III–IV: 5/21 (24%)	4/14 (29%) eligible	35.5% (1 y)	64.5%	1.1 (0.05–16.2)	72
Bu/CY (3) + ATG (3) TBI/CY (3) TBI/Mel (1)	Sibling (4) URD (6) T-cell depleted (2)	BM (10)	11.2 (1.1–27.7)	8/10[a]	CSP/MTX (5) CSP/MTX/ Steroids (2) Other (3)	II (3)/IV (3)	2/10	3/10	60% (5 y) EFS	7.6 (3.9–16.9)	39
Flu/Treo/Mel + Campath-1H (2) + ATG (1)	Sibling (1) URD (2)	BM (2) CB (1)	9.6 (1.5–17)	3/3	CSP/MTX (2) CSP/MMF (1)	II (1)	NR	1/3	2/3	2 1.3[b]	73
Campath-1H/ Flu/Mel (7)	Sibling (4) URD (3)	BM (4) PBSC (2) BM + CB (1)	8 (1–29)	7/7	CSP/MTX (6) CSP/steroids (1)	II (1)	NR	0/7	100%	1.5 (0.3–2.5)	74

Abbreviations: ATG, antithymocyte globulin; Bu, busulfan; BM, bone marrow; CB, cord blood; cGVHD, chronic graft-versus-host-disease; CSP, cyclosporine; CY, cyclophosphamide; EFS, event-free survival; Flu, fludarabine; f/u, follow-up; HCT, hematopoietic cell transplantation; Mel, melphalan; MMF, mycophenolate mofetil; MTX, methotrexate; NR, not reported; OS, overall survival; PBSC, peripheral blood stem cells; Pt, patient; TBI, total body irradiation; Treo, treosulfan; TRM, transplant-related mortality; URD, unrelated donor.

[a] Two patients died before engraftment.

[b] Follow-up of two living patients.

(N = 4) or unrelated peripheral blood stem cell (N = 2) or marrow (N = 1) grafts. Patients underwent HCT because of worsening cytopenias with increasing transfusion dependence (N = 5) and/or the appearance of clonal hematopoiesis (N = 6). With a median follow-up of 548 days (range, 93–920), all patients are alive with full donor engraftment. Viral infections were observed in four patients following HCT, likely related to the Campath-1H.

The rarity of the disease combined with an apparent lack of correlation between genotype and phenotype have contributed to the controversy on the role and optimal timing of HCT. A major challenge is identifying those patients who are at risk for MDS or leukemia development. SDS patients with leukemia have been treated with conventional chemotherapy alone; however, some patients fail to regenerate normal hematopoiesis or die from toxicities related to the chemotherapy given. As a result, HCT is the only definitive treatment for patients with bone marrow failure, MDS, or leukemia; however, it seems that patients with SDS may be at increased risk for transplant-related mortality. It is unclear whether the increased transplant-related mortality is related to complications of the underlying organ dysfunction or caused by an as yet undetermined genetically mediated susceptibility to certain conditioning agents. As a result, there is no clear consensus on when a patient with SDS should undergo HCT.

HCT studies for treatment of other genetic diseases, such as Wiskott-Aldrich syndrome and sickle cell disease, clearly show benefit when HCT is performed at a younger age, presumably because younger patients are healthier. SDS patients with MDS or leukemia at time of HCT seem to have worse outcomes compared with those with bone marrow failure alone. Thus, it seems reasonable that transplant be performed before complications of SDS develop.

Indications for HCT include severe persistent or symptomatic cytopenia; MDS with excess blasts (5%–20%); and overt leukemia with high-risk features. Particularly in the era of better supportive care and reduced-intensity conditioning regimens, one should consider HCT for those patients with AML and high-risk characteristics including evolution from MDS or abnormal cytogenetics, such as monosomy 7 (-7), monosomy 5 (-5), deletion of q arm of chromosome 5 (del5q), or complex cytogenetics with multiple cytogenetic abnormalities. In addition, molecular alterations including internal tandem duplication of the FLT3 gene (FLT3/ITD), a gene involved in regulation of stem cell differentiation, should also be considered. AML-like treatment has not been shown to provide a curative treatment approach for patients with MDS, and HCT remains the treatment of choice for clinically significant MDS. In general, there is a significant survival benefit when HCT is performed at an earlier phase of disease.[75] For those patients with marrow failure alone, the indications for HCT may include severe persistent or symptomatic cytopenias or a history of frequent life-threatening infections secondary to intractable neutropenia. These general guidelines, however, need to take into consideration donor source and histocompatibility.

SUMMARY

SDS is a rare autosomal-recessive multisystem disorder with varying phenotypic presentation. The identification of the SBDS gene has greatly expanded diagnostic capabilities; however, mechanistic and biologic studies defining SBDS gene function are needed to advance understanding of the molecular pathogenesis of marrow failure and leukemia. To date, studies have not shown any correlation between hematologic or skeletal phenotype and the SBDS genotype.[30,76] The complete clinical phenotype, natural history, and risk factors associated with the development of future complications, such as aplastic anemia, MDS, or leukemia, need to be elucidated to better determine the optimal timing of therapeutic intervention. Collaborative efforts are currently underway to develop a longitudinal data registry and tissue repository specifically for patients with SDS for clinical and scientific studies. Equally important is the development of clinical trials addressing pertinent clinical challenges, such as optimal HCT regimens. These efforts will advance the ability to diagnose and better treat patients with SDS.

REFERENCES

1. Boocock GR, Morrison JA, Popovic M, et al. Mutations in SBDS are associated with Shwachman-Diamond syndrome. Nat Genet 2003;33:97–101.
2. Smith OP, Hann IM, Chessells JM, et al. Haematological abnormalities in Shwachman-Diamond syndrome. Br J Haematol 1996;94:279–84.
3. Mack DR, Forstner GG, Wilschanski M, et al. Shwachman syndrome: exocrine pancreatic dysfunction and variable phenotypic expression. Gastroenterology 1996;111:1593–602.
4. Aggett PJ, Cavanagh NP, Matthew DJ, et al. Shwachman's syndrome: a review of 21 cases. Arch Dis Child 1980;55:331–47.
5. Cipolli M, D'Orazio C, Delmarco A, et al. Shwachman's syndrome: pathomorphosis and long-term outcome. J Pediatr Gastroenterol Nutr 1999;29:265–72.
6. Lesesve JF, Dugue F, Gregoire MJ, et al. Shwachman-Diamond syndrome with late-onset neutropenia and fatal acute myeloid leukaemia without maturation: a case report. Eur J Haematol 2003;71:393–5.
7. Woods WG, Krivit W, Lubin BH, et al. Aplastic anemia associated with the Shwachman syndrome: in vivo and in vitro observations. Am J Pediatr Hematol Oncol 1981;3:347–51.
8. Woods WG, Roloff JS, Lukens JN, et al. The occurrence of leukemia in patients with the Shwachman syndrome. J Pediatr 1981;99:425–8.
9. Dror Y, Squire J, Durie P, et al. Malignant myeloid transformation with isochromosome 7q in Shwachman-Diamond syndrome. Leukemia 1998;12:1591–5.
10. Donadieu J, Leblanc T, Bader MB, et al. Analysis of risk factors for myelodysplasias, leukemias and death from infection among patients with congenital neutropenia. Experience of the French Severe Chronic Neutropenia Study Group. Haematologica 2005;90:45–53.
11. Dror Y. Shwachman-Diamond syndrome. Pediatr Blood Cancer 2005;45:892–901 [review].
12. Dror Y, Durie P, Ginzberg H, et al. Clonal evolution in marrows of patients with Shwachman-Diamond syndrome: a prospective 5-year follow-up study. Exp Hematol 2002;30:659–69.
13. Maserati E, Minelli A, Pressato B, et al. Shwachman syndrome as mutator phenotype responsible for myeloid dysplasia/neoplasia through karyotype instability and chromosomes 7 and 20 anomalies. Genes Chromosomes Cancer 2006;45:375–82.
14. Dror Y, Freedman MH. Shwachman-Diamond syndrome marrow cells show abnormally increased apoptosis mediated through the Fas pathway. Blood 2001;97:3011–6.
15. Austin KM, Gupta ML, Coats SA, et al. Mitotic spindle destabilization and genomic instability in Shwachman-Diamond syndrome. J Clin Invest 2008;118:1511–8.
16. Grinspan ZM, Pikora CA. Infections in patients with Shwachman-Diamond syndrome. Pediatr Infect Dis J 2005;24:179–81 [review].

17. Aggett PJ, Harries JT, Harvey BA, et al. An inherited defect of neutrophil mobility in Shwachman syndrome. J Pediatr 1979;94:391–4.
18. Dror Y, Ginzberg H, Dalal I, et al. Immune function in patients with Shwachman-Diamond syndrome. Br J Haematol 2001;114:712–7.
19. Stepanovic V, Wessels D, Goldman FD, et al. The chemotaxis defect of Shwachman-Diamond syndrome leukocytes. Cell Motil Cytoskeleton 2004;57:158–74.
20. Rothbaum RJ, Williams DA, Daugherty CC. Unusual surface distribution of concanavalin A reflects a cytoskeletal defect in neutrophils in Shwachman's syndrome. Lancet 1982;2:800–1.
21. Kornfeld SJ, Kratz J, Diamond F, et al. Shwachman-Diamond syndrome associated with hypogammaglobulinemia and growth hormone deficiency. J Allergy Clin Immunol 1995;96:247–50.
22. Ip WF, Dupuis A, Ellis L, et al. Serum pancreatic enzymes define the pancreatic phenotype in patients with Shwachman-Diamond syndrome. J Pediatr 2002;141: 259–65.
23. Toiviainen-Salo S, Raade M, Durie PR, et al. Magnetic resonance imaging findings of the pancreas in patients with Shwachman-Diamond syndrome and mutations in the SBDS gene. J Pediatr 2008;152:434–6.
24. Maki M, Sorto A, Hallstrom O, et al. Hepatic dysfunction and dysgammaglobulinaemia in Shwachman-Diamond syndrome. Arch Dis Child 1978;53:693–4.
25. Ginzberg H, Shin J, Ellis L, et al. Shwachman syndrome: phenotypic manifestations of sibling sets and isolated cases in a large patient cohort are similar. J Pediatr 1999;135:81–8.
26. Bodian M, Sheldon W, Lightwood R. Congenital hypoplasia of the exocrine pancreas. Acta Paediatr 1964;53:282–93.
27. Brueton MJ, Mavromichalis J, Goodchild MC, et al. Hepatic dysfunction in association with pancreatic insufficiency and cyclical neutropenia. Shwachman-Diamond syndrome. Arch Dis Child 1977;52:76–8.
28. Bunin N, Leahey A, Dunn S. Related donor liver transplant for veno-occlusive disease following T-depleted unrelated donor bone marrow transplantation. Transplantation 1996;61:664–6.
29. Danks DM, Haslam R, Mayne V, et al. Metaphyseal chondrodysplasia, neutropenia, and pancreatic insufficiency presenting with respiratory distress in the neonatal period. Arch Dis Child 1976;51:697–702.
30. Makitie O, Ellis L, Durie PR, et al. Skeletal phenotype in patients with Shwachman-Diamond syndrome and mutations in SBDS. Clin Genet 2004;65:101–12.
31. Toiviainen-Salo S, Mayranpaa MK, Durie PR, et al. Shwachman-Diamond syndrome is associated with low-turnover osteoporosis. Bone 2007;41:965–72.
32. Savilahti E, Rapola J. Frequent myocardial lesions in Shwachman's syndrome: eight fatal cases among 16 Finnish patients. Acta Paediatr Scand 1984;73: 642–51.
33. Sacrez R, Klein F, Hoffmann B, et al. [Hypoplasia of exocrine pancreas: associated myoendocardial fibrosis in 1 of 2 brothers]. Ann Pediatr (Paris) 1969;16: 43–8 [in French].
34. Nivelon JL, Michiels R, Martres-Lassauniere MN, et al. [Myocardial fibrosis in Shwachman's syndrome: pathogenic discussion of cardiac complications]. Pediatrie 1978;33:461–9 [French].
35. Nezelof C, LeSec G. Multifocal myocardial necrosis and fibrosis in pancreatic diseases of children. Pediatrics 1979;63:361–8.
36. Graham AR, Walson PD, Paplanus SH, et al. Testicular fibrosis and cardiomegaly in Shwachman's syndrome. Arch Pathol Lab Med 1980;104:242–4.

37. Toiviainen-Salo S, Pitkanen O, Holmstrom M, et al. Myocardial function in patients with Shwachman-Diamond syndrome: aspects to consider before stem cell transplantation. Pediatr Blood Cancer 2008;51:461–7.

38. Fleitz J, Rumelhart S, Goldman F, et al. Successful allogeneic hematopoietic stem cell transplantation (HSCT) for Shwachman-Diamond syndrome. Bone Marrow Transplant 2002;29:75–9 [review].

39. Donadieu J, Michel G, Merlin E, et al. Hematopoietic stem cell transplantation for Shwachman-Diamond syndrome: experience of the French neutropenia registry. Bone Marrow Transplant 2005;36:787–92.

40. Tsai PH, Sahdev I, Herry A, et al. Fatal cyclophosphamide-induced congestive heart failure in a 10-year-old boy with Shwachman-Diamond syndrome and severe bone marrow failure treated with allogeneic bone marrow transplantation. Am J Pediatr Hematol Oncol 1990;12:472–6 [erratum appears in Am J Pediatr Hematol Oncol 1991 Summer;13(2):248].

41. Raj AB, Bertolone SJ, Barch MJ, et al. Chromosome 20q deletion and progression to monosomy 7 in a patient with Shwachman-Diamond syndrome without MDS/AML. J Pediatr Hematol Oncol 2003;25:508–9.

42. Goobie S, Popovic M, Morrison J, et al. Shwachman-Diamond syndrome with exocrine pancreatic dysfunction and bone marrow failure maps to the centromeric region of chromosome 7. Am J Hum Genet 2001;68:1048–54.

43. Austin KM, Leary RJ, Shimamura A. The Shwachman-Diamond SBDS protein localizes to the nucleolus. Blood 2005;106:1253–8.

44. Woloszynek JR, Rothbaum RJ, Rawls AS, et al. Mutations of the SBDS gene are present in most patients with Shwachman-Diamond syndrome. Blood 2004;104: 3588–90.

45. Zhang S, Shi M, Hui CC, et al. Loss of the mouse ortholog of the Shwachman-Diamond syndrome gene (Sbds) results in early embryonic lethality. Mol Cell Biol 2006;26:6656–63.

46. Dror Y, Freedman MH. Shwachman-Diamond syndrome: an inherited preleukemic bone marrow failure disorder with aberrant hematopoietic progenitors and faulty marrow microenvironment. Blood 1999;94:3048–54.

47. Elghetany MT, Alter BP. p53 protein overexpression in bone marrow biopsies of patients with Shwachman-Diamond syndrome has a prevalence similar to that of patients with refractory anemia. Arch Pathol Lab Med 2002;126:452–5.

48. Rawls AS, Gregory AD, Woloszynek JR, et al. Lentiviral-mediated RNAi inhibition of Sbds in murine hematopoietic progenitors impairs their hematopoietic potential. Blood 2007;110:2414–22.

49. Venkatasubramani N, Mayer AN. A zebrafish model for the Shwachman-Diamond syndrome (SDS). Pediatr Res 2008;63:348–52.

50. Shammas C, Menne TF, Hilcenko C, et al. Structural and mutational analysis of the SBDS protein family: insight into the leukemia-associated Shwachman-Diamond Syndrome. J Biol Chem 2005;280:19221–9.

51. Savchenko A, Krogan N, Cort JR, et al. The Shwachman-Bodian-Diamond syndrome protein family is involved in RNA metabolism. J Biol Chem 2005;280:19213–20.

52. Ganapathi KA, Austin KM, Lee CS, et al. The human Shwachman-Diamond syndrome protein, SBDS, associates with ribosomal RNA. Blood 2007;110: 1458–65.

53. Hesling C, Oliveira CC, Castilho BA, et al. The Shwachman-Bodian-Diamond syndrome associated protein interacts with HsNip7 and its down-regulation affects gene expression at the transcriptional and translational levels. Exp Cell Res 2007;313:4180–95.

54. Menne TF, Goyenechea B, Sanchez-Puig N, et al. The Shwachman-Bodian-Diamond syndrome protein mediates translational activation of ribosomes in yeast. Nat Genet 2007;39:486–95.
55. Basu U, Si K, Warner JR, et al. The Saccharomyces cerevisiae TIF6 gene encoding translation initiation factor 6 is required for 60S ribosomal subunit biogenesis. Mol Cell Biol 2001;21:1453–62.
56. Ceci M, Gaviraghi C, Gorrini C, et al. Release of eIF6 (p27BBP) from the 60S subunit allows 80S ribosome assembly. Nature 2003;426:579–84.
57. Senger B, Lafontaine DL, Graindorge JS, et al. The nucle(ol)ar Tif6p and Efl1p are required for a late cytoplasmic step of ribosome synthesis. Mol Cell 2001;8: 1363–73.
58. Ganem NJ, Storchova Z, Pellman D. Tetraploidy, aneuploidy and cancer. Curr Opin Genet Dev 2007;17:157–62 [Review] [52 refs].
59. Grisendi S, Bernardi R, Rossi M, et al. Role of nucleophosmin in embryonic development and tumorigenesis. Nature 2005;437:147–53.
60. Oeffinger M, Fatica A, Rout MP, et al. Yeast Rrp14p is required for ribosomal subunit synthesis and for correct positioning of the mitotic spindle during mitosis. Nucleic Acids Res 2007;35:1354–66.
61. Rothbaum R, Perrault J, Vlachos A, et al. Shwachman-Diamond syndrome: report from an international conference. J Pediatr 2002;141:266–70 (review).
62. Rosenberg PS, Alter BP, Bolyard AA, et al. The incidence of leukemia and mortality from sepsis in patients with severe congenital neutropenia receiving long-term G-CSF therapy. Blood 2006;107:4628–35.
63. Hsu JW, Vogelsang G, Jones RJ, et al. Bone marrow transplantation in Shwachman-Diamond syndrome. Bone Marrow Transplant 2002;30:255–8 (case report).
64. Vibhakar R, Radhi M, Rumelhart S, et al. Successful unrelated umbilical cord blood transplantation in children with Shwachman-Diamond syndrome. Bone Marrow Transplant 2005;36:855–61.
65. Mitsui T, Kawakami T, Sendo D, et al. Successful unrelated donor bone marrow transplantation for Shwachman-Diamond syndrome with leukemia. Int J Hematol 2004;79:189–92 (review).
66. Park SY, Chae MB, Kwack YG, et al. Allogeneic bone marrow transplantation in Shwachman-Diamond syndrome with malignant myeloid transformation: a case report. Korean J Intern Med 2002;17:204–6.
67. Faber J, Lauener R, Wick F, et al. Shwachman-Diamond syndrome: early bone marrow transplantation in a high risk patient and new clues to pathogenesis. Eur J Pediatr 1999;158:995–1000 (review).
68. Okcu F, Roberts WM, Chan KW. Bone marrow transplantation in Shwachman-Diamond syndrome: report of two cases and review of the literature. Bone Marrow Transplant 1998;21:849–51 [review].
69. Smith OP, Chan MY, Evans J, et al. Shwachman-Diamond syndrome and matched unrelated donor BMT. Bone Marrow Transplant 1995;16:717–8.
70. Barrios N, Kirkpatrick D, Regueira O, et al. Bone marrow transplant in Shwachman Diamond syndrome. Br J Haematol 1991;79:337–8.
71. Arseniev L, Diedrich H, Link H. Allogeneic bone marrow transplantation in a patient with Shwachman-Diamond syndrome. Ann Hematol 1996;72:83–4.
72. Cesaro S, Oneto R, Messina C, et al. Haematopoietic stem cell transplantation for Shwachman-Diamond disease: a study from the European Group for Blood and Marrow Transplantation. Br J Haematol 2005;131:231–6.
73. Sauer M, Zeidler C, Meissner B, et al. Substitution of cyclophosphamide and busulfan by fludarabine, treosulfan and melphalan in a preparative regimen for

children and adolescents with Shwachman-Diamond syndrome. Bone Marrow Transplant 2007;39:143–7.

74. Bhatla D, Davies SM, Shenoy S, et al. Reduced-intensity conditioning is effective and safe for transplantation of patients with Shwachman-Diamond syndrome. Bone Marrow Transplant 2008;42:159–65.

75. Yusuf U, Frangoul HA, Gooley TA, et al. Allogeneic bone marrow transplantation in children with myelodysplastic syndrome or juvenile myelomonocytic leukemia: the Seattle experience. Bone Marrow Transplant 2004;33:805–14.

76. Kuijpers TW, Alders M, Tool AT, et al. Hematologic abnormalities in Shwachman Diamond syndrome: lack of genotype-phenotype relationship. Blood 2005;106: 356–61.

Diagnosis and Management of Acquired Pure Red Cell Aplasia

Kenichi Sawada, MD, PhD[a,b,]*, Makoto Hirokawa, MD, PhD[c],
Naohito Fujishima, MD, PhD[a]

KEYWORDS

- Pure red cell aplasia • Diagnosis • Management
- Corticosteroids • Cyclosporine • Cyclophosphamide

Pure red cell aplasia (PRCA), a disorder first described in 1922 by Kaznelson, is a syndrome characterized by severe normochromic, normocytic anemia associated with reticulocytopenia and absence of erythroblasts from an otherwise normal bone marrow. PRCA may appear as a congenital disorder or occur as an acquired syndrome. The acquired form of PRCA presents either as an acute self-limited disease, predominantly seen in children, or as a chronic illness that is more frequently seen in adults. It may present as a primary hematologic disorder in the absence of any other disease, or secondary to various underlying diseases including parvovirus B19 infection, large granular lymphocyte (LGL) leukemia and other lymphoproliferative disorders, thymoma, autoimmune diseases, the use of offensive drugs, and ABO-incompatible allogeneic stem cell transplantation. Depending on the cause, the course can be acute and self-limiting or chronic with rare spontaneous remissions.[1,2] PRCA is comprised of heterogeneous disorders and the treatment should be based on the underlying pathophysiologic mechanisms. Primary or secondary PRCA not responding to treatment of the underlying diseases is treated as an immunologically mediated disease, based on a number of studies implicating a pathologic role of serum

This work was supported by a research grant from the Idiopathic Disorders of Hematopoietic Organs Research Committee of the Ministry of Health, Labor and Welfare of Japan and a fund from the "Global Center of Excellence Program" of the Ministry of Education, Science, Technology, Sports, and Culture of Japan.

[a] Division of Hematology, Department of Medicine, Akita University School of Medicine, Hondo 1-1-1, Akita 018-8543, Japan

[b] Division of Nephrology, Department of Medicine, Akita University School of Medicine, Hondo 1-1-1, Akita 018-8543, Japan

[c] Oncology Center, Akita University School of Hospital, Hondo 1-1-1, Akita 018-8543, Japan

* Corresponding author. Department of Medicine, Division of Hematology, Akita University School of Medicine, Hondo 1-1-1, Akita 018-8543, Japan.

E-mail address: ksawada@doc.med.akita-u.ac.jp (K. Sawada).

autoantibodies, natural killer (NK) cell–mediated, or T lymphocyte–mediated effects impairing various stages and mechanisms of erythropoiesis.

ETIOLOGY AND PATHOGENESIS
Parvovirus B19–Associated Pure Red Cell Aplasia

Parvovirus B19 is the smallest DNA virus containing single-stranded DNA genome, and has a limited tissue-tropism. The blood group P antigen (globoside) is used as primary receptor for virus entry and the virus replication is restricted to human erythroid progenitor cells.[3] In the absence of documented immunodeficiency, the B19 parvovirus causes erythema infectiosum in children, aplastic crisis in hemolytic disorders, and fetal death in pregnancy. In immunocompromised hosts, such as recipients of organ transplantation, patients infected with HIV, or those receiving chemotherapy, acute or chronic anemia can develop following parvovirus B19 infection because of the lack of production of specific antibodies.[4]

Pure Red Cell Aplasia Mediated by T Cells and Natural Killer Cells

The expansion of LGLs is the disorder most commonly associated with PRCA.[5–7] These LGLs may be of T-cell type or of NK-cell type. T-LGLs express CD3 and a T-cell receptor of $\alpha\beta$-type in most cases or $\gamma\delta$-type. In contrast, NK-LGLs, recently defined as chronic lymphoproliferative disorders of NK cells,[8] are CD3$^-$ and do not express a T-cell receptor at the cell surface. Triggering of cytolysis by LGLs against erythroblasts could occur (1) by the T-cell receptor that could recognize unknown ligands expressed by erythroid progenitors,[9] (2) by antibodies against red cell progenitors binding to CD16 on the LGLs (Tg cells),[10] or (3) by "lack of inhibition" by diminished HLA class I expression.[9,11] Functional inhibitory MHC class I receptors referred to as "killer cell inhibitory receptors" inhibit the lytic machinery of the killer cell when the target cell expresses the HLA class I antigen to which the particular killer cell inhibitory receptor binds. This mechanism probably induced the PRCA in the patient with the $\gamma\delta$ T-LGL proliferation.[11] The killer cell inhibitory receptors inhibited cytolysis by the LGLs of myeloid cells that express normal HLA class I levels, but not the cytolysis of red-cell progenitors that are in the process of progressively losing HLA class I.

Antibody-Dependent Pure Red Cell Aplasia

Krantz and Kao,[12] for the first time, reported that plasma from a patient with PRCA inhibited heme synthesis by the patient's own bone marrow cells in vitro. The serum of patients with antierythropoietin antibody-related PRCA also inhibited the growth of erythroid progenitor cells in vitro.[13] PRCA caused by autoantibodies against endogenous erythropoietin could occur,[12,13] but is quite rare in patients who have never been treated with recombinant human erythropoietin. Recombinant human erythropoietin–related PRCA reached peak incidence mainly in Europe in 2001 to 2002, largely related to a change of formulation and because of uncoated rubber stoppers in a particular recombinant human erythropoietin product and subcutaneous administration.[14]

Antibody-dependent PRCA can also occur in allogeneic hematopoietic stem cell transplantation. Delayed hemolysis and PRCA have been reported in patients receiving allogeneic hematopoietic stem cell grafts from ABO major mismatched donors.[15] PRCA results from the pre-existing isohemagglutinin antibodies, anti-IgA isoagglutinin in particular, reacting with incompatible blood antigens on erythroid progenitors, and times to disappearance of isoagglutinins correlates directly with times to recovery of reticulocytes. Incompatible isohemagglutinin can also be produced by long-lived plasma cells derived from the host.[15]

Pure Red Cell Aplasia Associated with Thymoma

Thymomas are epithelial tumors of the thymus, and are associated with paraneoplastic autoimmune diseases, of which myasthenia gravis is the most common. The role for thymoma in the pathogenesis of PRCA remains uncertain but it seems reasonable to assume that thymomas are less capable than normal thymic epithelial cells of suppressing the formation or activity of autoreactive T-cell clones. That such clones are established at the time of PRCA diagnosis probably accounts for the lack of efficacy of thymoma resection in most patients with thymoma-related PRCA.[16,17] Indeed, a significant fraction of patients develop PRCA after thymectomy.[17,18] There is clear evidence that thymoma-associated PRCA is mediated through autoimmune mechanisms. Immunosuppressive therapy is useful[6,19] and an oligoclonal T-cell expansion has been reported in some of the patients with thymoma-associated PRCA.[20–22]

Erythroid Hypoplasia-Aplasia Associated with Myelodysplastic Syndrome

Acquired PRCA may present as an initial manifestation of a preleukemic syndrome.[9] The exact prevalence of erythroid hypoplasia in myelodysplastic syndrome is not known. In a series of 360 cases of myelodysplastic syndrome diagnosed in a single institute, six (1.6%) were found to have myelodysplastic syndrome with erythroid hypoplasia-aplasia.[23]

Pure Red Cell Aplasia Associated with Other Causes

PRCA has been reported in association with more than 50 drugs, various hematologic malignancies, solid tumors, infections, autoimmune diseases including collagen vascular diseases, pregnancy, and severe renal failure.[2] Although the pathogenesis of PRCA in most cases is largely unknown, a careful assessment of the increase of LGLs is critical in most of cases, because chronic lymphoproliferative disorders of NK cells may occur in association with solid and hematologic tumors, vasculitis, neuropathy, and autoimmune disorders.[8,24]

DIAGNOSIS AND INITIAL EVALUATION

The bone marrow examination (a smear, biopsy, or both) is required to establish that the missing hematopoietic element is the erythron. Unfortunately, today there is no clinical or laboratory tests that can differentiate between chronic and self-limited disease. Evaluations for the possible causes of PRCA should include taking a careful history of drug use and infections; obtaining liver and renal function tests; tests for autoantibodies (eg, antinuclear and antierythropoietin antibodies);[25] additional bone marrow examination to include cytogenetic analysis; T-cell receptor analysis; peripheral-blood flow cytometry (CD2, CD3, CD4, CD5, CD8, CD16, CD56, and CD57); virologic examination including parvovirus B19 DNA; and CT or MRI examinations to rule out the presence of thymoma or other lymphoid neoplasms.

A careful assessment of the increase of LGLs is especially critical and an analysis of immunophenotype and T-cell receptor rearrangement of lymphocytes may be essential to rule out LGL leukemia. Because the diagnosis of LGL leukemia is somewhat difficult in patients without lymphocytosis, this group of patients can be misdiagnosed as idiopathic PRCA, although LGL leukemia-associated PRCA may require a different treatment for the primary disease.[26]

Most recently, the characteristics of the morphology and immunophenotypes of T-LGL leukemia and chronic lymphoproliferative disorders of NK cells are defined by the World Health Organization (**Table 1**).[8,27]

Table 1
The morphology and immunophenotypes of T large granular lymphocyte leukemia and chronic lymphoproliferative disorders of natural killer cells

	T-LGL Leukemia	CLPD-NK
Morphology	LGL with moderate to abundant cytoplasm and fine to coarse azurophilic granules	Intermediate in size with round nuclei with condensed chromatin and moderate amounts of slightly basophilic cytoplasm containing fine or coarse azurophilic granules
Immunophenotypes	Typically CD3+, CD8+, and TCRαβ+. Uncommon variants include CD4+, TCRαβ+, and TCRγδ+ cases; approximately 60% of the latter express CD8, the remainder are CD4-CD8-. Abnormally diminished CD5 or CD7 is common. CD57 and CD16 are expressed in over 80% of the cases	Surface CD3 is negative. CD16 is positive, whereas weak CD56 expression is frequent. There may be diminished or lost expression of CD2, CD7, and CD57; also seen are aberrant coexpression of CD5 and abnormal uniform expression of CD8. Expression of KIR family of NK-cell receptors is abnormal

Abbreviations: CLPD-NK, chronic lymphoproliferative disorders of NK cells; KIR, killer cell inhibitory receptor; LGL, large granular lymphocyte; NK, natural killer cells; TCR, T-cell receptor.

Data from Villamor N, Morice WG, Chan WC, et al. Chronic lymphoproliferative disorders of NK cells. In: Swerdlow S, Campo E, Harris NL, editors. WHO classification of tumors of haematopoietic and lymphoid tissues, 4th edition. Lyon (France): WHO press; 2008. p. 274–5; and Chan WC, Foucar K, Morice WG, et al. T-cell large granular lymphocyte leukaemia. In: Swerdlow S, Campo E, Harris NL, editors. WHO classification of tumors of haematopoietic and lymphoid tissues, 4th edition. Lyon (France): WHO Press; 2008. p. 272–3.

Immunosuppressive Therapy

Immunosuppressive therapy should be considered in patients with thymoma, or in patients with antierythropoietin antibodies, or if there is no sign of recovery of erythropoiesis approximately 1 month after having diagnosed as PRCA in a patient who has received definitive therapy for an associated disease. Remissions have been achieved by treatment with corticosteroids (CS), cyclophosphamide (CY), cyclosporine A (CsA), antithymocyte globulin, splenectomy, and plasmapheresis.[2] More recently, the efficacies of the anti-CD20 monoclonal antibody rituximab[28] and anti-CD52 monoclonal antibody alemtuzumab[29] to induce remissions of therapy-resistant PRCA have also been reported. Androgen therapy may also play a role in selected cases.[30] The efficacy of CS, CY, and CsA for patients with primary or secondary PRCA has been reported to be between 30% and 62%, 7% and 20%, and 65% and 87%, respectively.[1,7,16,31–33] The efficacy of a combination of CY and CS for refractory patients has been reported to be between 40% and 60%.[1,16,31] CS, CsA, and CY plus CS are almost equally effective for inducing remissions of PRCA, but there is a concern regarding the long-term efficacy and adverse events of these drugs. Because the disease is so rare no prospective studies have been conducted, so no particular immunosuppressive approach can be considered best. Because the number of patients treated with CsA has accumulated during the past two decades, a large cohort study has been recently done.[34]

Corticosteroids

CS were the first immunosuppressive drugs used in the treatment of PRCA and so far have been considered the treatment of first choice, especially in young adults.[1,2,6,31]

The details of CS therapy are described elsewhere.[1,2] Prednisone is given orally at a dose of 1 mg/kg/d until remission is induced. In approximately 40% of patients, remission usually occurs within 4 weeks, so continuation of a trial with prednisone longer than 12 weeks is not recommended.[31] Once the hematocrit reaches a level of 35%, the dose of prednisone can be tapered very slowly, and the drug can eventually be discontinued, preferably after 3 to 4 months.[1,2]

One of the important drawbacks of CS is that relapse is common: 80% of patients relapsed, as the dosage was tapered, during the 24 months after remission.[31] The principal reason for discontinuing the drug, despite subsequent recurrence of anemia, was the presence of unacceptable side effects, such as myopathy, infection, hyperglycemia, and compression fractures at the dose required to maintain remission. Treatment of relapses was successful with 10 (77%) of 13 patients entering a second or third remission; the median survival in patients with primary idiopathic PRCA was 14 years.[31]

Cyclosporin A

Raghavachar[32] reported that the overall response rate to CsA is excellent (65%) and proposed that CsA should be the first drug to be given in acquired PRCA. Comparable results of CsA treatment have been reported by other investigators, ranging from 65% to 87%.[1,7,16,33,34]

Recently, the Japan PRCA Collaborative Study Group conducted a nationwide survey in Japan between 1990 and 2006.[34] From a total of 185 patients consisting of 73 primary idiopathic and 112 secondary PRCA cases, 62 patients with primary idiopathic PRCA were evaluated, which is the largest and the longest follow-up study so far. Although a retrospective one, this study for the first time answered many of the unknown questions concerning CsA therapy. The remission induction therapies for these patients by CsA and CS produced remissions in 74% and 60% of patients, respectively. The initial dose of CsA for the responding patients was 4.8 ± 1.2 mg/kg (mean $\pm$ SD, N = 23) with a range of 2.9 to 7.6 mg/kg body weight. Salvage immunosuppressive treatment achieved remissions in 58 patients (94%). Forty-one and 15 patients were maintained on CsA $\pm$ CS (CsA-containing group) or CS alone (CS group), respectively. The median relapse-free survival in the CsA-containing group was 103 months, longer than that seen in the CS group (33 months), with statistical significance ($P<.01$). Combined CsA therapy can sustain a longer duration of initial remission than CS; however, discontinuation of maintenance therapy was strongly correlated with relapse ($P<.001$) and caused relapses with a median of 3 months with a range of 1.5 to 40 months. Tötterman and colleagues[35] also reported that PRCA patients did not remain in remission after CsA was stopped. In contrast, 88% of relapses in the CS-group occurred during maintenance prednisolone therapy.[34] Maintenance therapy with CsA decreases the relapse of anemia and the risk of transfusion-related adverse events. Because organ transplantations have shown that long-term immunosuppression is associated with posttransplant malignancies,[36] continuous and careful follow-up is required for patients receiving long-term CsA therapy.

Cytotoxic Immunosuppressive Drugs

CY has been the principal alkylating agent used as an immunosuppressive drug in PRCA. The details of CY therapy are described elsewhere.[1,2] The duration of remission induced by CY seems to be prolonged as compared with remissions induced by CS.[31,37] LGL leukemia-associated PRCA has been primarily treated with chemotherapy, such as CY with or without CS, CsA, CS, or methotrexate.[7,37–40] The combination of CY plus CS is associated with a longer duration of response than CS alone.[7,37,38] The overall response to initial CY ± CS therapy has been reported to be 66% to 100% and the median duration of response is 32 to 53 months.[37,41]

In one study, none of the patients with a response to cytotoxic agents had relapses,[7] but in the other studies, a substantial number of patients relapsed when the CY was withdrawn.[31,41] In a report of 14 patients with LGL leukemia-associated PRCA, the maintenance CY therapy was discontinued in five patients, and two patients relapsed at 21 and 39 months after the discontinuation. Three patients have still maintained remission after the discontinuation of CY, but the relapse-free survival after the discontinuation was still only 0, 6, and 11 months.[41] Considering that a relapse can occur even 39 months after the discontinuation of CY, these observation periods may be insufficient to conclude that PRCA associated with LGL leukemia can be cured by CY.

Although CY seems to be a key drug for remission induction of LGL leukemia-associated PRCA, recognition of a variety of toxicities, particularly concerns about the long-term risk of malignancy and gonadal toxicity, often lead clinicians to consider less toxic alternative medications whenever possible.[42,43] Myelodysplastic syndromes may occur in up to 8% of patients.[42] In long-term follow-up of 145 patients treated with

Table 2
Treatment of pure red cell aplasia

Agent	% Response Rate (CR + PR)[a]	Mean Time to Response	Need for Maintenance Therapy	Feasibility of Long-Term Maintenance
CS (methyl-prednisolone/ prednisone/ prednisolone)	30–62	2.5 wk[b]	Required[b] (most patients relapsed during the taper of CS)	Unacceptable for the dose to maintain remission
CsA	65–87	12 wk in patients with primary acquired PRCA[c] (65% of patients achieved remission within 2 wk)	Required in patients with primary acquired PRCA (86% relapsed after discontinuation of CsA whereas 11% relapsed during the maintenance of CsA)	May be durable but needs careful monitoring
CY	7–20 (CY + CS: 46–56)	11 wk[b]	May be required in patients with LGL leukemia associated PRCA[d]	Unacceptable

Abbreviations: CR, complete response; CS, corticosteroids; CsA, cyclosporine A; CY, cyclophosphamide; LGL, large granular lymphocyte; PR, partial response; PRCA, pure red cell aplasia.
  [a] References are indicated in the text.
  [b] Referenced by Clark et al.[31]
  [c] Referenced by Sawada et al.[34]
  [d] Referenced by Fujishoma et al.[41]

prolonged oral CY for Wegener's granulomatosis, there was a 4.8% incidence of bladder cancer.[43] Strategies that reduce the duration of CY exposure can minimize the long-term risks. The best role of CY therapy for PRCA might be to induce remissions using oral treatment lasting not longer than 6 months, with a switch to a less toxic medication, such as CsA, for maintenance,[41] although no controlled studies exist and this is purely speculative.

Biologic Treatment in Pure Red Cell Aplasia

There are a few reports regarding the efficacy of antithymocyte globulin, alemtuzumab, and rituximab for treatment of refractory PRCA.[5,28,29] Although monoclonal antibodies directed against malignant lymphocyte clones may be potentially effective for PRCA associated with lymphoproliferative diseases, long-term efficacy is unknown. Intravenous immunoglobulin contains neutralizing antibody against parvovirus B19 and has been reported to be effective for chronic B19 infection–related anemia in immunocompromised hosts.[4]

Table 3
Table caption

Agent	Relapse-Free Survival (RFS)	Median Overall Survival (OS)
CS (methyl-prednisolone/ prednisone/prednisolone)	80% of patients relapse within the 24 mo after remission during dose-reduction[b] Median RFS: 33 mo in patients with primary acquired PRCA[c] (88% of patients relapse during CS maintenance)	14-year OS in patients with primary acquired PRCA treated with CS or with various combinations except for CsA[b]
CsA	Median RFS: 103 mo in patients with primary acquired PRCA[c] (including the patients who relapsed after the discontinuation of CsA)	12-y OS in patients with primary acquired PRCA responded to CsA
CY (CY plus CS)	The duration of remission induced by CY seems to be prolonged as compared with patients induced by CS[a] Median RFS in patients with LGL-leukemia associated PRCA: 53 mo under CY maintenance therapy, whereas 123 mo under CsA maintenance therapy[d]	The estimated 10-y OS was 86% in patients with LGL leukemia-associated PRCA treated with CY or CsA[d]

The patients with primary acquired PRCA and secondary PRCA are included if not indicated.
Abbreviations: CS, corticosteroids; CsA, cyclosporine A; CY, cyclophosphamide; LGL, large granular lymphocyte; OS, overall survival; PRCA, pure red cell aplasia; RFS, relapse-free survival.
[a] References are indicated in the text.
[b] Referenced by Clark et al.[31]
[c] Referenced by Sawada et al.[34]
[d] Referenced by Fujishoma et al.[41]

PROPOSALS FOR FIRST-LINE THERAPY AND MAINTENANCE THERAPY IN PRIMARY ACQUIRED PURE RED CELL APLASIA

There are several options for inducing remission of PRCA, but many patients with acquired PRCA require immunosuppressive therapy to maintain remissions. As summarized in **Tables 2** and **3**, CS, CsA, and CY plus CS are almost equally effective for inducing remissions of PRCA, but the most important difference between these agents is the feasibility of long-term maintenance. Considering the recurrent nature of acquired PRCA, CsA is suggested as the first-line therapy for these patients. Maintenance therapy by CsA is requisite for most patients to prevent relapse. Because nephrotoxicity constitutes the major limiting side effect of CsA, carefully reducing the dosage to the minimum required for maintenance of remission is appropriate. The mean maintenance dose of CsA in Japanese patients who were continuing their first remission for more than 24 months was 2.2 ± 0.8 mg/kg/d with a range of 1.1 to 3.8 mg/kg/d, 40% of the initial dose,[34] which suggests difficulty in reducing CsA under this dosage to maintain remissions. Adequate prevention and treatment of infections secondary to immunosuppression are also requisite for successful management of these patients. Specifically, *Pneumocystis carinii* (*jiroveci*) pneumonia is a widely recognized opportunistic infection in immunocompromised patients. The success of daily and intermittent prophylactic dosing of trimethoprim-sulfamethoxazole has been recognized. Current recommendations for trimethoprim-sulfamethoxazole dosing for *P carinii* (*jiroveci*) pneumonia prophylaxis are based on either daily dosing or dosing 2 or 3 consecutive days per week.[44,45]

SUMMARY

PRCA is a syndrome characterized by a severe normocytic anemia, reticulocytopenia, and absence of erythroblasts from an otherwise normal bone marrow. It may present as a primary hematologic disorder in the absence of any other disease, or secondary to various diseases and clinical settings. Depending on the cause, the course can be acute and self-limiting or chronic with rare spontaneous remissions. Primary or secondary PRCA not responding to treatment of the underlying diseases is treated as an immunologically mediated disease. In general, remission can be easily achieved in most patients. The efficacy of CS, CY, CY plus CS, and CsA for patients with primary or secondary PRCA has been reported to be between 30% and 62%, 7% and 20%, 40% and 60%, and 65% and 87%, respectively. Of note is that many patients with acquired PRCA require immunosuppressive therapy to maintain remissions. Although relapsed patients can be retreated with the same agents, such as CS or CS plus CY, the cumulative side effects and toxicity become unacceptable. Maintenance CsA therapy could be a candidate for most patients to prevent relapse. Because nephrotoxicity constitutes the major limiting side effect of CsA, careful and progressive decrease of the dosage to the minimum required for maintenance of remission is appropriate. Adequate prevention and treatment of infections secondary to immunosuppression are also requisite for successful management of these patients.

REFERENCES

1. Dessypris EN. Pure red cell aplasia. London. Baltimore (MD): The Johns Hopkins University Press; 1988. p. 41–113.
2. Dessypris EN, Lipton JM. Red cell aplasia. In: Greer JP, Foerster J, Lukens JN, et al, editors. Wintrobe's clinical hematology. 11th edition. Philadelphia: Lippincott Williams & Wilkins; 2004. p. 1421–7.

3. Brown KE, Anderson SM, Young NS. Erythrocyte P antigen: cellular receptor for parvovirus B19. Science 1993;262(5130):114–7.
4. Ramratnam B, Gollerkeri A, Schiffman FJ, et al. Management of persistent B19 parvovirus infection in AIDS. Br J Haematol 1995;91(1):90–2.
5. Abkowitz JL, Powell JS, Nakamura JM, et al. Pure red cell aplasia: response to therapy with anti-thymocyte globulin. Am J Hematol 1986; 23(4):363–71.
6. Charles RJ, Sabo KM, Kidd PG, et al. The pathophysiology of pure red cell aplasia: implications for therapy. Blood 1996;87(11):4831–8.
7. Lacy MQ, Kurtin PJ, Tefferi A. Pure red cell aplasia: association with large granular lymphocyte leukemia and the prognostic value of cytogenetic abnormalities. Blood 1996;87(7):3000–6.
8. Villamor N, Morice WG, Chan WC, et al. Chronic lymphoproliferative disorders of NK cells. In: Swerdlow S, Campo E, Harris NL, editors. WHO classification of tumors of haematopoietic and lymphoid tissues. 4th edition. Lyon (France): WHO press; 2008. p. 274–5.
9. Fisch P, Handgretinger R, Schaefer HE. Pure red cell aplasia. Br J Haematol 2000;111(4):1010–22.
10. Mangan KF, Chikkappa G, Farley PC. Tg (T gamma) cells suppress growth of erythroid colony-forming units in vitro in the pure red cell aplasia of B-cell chronic lymphocytic leukemia. J Clin Invest 1982;70(6):1148–56.
11. Handgretinger R, Geiselhart A, Moris A, et al. Pure red-cell aplasia associated with clonal expansion of granular lymphocytes expressing killer-cell inhibitory receptors. N Engl J Med 1999;340(4):278–84.
12. Krantz SB, Kao V. Studies on red cell aplasia. I. Demonstration of a plasma inhibitor to heme synthesis and an antibody to erythroblast nuclei. Proc Natl Acad Sci U S A 1967;58(2):493–500.
13. Casadevall N, Nataf J, Viron B, et al. Pure red-cell aplasia and antierythropoietin antibodies in patients treated with recombinant erythropoietin. N Engl J Med 2002;346(7):469–75.
14. Bennett CL, Luminari S, Nissenson AR, et al. Pure red-cell aplasia and epoetin therapy. N Engl J Med 2004;351(14):1403–8.
15. Bolan CD, Leitman SF, Griffith LM, et al. Delayed donor red cell chimerism and pure red cell aplasia following major ABO-incompatible nonmyeloablative hematopoietic stem cell transplantation. Blood 2001;98(6):1687–94.
16. Mamiya S, Itoh T, Miura AB. Acquired pure red cell aplasia in Japan. Eur J Haematol 1997;59(4):199–205.
17. Thompson CA, Steensma DP. Pure red cell aplasia associated with thymoma: clinical insights from a 50-year single-institution experience. Br J Haematol 2006;135(3):405–7.
18. Hirokawa M, Sawada K, Fujishima N, et al. Long-term response and outcome following immunosuppressive therapy in thymoma-associated pure red cell aplasia. Haematologica 2008;93(1):27–33.
19. Garcia Vela JA, Monteserin MC, Oña F, et al. Cyclosporine A used as a single drug in the treatment of pure red cell aplasia associated with thymoma. Am J Hematol 1993;42(2):238–9.
20. Mangan KF, Volkin R, Winkelstein A. Autoreactive erythroid progenitor-T suppressor cells in the pure red cell aplasia associated with thymoma and panhypogammaglobulinemia. Am J Hematol 1986;23(2):167–73.
21. Masuda M, Arai Y, Okamura T, et al. Pure red cell aplasia with thymoma: evidence of T-cell clonal disorder. Am J Hematol 1997;54(4):324–8.

22. Fujishima N, Hirokawa M, Fujishima M, et al. Oligoclonal T cell expansion in blood but not in the thymus from a patient with thymoma-associated pure red cell aplasia. Haematologica 2006;91(Suppl 12):e128–31.

23. Williamson PJ, Oscier DG, Bell AJ, et al. Red cell aplasia in myelodysplastic syndrome. J Clin Pathol 1991;44(5):431–2.

24. Oshimi K, Yamada O, Kaneko T, et al. Laboratory findings and clinical courses of 33 patients with granular lymphocyte-proliferative disorders. Leukemia 1993;7(6): 782–8.

25. Hara A, Wada T, Kitajima S, et al. Combined pure red cell aplasia and autoimmune hemolytic anemia in systemic lupus erythematosus with anti-erythropoietin autoantibodies. Am J Hematol 2008;83(9):750–2.

26. Lai DW, Loughran TP Jr, Maciejewski JP, et al. Acquired amegakaryocytic thrombocytopenia and pure red cell aplasia associated with an occult large granular lymphocyte leukemia. Leuk Res 2008;32(5):823–7.

27. Chan WC, Foucar K, Morice WG, et al. T-cell large granular lymphocyte leukaemia. In: Swerdlow S, Campo E, Harris NL, editors. WHO classification of tumors of haematopoietic and lymphoid tissues. 4th edition. Lyon (France): WHO Press; 2008. p. 272–3.

28. Ghazal H. Successful treatment of pure red cell aplasia with rituximab in patients with chronic lymphocytic leukemia. Blood 2002;99(3):1092–4.

29. Willis F, Marsh JCW, Bevan DH, et al. The effect of treatment with Campath-1H in patients with autoimmune cytopenias. Br J Haematol 2001;114(4):891–8.

30. Sánchez de la Nieta MD, Caparrós G, Rivera F. Epoetin-induced pure red cell aplasia successfully treated with androgens. J Nephrol 2006;19(2):220–1.

31. Clark AD, Dessypris E, Krantz SB. Studies on pure red cell aplasia. XI. Results of immunosuppressive treatment of 37 patients. Blood 1984;63(2):277–86.

32. Raghavachar A. Pure red cell aplasia: review of treatment and proposal for a treatment strategy. Blut 1990;61(2–3):47–51.

33. Marmont AM. Therapy of pure red cell aplasia. Semin Hematol 1991;28(4): 285–97.

34. Sawada K, Hirokawa M, Fujishima N, et al. Long-term outcome of patients with acquired primary idiopathic pure red cell aplasia receiving cyclosporine A: a nationwide cohort study in Japan for the PRCA Collaborative Study Group. Haematologica 2007;92(8):1021–8.

35. Tötterman TH, Höglund M, Bengtsson M, et al. Treatment of pure red-cell aplasia and aplastic anaemia with ciclosporin: long-term clinical effects. Eur J Haematol 1989;42(2):126–33.

36. Cattran DC, Greenwood C, Ritchie S, et al. A controlled trial of cyclosporine in patients with progressive membranous nephropathy. Canadian Glomerulonephritis Study Group. Kidney Int 1995;47(4):1130–5.

37. Go RS, Li CY, Tefferi A, et al. Acquired pure red cell aplasia associated with lymphoproliferative disease of granular T lymphocytes. Blood 2001;98(2): 483–5.

38. Dhodapkar MV, Li CY, Lust JA, et al. Clinical spectrum of clonal proliferations of T-large granular lymphocytes: a T-cell clonopathy of undetermined significance? Blood 1994;84(5):1620–7.

39. Loughran TP Jr, Kidd PG, Starkebaum G. Treatment of large granular lymphocyte leukemia with oral low-dose methotrexate. Blood 1994;84(7):2164–70.

40. Osuji N, Matutes E, Tjonnfjord G, et al. T-cell large granular lymphocyte leukemia: a report on the treatment of 29 patients and a review of the literature. Cancer 2006;107(3):570–8.

41. Fujishima N, Sawada K, Hirokawa M, et al. Long-term responses and outcomes following immunosuppressive therapy in large granular lymphocyte leukemia-associated pure red cell aplasia: a Nationwide Cohort Study in Japan for the PRCA Collaborative Study Group. Haematologica 2008;93(10):1556–9.
42. Reinhold-Keller E, Beuge N, Latza U, et al. An interdisciplinary approach to the care of patients with Wegener's granulomatosis: long-term outcome in 155 patients. Arthritis Rheum 2000;43(5):1021–32.
43. Talar-Williams C, Hijazi YM, Walther MM, et al. Cyclophosphamide-induced cystitis and bladder cancer in patients with Wegener granulomatosis. Ann Intern Med 1996;124(5):477–84.
44. Lindemulder S, Albano E. Successful intermittent prophylaxis with trimethoprim/sulfamethoxazole 2 days per week for Pneumocystis carinii (jiroveci) pneumonia in pediatric oncology patients. Pediatrics 2007;120(1):e47–51.
45. Thomas CF, Limper AH. Pneumocystis pneumonia. N Engl J Med 2004;350(24):2487–98.

Diamond-Blackfan Anemia: Diagnosis, Treatment, and Molecular Pathogenesis

Jeffrey M. Lipton, MD, PhD[a,b,c,]*, Steven R. Ellis, PhD[d,e]

KEYWORDS

- Diamond-Blackfan anemia • Pure red cell aplasia
- Ribosome biogenesis
- Inherited bone marrow failure syndrome
- Cancer predisposition

Diamond-Blackfan anemia (DBA; MIM #20,590,0) is one of a rare group of genetic disorders, known as the "inherited bone marrow failure syndromes."[1] These disorders have in common proapoptotic hematopoiesis, bone marrow failure, birth defects,[2] and in most a predisposition to cancer.[3] Interest in these disorders has grown dramatically as the study of each has clarified, or revealed for the first time, new molecular events in development or cellular function. Significant expectations await the complete elucidation of these events. In particular, DBA has revealed itself as a "ribosomapathy" (reviewed in[4]).

DBA was first reported by Josephs[5] in 1936 and more completely described by Diamond and Blackfan[6] in 1938. The diagnostic criteria for DBA published in 1976 consist of presentation of anemia before the first birthday with near normal or slightly

This work was supported by grants from the Daniella Maria Arturi Foundation, Diamond Blackfan Anemia Foundation, Pediatric Cancer Foundation, National Institutes of Health R01 HL 079571 and R01HL 079583, and the Feinstein Institute for Medical Research at the NSLIJ General Clinical Research Center M01 RR018535.

[a] Elmezzi Graduate School of Molecular Medicine, The Feinstein Institute for Medical Research, Manhasset, NY, USA
[b] Department of Pediatrics, Albert Einstein College of Medicine, Bronx, NY, USA
[c] Hematology-Oncology and Stem Cell Transplantation, Schneider Children's Hospital, 269-01 76th Avenue, New Hyde Park, NY 11040, USA
[d] Department of Biochemistry, University of Louisville, Health Sciences Research Tower, Louisville, KY 40202, USA
[e] Department of Molecular Biology, University of Louisville, Health Sciences Research Tower, Louisville, KY 40202, USA
* Corresponding author.
E-mail address: jlipton@lij.edu (J.M. Lipton).

Hematol Oncol Clin N Am 23 (2009) 261–282
doi:10.1016/j.hoc.2009.01.004
0889-8588/09/$ – see front matter © 2009 Elsevier Inc. All rights reserved.

decreased neutrophil counts, variable platelet counts, reticulocytopenia, macrocytosis, and normal marrow cellularity with a paucity of red cell precursors.[7] These criteria have, until recently, remained the accepted standard.

In addition to macrocytosis, the presence of elevated fetal hemoglobin levels and an elevation in erythrocyte adenosine deaminase enzyme activity are important supporting features associated with DBA. The presence of macrocytosis and elevated fetal hemoglobin levels, each believed to be a consequence of "stress erythropoiesis" and skipped erythroid cell divisions, is not unique to DBA but is observed in most incidences of bone marrow failure. These features are also found in recovery from anemia, such as that caused by iron deficiency when erythropoietin levels are elevated. An explanation for the elevated erythrocyte adenosine deaminase enzyme activity in DBA has remained frustratingly obscure for over 25 years since the original observation.[8]

The careful analysis of DBA-affected pedigrees for the presence of members with macrocytosis, elevated fetal hemoglobin levels, or increased erythrocyte adenosine deaminase enzyme activity (elevated in 85% of patients with DBA) and congenital anomalies strongly suggested a greater number of autosomal-dominant cases than previously thought.[9] With the discovery of the first gene mutated in DBA,[10,11] it became evident that the penetrance of autosomal-dominant DBA is quite variable with regard to both hematologic and nonhematologic manifestations. Indeed, as a consequence of mutational analysis in family members of probands the estimated incidence of familial, autosomal-dominant DBA has increased from approximately 10% to 15% to 45%.[12] Although the diagnostic criteria for classical DBA remain unchanged, there are numerous patients not meeting these criteria for whom a "nonclassical" DBA diagnosis is appropriate.[13] Consequently, a diagnosis of DBA may now be suitable, for example, in individuals with little or no anemia, macrocytosis only, a presentation in adulthood,[14] a phenotypically normal parent of an affected offspring, and individuals with congenital anomalies or short stature and minimal or no evidence of abnormal erythropoiesis.[13] Registry data must be interpreted with an understanding of the ascertainment bias introduced by this clinical heterogeneity. Nevertheless, recent advances in the understanding of DBA, in part as a result of data from international DBA registries,[9,15,16,17] are resulting in more sophisticated diagnostic criteria and improvements in clinical care.[13]

PATHOPHYSIOLOGY AND GENETICS

Diamond-Blackfan anemia is a disorder of ribosome biogenesis and the only known disorder characterized by mutations in structural ribosomal proteins. Evidence supporting DBA as an intrinsic disorder of erythropoiesis rather than the result of immune-mediated red cell failure first appeared in 1976 when the group from Toronto[18] suggested that some patients with DBA had decreased numbers of erythroid colony-forming units. Investigators in Boston[19] extended this observation and suggested a block in erythroid maturation before the less mature erythroid burst forming unit stage. These findings may not, however, be true in all instances because later studies showed that both erythroid burst-forming units and erythroid colony-forming units colonies are present, often in normal numbers, in the marrow of young DBA patients but their differentiation to mature erythrocytes is defective, further supporting DBA to be the result of an intrinsic progenitor defect.[20] Interestingly, Chan and colleagues[21] demonstrated that the growth in vitro of DBA progenitor cells in semisolid media could be enhanced by the addition of corticosteroids similar to the in vivo response.[19]

Studies exploring the pathophysiology of DBA had, until recently, been hampered by the fact that there were no available animal models for this disease. *RPS19* was the first DBA gene identified, and mutations in this gene account for approximately 25% of DBA cases. The initial *RPS19* knockout mouse was homozygous lethal and the hemizygote lacked a DBA phenotype.[22] Moreover, no naturally occurring animal models of DBA were known to exist because the anemic and macrocytic W/W[v] and Sl/Sl[d] mice did not respond to steroids and had mutations in genes for c-kit and kit ligand (now known not to be involved in the molecular pathology of DBA), respectively.[23] In the past year, however, two groups have been able to knockdown *rps19* in zebrafish using antisense morpholino oligonucleotides, each recapitulating the hematologic phenotype and producing malformations.[24,25] Uechi and colleagues[25] extended this observation to other ribosomal proteins demonstrating defective erythropoiesis in 3 of 20 knockdowns, one being *rpl35a*, recently described to be mutated in humans with DBA.[26] Also within the past year, McGowan and colleagues[27] identified *rps19* and *rps20* as genes mutated in mice with a dark skin phenotype. Further studies revealed that the *rps19*[Dsk3] mouse recapitulated the human DBA phenotype insofar as a hypoproliferative, proapoptotic anemia with growth retardation. Based on available data it is now widely accepted that DBA results from an intrinsic cellular defect in which erythroid progenitors and precursors are highly sensitive to death by apoptosis.[20,28,29,30] The observation that phenotypes observed in zebrafish and mouse models of DBA can be partially or fully rescued by mutations in p53 strongly suggests that p53 stabilization and activation plays an important role in the proapoptotic phenotype of cells with ribosomal protein haploinsufficiency.

Considerable attention, facilitated by new zebrafish and mouse models of DBA, has been directed toward this "ribosomal stress hypothesis" reviewed recently by Dianzani and Loreni[4] in which decreased ribosome protein synthesis activates p53, inducing downstream events resulting in cell cycle arrest or apoptosis. This in turn results in the DBA phenotype of anemia, poor growth, and congenital malformations. Furthermore, the relationship of the nucleolus and defective ribosome synthesis to p53-mediated apoptosis suggests a role for interdicting mutations in p53 and distal pathways in oncogenesis in DBA.[31]

In addition to *RPS19*, five other ribosomal protein genes have been shown to be mutated in patients with DBA.[26,32,33,34] Mutations in these genes account for approximately 50% of DBA cases. Work being done by investigators in collaboration with the NHLBI Resequencing and Genotyping Service (http://rsng.nhlbi.nih.gov/scripts/about.cfm) to sequence each of the 80 ribosomal protein genes in patients from the North American DBA registry will no doubt identify additional DBA genes. The genes identified to date encode proteins of both the 40S ribosomal subunit (RPS17, RPS19, and RPS24) and the 60S subunit (RPL5, RPL11, and RPL35A). Many of these proteins have been shown to be required for the maturation of their respective ribosomal subunits in both yeast and mammalian cells.[26,34,35,36,37]

There are several potential mechanisms whereby abortive ribosome assembly or nucleolar stress could signal to p53 activation. One of the more intriguing of these mechanisms from the perspective of DBA pathophysiology involves the interaction of certain ribosomal proteins with MDM2 (Murine Double Minute), a potent regulator of p53 levels and activity. MDM2 is a RING finger ubiquitin ligase that interacts with and promotes the degradation of p53. Three proteins of the 60S subunit (RPL5, RPL11, and RPL23) have been shown to bind to MDM2 reducing its ubiquitin ligase activity, which in turn results in p53 stabilization.[38,39,40,41,42] The interaction of these proteins with MDM2 has been studied most frequently in the context of drugs that either inhibit RNA polymerase I transcription or have a general effect on the assembly of both 40S and 60S ribosomal subunits. Under these treatments, ribosome assembly is inhibited at very early stages of a complex hierarchical process whereby proteins that bind directly to rRNA facilitate the subsequent binding of other ribosomal proteins, a process facilitated in eukaryotic cells by a host of accessory factors.[43,44] Disruption of ribosome assembly early in the process results in the diversion of ribosomal proteins from ribosomal subunits to other fates within cells. In many cases it is thought that free ribosomal proteins are rapidly degraded to avoid the presumed toxicity associated with the release of small highly basic proteins into the cell.[45] In recent years, however, it has become clear that ribosomal proteins diverted from their normal fates as components of the ribosome can be important signaling molecules as seen in these studies linking abortive ribosome assembly to p53 activation and stabilization.

There are a number of caveats associated with trying to apply the pathway outlined previously linking abortive ribosome assembly to p53 activation to the context of the ribosomal protein haploinsufficiency in DBA. In contrast to the studies using drugs that inhibit the assembly of both ribosomal subunits, a ribosomal protein deficiency primarily affects only its corresponding ribosomal subunit.[26,36] Although there are good candidates for ribosomal protein signaling molecules derived from the 60S subunit, only one protein of the 40S subunit (RPS7) has been shown to interact with MDM2 and this interaction is much weaker than that observed for the large ribosomal subunit proteins mentioned.[46] Also, curiously, two recently identified "DBA genes" encode the signaling ribosomal proteins RPL5 and RPL11.[34] What makes this observation puzzling is that RPL5 and RPL11 have been shown to bind synergistically to MDM2, perhaps as a complex with 5S rRNA,[47] and so each protein must be present for maximal signaling through MDM2 (**Fig. 1**). The finding of *RPL5* and *RPL11* as DBA genes may suggest that this signaling pathway may not need to operate at maximal efficiency to elicit the proapoptotic phenotype associated with ribosomal protein haploinsufficiency. Finally, this pathway does not provide a ready rationale for the acute sensitivity of the erythroid lineage to the effects of ribosomal protein haploinsufficiency. One could, however, argue that abortive assembly in the context of the large demands for ribosome synthesis during erythroid development could unleash a relatively high concentration of wayward ribosomal proteins to trigger this and other signaling pathways leading to growth arrest or apoptosis.

As noted, there are other pathways by which nucleolar stress may signal to p53 activation and play a role in DBA pathophysiology. In this context, the tumor suppressor protein ARF is also known to interact with MDM2 to promote p53 stabilization.[48] ARF is also known to bind nucleophosmin (B23), a protein involved in ribosome biogenesis and export.[49] The relative stoichiometry of ARF and its binding partners MDM2 and B23 is thought to play a critical role in linking cell cycle regulation with ribosome synthesis.[50] The extent to which this pathway cooperates with the pathway involving liberated ribosomal proteins in nucleolar stress signaling has not been determined. It is possible that the contribution of each pathway to p53 stabilization and activation may vary depending on the nature of the nucleolar stress.

A CLINICALLY HETEROGENEOUS SYNDROME: PERHAPS DIAMOND-BLACKFAN "ANEMIA" IS A MISAPPELLATION AND IT SHOULD BE DESIGNATED AS DIAMOND-BLACKFAN SYNDROME

Congenital Anomalies

Birth defects have long been known to be a feature of DBA. A distinct facial appearance and triphalangeal thumbs have been classically described in DBA as the Cathie facies[51] and Aase syndrome,[52] respectively. A cute snub nose and wide-spaced eyes as originally described by Cathie and other craniofacial anomalies, some quite severe,

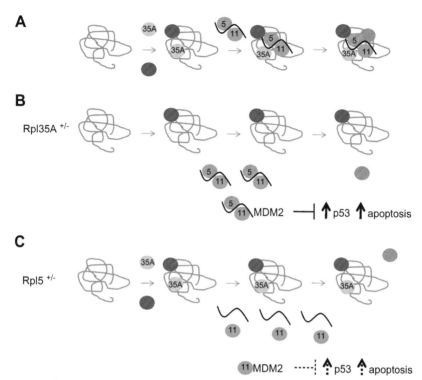

Fig. 1. Hypothetic model for abortive ribosome assembly and p53 activation relevant to DBA. (*A*) 60S subunit assembly in healthy individuals. (*B*) DBA patients haploinsufficient for RPL35A. (*C*) DBA patients haploinsufficient for RPL5. Ribosomal RNAs are shown with twisted lines and ribosomal proteins are shown with circles. Relevant ribosomal proteins are indicted with their numerical designation in the center. The effects of ribosomal proteins on the level or activity of MDM2 and p53 are shown below the assembly pathways. The solid bars indicate that the 5S rRNA-Rpl5-Rpl11 ternary complex may bind more strongly to MDM2, and have a more substantial effect on p53 stabilization that Rpl11 alone (*dashed bars*).

are the most common physical anomalies described in DBA. Abnormal thumbs are classic.[53] In all, congenital anomalies were found in 30% to 47% of the patients in the Italian,[16] French,[15] United Kingdom,[12] and North American registries.[54] Additional anomalies of the upper limb and hand, genitourinary system, and heart each are described in as many as 30% to 40% of these patients.[54] The prevalence of genitourinary and cardiac anomalies may be underestimated when abdominal-pelvic and cardiac ultrasonography is not routinely performed in asymptomatic patients. More than one anomaly is described in about a quarter of all patients. Short stature is clearly constitutional, a function of the ribosomapathy, in many patients. An accurate assessment of the etiology of linear growth retardation is complicated, however, in patients who may be anemic, iron-overloaded, or taking corticosteroids, all from a very young age. A representative table of malformations has been published.[15]

A disorder of craniofacial morphogenesis linked to diminished ribosome biogenesis, Treacher Collins syndrome (TCS; MIM #154,500) provides additional evidence linking DBA to defective ribosome synthesis. TCS is characterized in classical cases by "bilateral downslanting palpebral fissures, frequently accompanied by colobomas of the lower eyelids and a paucity of eyelashes medial to the defect, abnormalities of the external ears, atresia of the external auditory canal and bilateral conductive hearing loss, hypoplasia of the zygomatic complex and mandible and cleft palate."[55] As in DBA the disorder is inherited as an autosomal-dominant trait. The incidence is of the same order of magnitude at about 1 in 50,000 live births for TCS[56] and 1 in 100,000 for DBA.[15] Case ascertainment of mild phenotypes in both disorders is clearly a cause for underreporting. Additional similarities between TCS and DBA exist. Orofacial clefts have been reported in 3% of cases of DBA in the literature[57] and in 5.7% of cases from the Diamond Blackfan Anemia Registry.[9] Gripp and colleagues[2] identified first cousins, male children of sisters, with bilateral microtia and cleft palate consistent with TCS, but with hematologic abnormalities consistent with DBA. The proband had been previously enrolled in the Diamond Blackfan Anemia Registry of North America (DBAR), a database of now over 500 patients,[9,54] whereas his cousin with similar facial anomalies had not developed classic DBA at the time of the report. The cousin's relevant hematologic parameters were significant for macrocytosis, elevated fetal hemoglobin level, and increased erythrocyte adenosine deaminase enzyme activity, and consistent with a nonclassical hematologic DBA phenotype. Physical and hematologic evaluations of the patients' mothers were normal. Both mothers seem to be obligate heterozygotes for this dominantly inherited disorder, with neither demonstrating any hematologic evidence of DBA or even minimal congenital anomalies. This multiplex family demonstrates the extremely variable penetrance and expressivity of this DBA gene. In all, the described proband and 2 other of the 21 patients with DBA and a cleft palate reported to the DBAR were originally diagnosed with "classical" TCS. None of these three had mutations in TCOF1 (5q32-q33.1); however, the gene mutated in 90% of patients with TCS.[58] Indeed, in the absence of hematologic manifestations a number of the DBA patients would likely be considered as nonclassical TCS. A distinct minority of DBA patients are phenocopies of TCS (**Fig. 2**). All the patients met the criteria for a diagnosis of DBA (either classical or nonclassical); however, none of those with craniofacial anomalies had RPS19 mutations (DBAR, unpublished data). In addition to these observations from the DBAR, no other investigators[12,59] have identified patients with cleft palate or microtia and an RPS19 mutation.[12,59] Intriguingly, a possible genotype-phenotype correlation has recently been identified when a "TCS-like" phenotype in DBA, not associated with mutations in RPS19 or TCOF1, was identified in four of seven patients mutated at RPL5.[34] The discovery of the remaining DBA genes will enable further genotyping of this important subset of patients. Other patients with DBA and craniofacial anomalies have not yet been evaluated for TCOF1 mutations, nor have extensive hematologic evaluations of patients with TCS been reported. It is probable that a substantial minority of patients with TCS have a DBA genotype.

TCOF1 encodes the nucleolar phosphoprotein treacle,[58,59,60] mutated in TCS. Analogous to RPL5 in DBA,[34] TCS results most likely from treacle haploinsufficiency.[61] Treacle has been reported to interact with upstream binding factor, a known transcription regulator of RNA polymerase I, which participates in the initiating event in ribosomal DNA (rDNA) transcription, generating the 47S pre-rRNA.[62] Treacle is also involved in other early steps in ribosome synthesis, linking rDNA transcription to pre-rRNA posttranscriptional methylation.[63] Treacle haploinsufficiency would inhibit early events in the ribosome biosynthetic pathway, having a profound effect on ribosome synthesis. Comparable with proapoptotic erythropoiesis in DBA, the mechanism for the disruption of craniofacial structures in TCS seems to be increased apoptosis in the neural crest cells of the prefusion neural folds just before fusion during embryogenesis.[64] Intriguingly, just as in animal models of DBA, the "neurocristopathy" in the mouse model of TCS can be prevented by inhibition of p53.[65]

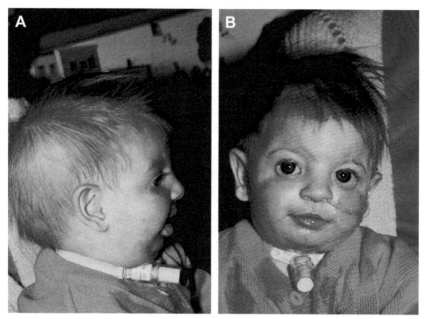

Fig. 2. (*A, B*) Patient with Diamond-Blackfan anemia originally diagnosed with Treacher Collins syndrome. Note absent lower eyelashes, down slanting palpebral fissures, deformed external ears, malar hypoplasia, and micrognathia.

The molecular underpinnings of DBA and TCS share certain common features, just as do their clinical presentations. The remarkable observation that a subset of DBA patients with orofacial abnormalities cluster together with mutations in *RPL5* demonstrates that not all ribosomal protein genes behave identically in disrupting craniofacial development. Identification of the potential ties that bind *TCOF1* with *RPL5* and other currently unknown DBA genes that disrupt orofacial development promises to be a fascinating area of investigation. These studies suggest that there may be other genotype-phenotype relationships buried within the DBA registries. Moreover, as with TCS other syndromes with congenital anomalies shared with DBA patients may be shown to have ribosome biogenesis defects as their molecular bases. A recent survey of patients who were diagnosed or had undergone repair of common DBA-associated anomalies, namely congenital heart disease (atrial septal defect, ventricular septal defect, coarctation of the aorta, and multiple defects), radial ray anomalies (bifid, subluxed, triphalangeal, or hypoplastic thumbs and flat thenar muscles), and orofacial clefts, demonstrated approximately 2% to 3% had otherwise unexplained macrocytosis (DBAR, unpublished data). Although this was not a controlled study it is probable that unrecognized cases of DBA and perhaps other inherited bone marrow failure syndromes exist undiagnosed in the general population. Furthermore, there is a reasonable possibility that other mutations in the complex process of ribosome assembly not related to either ribosomal proteins or hematopoiesis may account for a portion of these malformations.

CANCER: DIAMOND-BLACKFAN ANEMIA IS A CANCER PREDISPOSITION SYNDROME

At least 30 cases of cancer in patients with DBA have been reported in the literature. Fifteen were hematopoietic malignancies. Of these, 10 were cases of acute myeloid leukemia, 3 were Hodgkin disease, 1 was non-Hodgkin lymphoma, and 1 was acute lymphoblastic leukemia. Three additional cases of myelodysplastic syndrome were not included in this total. Fifteen solid tumors have been reported: seven osteogenic sarcoma; two breast cancer; two hepatocellular carcinoma; and one each of colon carcinoma, gastric carcinoma, vaginal melanoma, and malignant fibrous histiocytoma (updated from Alter[66] and Yaris and colleagues).[67] A number of cases have been reported from international registries and a large institutional cohort.[15,54,68] Of over 500 patients registered in the DBAR at the time of the most recent analysis, there were 12 patients who were found to have a total of 14 malignancies. Some of these patients also appear as case reports in the literature. Three patients were diagnosed with osteogenic sarcoma; one with acute myeloid leukemia; three with myelodysplastic syndrome (including myelofibrosis with myeloid metaplasia); two with colon cancer; two with breast cancer; one with a soft tissue sarcoma; and two with squamous cell carcinoma (oral and vaginal). There is an individual who is a DBA affected relative of a registered patient with melanoma, who is not yet enrolled in the DBAR. Although cancer is relatively rare in DBA as compared with Fanconi anemia, the incidence seems to be well in excess of what would be expected for the age group represented. In particular, cases of breast and colon cancer have been described in very young adults.[3,15] The prognosis for patients with DBA and cancer is poor. This is caused in part by severe chemotherapy-induced myelosuppression.[3] The presence of these malignancies and the young age at diagnosis of many of these cancers seems to define DBA as a cancer predisposition syndrome. Before a true cancer incidence is determined, however, data from international DBA registries need to undergo a careful analysis as has been applied to Fanconi anemia[69] and severe congenital neutropenia.[70]

A mechanism leading to acute myeloid leukemia and myelodysplastic syndrome in Fanconi anemia has been postulated[71] and has been recently confirmed in a murine model of clonal selection.[72] In this model, outlined in more detail elsewhere in this issue, the existence of proapoptotic hematopoiesis exerts a selective pressure on the myeloid compartment. This results in the emergence of clones with apoptosis-contravening mutations, resulting in leukemia. It seems reasonable to suggest that a similar mechanism could exist for DBA. Several recent studies, including work already cited, have shown that nucleolar stress can induce p53-dependent cell cycle arrest or apoptosis.[73,74] Mutations in the p53 gene and MDM2 could potentially subvert this process providing a growth advantage to clones harboring p53 mutations, which at the same time could favor malignant outgrowth. Other mechanisms also exist that could explain the increased cancer incidence in DBA patients. Because DBA patients characterized to date have one remaining active ribosomal gene, mutations that enhance ribosomal protein gene expression could potentially compensate for the inactive allele. The oncogene c-Myc is known to up-regulate many components of the translational machinery in its role in stimulating cell growth and proliferation.[75,76] Activating mutations in c-Myc could compensate for a ribosomal protein deficiency allowing for the emergence of clones with a survival advantage predisposed to malignancy. Because many signaling pathways promoting cell growth and division regulate ribosome synthesis as a downstream target, numerous other targets also exist to explain the increased cancer incidence in DBA patients.[77] Finally, heterozygous mutations in 11 different ribosomal protein genes in zebrafish have recently been found in fish with peripheral nerve sheath tumors.[78] These dominantly inherited mutations seem to result from loss of function, raising the specter that under certain circumstances ribosomal protein genes may act as tumor suppressor loci (**Fig. 3**).

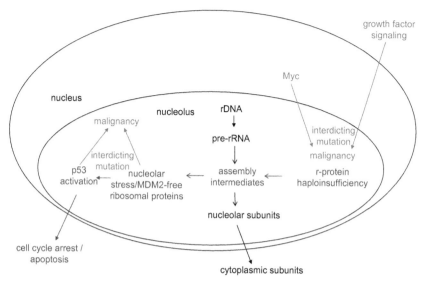

Fig. 3. Proposed mechanism for cancer predisposition in DBA. Ribosomal protein haploinsufficiency results in the accumulation of partially assembly intermediates that result in nucleolar stress signaling. Nucleolar stress, in turn, leads to p53 activation and either cell cycle arrest or apoptosis. These steps are outlined in red. Interdicting mutations that subvert the p53 pathway and favor the outgrowth of malignant clones are shown in green. Also shown in green are interdicting mutations that could enhance ribosomal protein synthesis and diminish nucleolar stress but because of the oncogenic nature of the genes involved could again favor the outgrowth of malignant clones.

RIBOSOME DYSFUNCTION AND RED BLOOD CELL DEVELOPMENT

Conventional wisdom describes selective red cell hypoplasia as the defining characteristic of DBA, which seems at odds with the fact that ribosomes are a ubiquitous feature of all cell types with the exception of mature erythrocytes. This uniquely hematologic prospective, however, disregards the existence of growth retardation and other congenital anomalies in DBA patients. Furthermore, in rare instances other significant hematologic cytopenias are also observed. How then does haploinsufficiency for RPS19, RPS24, RPS17, RPL35a, RPL5, and RPL11 manifest clinically by selectively affecting only certain tissues and most evidently red cell production? It has been argued that the high demand for ribosome synthesis associated with the proliferation and differentiation of red cell precursors may make these precursors unusually sensitive to the effects of a reduction in ribosome synthesis.[28,79,80] It is important to consider this point of view from the perspective of distinct features of red cell development between the fetus, the neonatal period, and the transition to adult erythropoiesis. Red cell production in rapidly growing fetuses in the third trimester is reported to be approximately three to five times that in the adult steady state.[81] If DBA is solely a consequence of the unusually high demands for ribosome synthesis in red cell progenitors, one would predict DBA to manifest initially during fetal development. Although there are instances of early fetal loss (perhaps attributable to erythroid failure) and hydrops fetalis in DBA, the median age at presentation of classical DBA is 8 weeks with 93% of DBA patients presenting during the first year of life.

A number of developmental and physiologic changes conspire to decrease red blood cell production shortly after birth. After birth, erythropoietin production decreases in response to high partial pressures of oxygen, a high hemoglobin level, and the switch to the lower O_2-affinity adult hemoglobin allowing more oxygen delivery to tissues.[81] Because erythropoietin provides proliferative, survival, and differentiation signals to erythroid progenitors, the fall in its production with birth contributes to a diminished erythron. There is also evidence to suggest that erythroid progenitors become less sensitive to erythropoietin in the transition from the fetal-neonatal state to the adult state.[82] Together, these changes lead to a transient physiologic anemia at 4 to 8 weeks after birth until a new steady-state of red cell production is reached. The failure to reach a new steady state results in an anemic presentation of DBA at 8 weeks, the time when new red cell production is required. It is also conceivable that the switch from primitive embryonic and fetal hematopoiesis derived from mesoderm to definitive fetal and adult erythropoiesis derived from liver and then bone marrow repopulating hematopoietic stem cells as described by Palis and Sege[81] is accompanied by more robust translation making them more vulnerable to ribosomal protein insufficiency. After birth when the demand for red cell production decreases, the demand for ribosome synthesis likely also decreases. Then, on the re-establishment of an erythroid drive and the establishment of a new steady state of ribosome synthesis and red cell production the presence of haploinsufficiency for critical ribosomal proteins becomes manifest. An important question relevant to DBA pathophysiology is, after 8 weeks of postnatal life, what effect these changes in developmental and physiologic signals have on ribosome synthesis and whether, as conditions change beyond this 8-week time point, a state is triggered where mutational inactivation of an allele of any of the implicated ribosomal protein genes limits ribosome synthesis in erythroid progenitors. Ribosome synthesis defects, in turn, could result in p53-dependent cell cycle arrest and enhanced apoptosis thereby explaining the ability of mutations in the p53 genes and compounds that inactivate p53 to rescue phenotypes in animal models of DBA.[24,27]

MAKING THE DIAGNOSIS OF DIAMOND-BLACKFAN ANEMIA

The median age at presentation and diagnosis of classical DBA are 8 weeks and 12 weeks, respectively.[54] Ninety-three percent of DBA patients present during the first year of life, but like the other inherited bone marrow failure syndromes, DBA may present in adulthood[13] when it is often misdiagnosed. The differential diagnosis of DBA in children presenting with red cell failure, anemia, reticulocytopenia, and decreased or absent marrow erythroid precursors is limited. In adults the diagnosis is less common, however, and the differential diagnosis includes a vast array of conditions, many of which rarely, if ever, are seen in children (**Box 1**). With awareness that mild DBA phenotypes may be missed in children and even more obvious cases misdiagnosed in adults, maintaining an index of suspicion is important. In the presence of a family history and in particular when a mutation is identified, the diagnosis of nonclassical DBA may be quite straightforward. Isolated macrocytosis, for example, should not be dismissed after more obvious etiologies (folate or B_{12} deficiencies) are ruled out. Of utmost importance, patients with characteristic birth defects must be carefully evaluated for DBA and other inherited bone marrow failure syndromes.

The differential diagnoses that need to be more commonly considered in children are highlighted in bold.

In children the more common disorder, transient erythroblastopenia of childhood (TEC), must be ruled out. TEC is an acquired, short-lived failure of red cell production usually of a month or so in duration. As in DBA, children with TEC often present with profound anemia. TEC, most likely a postinfectious, transient autoimmune

IgG-mediated disorder,[83] characteristically occurs in toddlers probably as the result of infections acquired through contact with playmates. As more infants are placed in day care settings, however, TEC seems to be presenting more often in children younger than 1 year of age. **Table 1** summarizes the salient features distinguishing the two disorders. Most important, a positive family history and congenital anomalies are not characteristic of TEC. Elevated fetal hemoglobin levels and macrocytosis, common presenting features in DBA, are only seen in TEC on recovery as a consequence of so-called "stress erythropoiesis." Of note, macrocytosis is often obscured in the newborn period by residual fetal erythrocytes and also can be masked by concomitant thalassemia minor or iron deficiency, and other cytopenias are found in both disorders. Although the mechanism is unknown, an elevated erythrocyte adenosine deaminase activity is found in about 85% of patients with DBA and none with TEC.[13] The two disorders can usually be distinguished. The use of limited packed red cell transfusions to achieve a hemoglobin level that does not inhibit erythroid recovery is recommended, particularly when the diagnosis is unclear. Once the diagnosis is made definitive treatment for DBA can commence.

When DBA is clinically diagnosed, or in cases where a DBA diagnosis is equivocal based on clinical presentation, mutational analysis of known genes should be performed to confirm the diagnosis. All immediate family members of the proband should be evaluated with a history and physical examination looking for evidence of a transient or mild to moderate chronic anemia and birth defects. In addition, a complete blood count with red cell indices, fetal hemoglobin levels, and erythrocyte adenosine deaminase enzyme activity should be performed in search of a mild phenotype. When the proband has a mutation in a known DBA gene, family members, even with normal evaluations, should be similarly tested. This information is of value with regard to reproductive choices and in the consideration of family members as potential hematopoietic stem cell donors. In the future the identification of a specific mutation may direct cancer-screening strategies or other clinical decisions. The deliberations of a consensus conference describing in great detail the current approach to diagnosis and treatment of DBA has recently been published.[13]

TREATMENT AND OUTCOMES
Corticosteroids and Red Cell Transfusions

Corticosteroids and red cell transfusions are the mainstays of therapy for DBA. Since 1951,[84] it has been known that the anemia of DBA can be ameliorated by corticosteroids. The response to corticosteroids perpetuated the erroneous notion of DBA as an autoimmune disease, even when only miniscule doses were required to maintain adequate erythropoiesis. Clinically, the almost unlimited use of corticosteroids, even when toxic doses were required, continued into the early twenty-first century. This seems to be caused largely by the persistent fear, in patients and physicians, of transfusion-acquired HIV and hepatitis C and the difficulty encountered in the almost daily subcutaneous administration of the iron chelator, deferoxamine.[85] Data from international registries has clarified the efficacy and toxicity of corticosteroid therapy. Data from the DBAR are representative.[54] As has been reported in the literature, 79% of patients were initially responsive to steroids, 17% were nonresponsive, and 4% of patients were never treated with steroids. Not surprising, nearly half of the patients had developed cushingoid features. With the disturbing finding that 22% and 12% of patients ever treated with steroids developed pathologic fractures and cataracts, respectively, however, the use of steroids has been modified. A snapshot of the DBAR reveals 37% of the patients receiving corticosteroids and 31% receiving red

Box 1
Classification of pure red cell aplasia

Inherited

Diamond-Blackfan anemia

Acquired pure red cell aplasia

Congenital

   Pearson syndrome

Primary

   Autoimmune (includes transient erythroblastopenia of childhood)

   Preleukemic

   Idiopathic

Secondary, associated with

   Thymoma

   Hematologic malignancies

      Chronic lymphocytic leukemia

      Large granular lymphocytic leukemia (Tγ lymphoproliferative disorder)

      Chronic myelocytic leukemia

      Acute lymphoblastic leukemia

   Hodgkin disease

   Non-Hodgkin lymphomas

   Multiple myeloma

   Waldenström macroglobulinemia

   Myelofibrosis with myeloid metaplasia

   Essential thrombocythemia

   Solid tumors

      Carcinoma of the stomach

      Adenocarcinoma of the breast

      Adenocarcinoma of bile duct

      Squamous cell carcinoma of the lung

      Epidermoid carcinoma of the skin

      Carcinoma of the thyroid

      Renal cell carcinoma

      Carcinoma of unknown primary site

      Kaposi sarcoma

   Infections

      Human B19 parvovirus

      HIV

      T-cell leukemia-lymphoma virus

      Epstein-Barr virus (infectious mononucleosis)

      Viral hepatitis

      Mumps

Cytomegalovirus

Atypical pneumonia

Meningococcemia

Staphylococcemia

Leishmaniasis

Chronic hemolytic anemias (usually associated with B19 parvovirus)

Collagen vascular diseases

Systemic lupus erythematosus

Rheumatoid arthritis

Mixed connective tissue disease

Sjögren's syndrome

Drugs and chemicals

Pregnancy

Severe renal failure

Severe nutritional deficiencies

Miscellaneous

Post-ABO incompatible bone marrow transplantation

Angioimmunoblastic lymphadenopathy

Autoimmune multiple endocrine gland insufficiency

Autoimmune hypothyroidism

Autoimmune chronic hepatitis

Anti-EPO antibodies posttreatment with EPO

Modified from Dessypris EN, Lipton JM. Red cell aplasia. In: Greer JP, Foerster J, Lukens JN, et al, editors. Wintrobe's clinical hematology. 11th edition. Philadelphia: Lippincott, Williams & Wilkins; 2003. p. 1421–37; with permission.

cell transfusions. Of the transfusion-dependent patients, 35% were never steroid responsive, 22% became steroid refractory over time, and 33% could not be weaned to an acceptable dose. Five percent never received steroid therapy and 5% are being transfused for unknown reasons.

Recently, there seems to be an increase in the number of patients judged as "unable to be weaned" and an increase in patients who never received steroids. The number of patients never on corticosteroids reflects the youngest cohort for whom corticosteroid administration is being delayed during the critical period of growth and development during the first year of life.[54] The ability to wean a patient is dependent to some extent on the side effects that the patient and the physician are willing to tolerate. Corticosteroids should commence with a corticosteroid-equivalent dose of prednisone, 2 mg/kg/d. Patients who fail to respond within a month are considered steroid refractory and must receive red cell transfusions. In general, a corticosteroid dose-equivalent of 0.5 mg/kg/d (≤ 1 mg/kg/d every other day) of prednisone is suggested as a maximum "maintenance" dose. Clearly, the recognition that the blood supply is safe combined with the recent availability of an oral iron chelator[86] seems to have permitted a more liberal use of packed red cell transfusions in patients rather than toxic doses of corticosteroids. Patients

Table 1
Differential diagnosis of Diamond-Blackfan anemia versus transient erythroblastopenia of childhood

	Diamond-Blackfan Anemia	Transient Erythroblastopenia of Childhood
Pure red cell aplasia	Present	Present
Age	Younger than 1 y	Older than 1 y
Inheritance	Sporadic and dominant inheritance. Mutation analysis as available.	Not inherited
Congenital anomalies	Present	Absent
Mean corpuscular volume	Elevated	Normal (may be elevated on recovery)
Fetal hemoglobin	Elevated	Normal (may be elevated on recovery)
Erythrocyte ADA activity	Elevated	Normal
Other cytopenias	May be present	May be present

All RBC characteristics except erythrocyte adenosine deaminase enzyme activity are helpful only when tested in a reticulocytopenic child. During recovery from transient erythroblastopenia of childhood, a transient wave of fetal-like erythropoiesis with elevated mean corpuscular volume and fetal hemoglobin may be detected.

Modified from Dessypris EN, Lipton JM. Red cell aplasia. In: Greer JP, Foerster J, Lukens JN, et al, editors. Wintrobe's clinical hematology. 11th edition. Philadelphia: Lippincott, Williams & Wilkins; 2003. p. 1421–37; with permission.

should be closely monitored for steroid toxicity and the drug discontinued rather than risk significant complications.

Although remissions had been reported in DBA, data on the fraction of patients who were able to sustain erythropoiesis for over 6 months without treatment have been sparse. The DBAR has provided some actuarial data.[54] About 20% of patients enter remission, most sustained. Of these about 75% do so before their tenth birthday. These data may reflect the bias to a younger age of patients in the DBAR, underestimating the actuarial likelihood of remission, because anecdotal observations suggest a surge in remissions in adolescent boys. Proportionally, an equal number of patients remit from both transfusion and steroid therapy. There are very few remitters, however, who had never responded to corticosteroids. Pregnancy[87] and the use of birth control pills contribute to relapse.

Stem Cell Transplantation

Although curative in DBA,[15,54,88] hematopoietic stem cell transplantation (SCT) remains the most controversial aspect of therapy. A recent series from the International Bone Marrow Transplant Registry and a compilation from the literature are consistent with findings from the DBAR.[89] At the last published evaluation 36 patients had undergone SCT; 21 HLA-matched related and 15 alternative donor SCT. The major indication for SCT was transfusion dependence. In addition, two patients had developed severe aplastic anemia and one significant thrombocytopenia. Two patients transplanted using a nonmyeloablative conditioning regimen, one receiving a matched-related umbilical cord and one receiving unrelated bone marrow, are alive and well. Most alternative donor transplants were performed using total body irradiation for conditioning, whereas busulfan-cyclophosphamide–containing regimens were typical of the matched-related transplants. Sixteen of the 21 HLA-matched sibling donor transplants are alive and red cell transfusion–independent. Of the 15 alternative donor SCTs, two patients received mismatched-related bone marrow, four patients unrelated cord blood, eight unrelated bone marrow, and one unrelated peripheral blood stem cells. Four of these 15 patients are alive. Of the 16 deaths, 15 were related to infection, graft-versus-host disease, or veno-occlusive disease of the liver with only one death, in the alternative donor group, occurring as a consequence of graft failure. In contrast to Fanconi anemia, dyskeratosis congenita, and Shwachman-Diamond syndrome, these deaths do not seem to be the consequence of intolerance to typical transplant conditioning regimens. The survival for allogeneic sibling versus alternative donor transplant is 72.7% ± 10.7% versus 19.1% ± 11.9% at greater than 5 years from SCT ($P = .01$) or 17.1% ± 10.8% (including a patient diagnosed with osteogenic sarcoma posttransplant [$P = .012$]). The survival rate for patients under the age of 10 years receiving matched-related SCT is greater than 90%. Unpublished data from the DBAR on over 50 patients continue to show a greater than 90% actuarial survival for young DBA patients transplanted using matched allogeneic related donors. This success has led to an increase in families looking to preimplantation genetic diagnosis with in vitro fertilization to "create" HLA-matched, non-*RPS19* mutated sibling donors. A number of patients worldwide have been successfully transplanted using umbilical cord–derived stem cells from donors produced in this way. A discussion of the complicated religious, ethical, and economic questions generated by this approach is beyond the scope of this article.[90,91] Unpublished data from the DBAR show the actuarial survival, since 2000, for all DBA patients transplanted using alternative donors to be approximately 80%, offering this option to carefully selected patients lacking a suitable matched-related donor.

Of the 36 deaths reported to the DBAR at the last evaluation 25 (70%) were treatment-related: 5 from infections (two *Pneumocystis jiroveci* pneumonia, one varicella pneumonia, one pseudomonas pneumonia–sepsis, one unknown infection); 5 from complications of iron overload; 1 from cardiac tamponade secondary to a vascular access device complication; and 14 from SCT complications. Only three of the deaths related to SCT were in patients with life-threatening cytopenias. Recent unpublished data show an expected increase in reported iron overload–related deaths as the DBAR population matures. This finding is of considerable concern. Just eight deaths were directly related to DBA: one from severe aplastic anemia and seven from malignancy (two of whom also received a SCT), and three deaths were from undetermined causes. Although SCT is potentially curative and reduces the risk of aplastic anemia, acute myeloid leukemia, and myelodysplastic syndrome, and the outcome for unrelated-donor SCT has improved considerably, reasonable restraint should be exercised in the use of this modality. The probability of remission must also be taken into account when high-risk SCT is being considered.

The last reported overall actuarial survival at greater than 40 years of age is 75.1% ± 4.8%; 86.7% ± 7% for corticosteroid-maintainable patients and 57.2% ± 8.9% for transfusion-dependent patients.[54] There is a statistically significant survival advantage for steroid-maintainable patients as compared with transfusion-dependent patients ($P = .007$). Seven transfusion-dependent patients died as a consequence of SCT-related complications. Clearly, the next analysis will reflect both the increase in iron overload–related and the decrease in alternative donor transplant–related deaths, respectively.

SUMMARY

The use of patient registries for rare diseases has been clearly demonstrated in DBA, and these valuable resources need to be supported. These databases have permitted the more precise description of congenital anomalies in DBA revealing the connection between DBA and TCS. Similarities between the two diseases were instrumental in recognizing DBA as a disorder of ribosome biosynthesis. Other disorders involving defects in ribosome assembly or function (cartilage hair hypoplasia, Shwachman-Diamond syndrome, and dyskeratosis congenita) have also been described (reviewed in)[79] and a new nosology of human disease is emerging. **Fig. 4** demonstrates the known defects in ribosome biosynthesis and function characterized by this new class of disorders. Motivated by newly recognized clinical relevance the study of ribosome biosynthesis and function is attracting more interested scientists.

Extensive work is ongoing in a number of laboratories using patient databases for DBA gene discovery. The complete genotyping of the patient databases should contribute to the discovery of most of the remaining DBA genes. Ultimately, the availability of a genetically based DBA diagnosis in the remaining 50% of patients not mutated at the known DBA genes will allow the diagnosis of previously undetectable mild phenotypes, facilitating reproductive choices and SCT donor selection.[92] The patient substrate provided by these registries will also allow for genotype-phenotype correlations that will shed light on scientific questions and at the same time suggest treatment and surveillance strategies. Within a few years an accurate cancer risk assessment will be available and perhaps cancer-prone genotypes will emerge. Furthermore, these registries have provided a clearer understanding of the epidemiology of DBA. Treatment options are already being modified based on new information

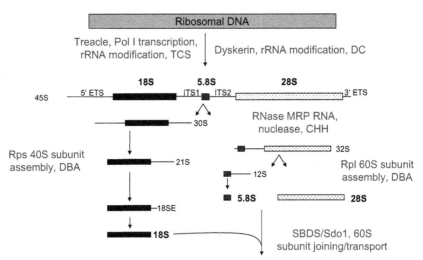

Fig. 4. Putative biochemical function for Treacle, Dyskerin, Rps19/Rps24, RMRP, and Sbds in ribosomal biogenesis. A simplified version of the human pre-rRNA processing pathway is shown. Functions are deduced from data for either yeast or human orthologs. Mature rRNA species (denoted in bold) are liberated from the 45S pre-rRNA primary transcript by a series of processing steps. 5′ and 3′ ETS represent external transcribed sequences found on the 5′ and 3′ ends of the primary transcript, respectively. ITS represents internal transcribed sequences present in the primary transcript that are not retained in mature rRNAs. The 18S rRNA is a component of the 40S ribosomal subunit. The 5.8S and 28S rRNAs, together with the 5S rRNA (not shown), are components of the 60S ribosomal subunit.

regarding the natural history of DBA. Prolonged use of corticosteroids, starting in infancy, has been curtailed as the result of this new knowledge. Packed red cell transfusions, rather than corticosteroids, are being used to avoid steroid-related growth retardation, developmental delay, pathologic fractures, cataracts, and other significant steroid-related side effects. Analyses of outcomes reveal that most patients succumb to complications that may be avoidable. The serious risk of death from transfusion-related iron overload has been clearly established. The extremely poor outcome previously reported with alternative donor hematopoietic SCT has improved dramatically. A greater than expected incidence of remission and a lower than expected incidence of aplastic anemia, myelodysplastic syndrome, and hematopoietic malignancy still support restraint in the use of alternative donor SCTs. In contrast, allogeneic matched-sibling SCT seems to have an acceptable outcome, justifying its use as frontline therapy. In such a rare disease as DBA controlled SCT clinical trials are virtually impossible to perform. Emerging therapies, such as SCT using reduced-intensity conditioning regimens in high-risk DBA patients, must be captured by the registries and provide a reasonable evaluation of the efficacy of this approach. As data mature the predisposition to nonhematopoietic malignancy in the context of SCT will also become known. The registries also provide the platform for clinical trials. The availability of tumor specimens, obtained from well-characterized patients, will allow for an investigation of the molecular biology of tumorigenesis in DBA. The recognition of nonclassical occult DBA phenotypes strongly suggests that patients with characteristic birth defects, certain cancers, or unexplained macrocytosis may have DBA. The clarification of these issues is critical with regard to patient follow-up, genetic counseling, and reproductive strategies. Preliminary work setting the stage for gene therapy trials is ongoing.[93]

The understanding of the molecular underpinnings of DBA has also pointed the way to new potential therapies. The observation that DBA is a "ribosome deficiency" disease has led Pospisilova and colleagues[94] to test the efficacy of nutritional supplementation with the amino acid leucine as a potential therapy for DBA. This approach is based on the documented role of this amino acid in up-regulating components of the protein synthetic machinery in skeletal muscle.[95] Positive results have so far been reported in a single patient.[94] A clinical trial for the efficacy of leucine supplementation in ameliorating the bone marrow failure in DBA is currently being designed in the United States. The finding that inhibitors of p53 can reverse phenotypes in mouse models of DBA and TCS also points to new treatment modalities.[24,27,65,96] Although p53 inhibitors pose an unacceptable risk for cancer in patient populations, perhaps small molecule inhibitors of the signaling pathways linking abortive ribosome assembly to p53 activation can provide clinical benefit without increasing cancer risk. Finally, the recent observation that the loss of a small subunit ribosomal protein gene, RPS14, is responsible for the refractory anemia in 5q⁻ syndrome has raised the possibility that lenalidomide may have some potential clinical benefit in DBA.[97]

The study of DBA, since its first description 70 years ago, has yielded extraordinary opportunities to understand the biology of hematopoiesis, oncogenesis, and morphogenesis. As important, significant improvements in patient care have emerged and should continue with a greater knowledge of disease mechanism.

ACKNOWLEDGMENTS

There has been considerable progress made in the understanding of DBA since the identification of the first gene mutated in this disorder in 1997. The commitment of the patients with DBA, their families, their clinicians, and the dedicated scientists, clinical- and laboratory-based, with whom we have the privilege to work is largely responsible for this progress. Improvement in the quantity and quality of life for patients with DBA is one of the great successes of twenty-first century translational medicine. The authors thank Adrianna Vlachos, MD, Johnson Liu, MD, Eva Atsidaftos, MA, and Hanna Gazda, MD, for their invaluable advice and assistance. One of us (JML) thanks David G. Nathan, MD, and Blanche Alter, MD, MPH, for their introduction to the field of bone marrow failure. A considerable debt of gratitude is owed to Marie and Manny Arturi and the Diamond Blackfan Anemia Foundation, who have supported and sustained the science and the scientists who work in this area. Indeed, the marriage of laboratory and clinical science to the management of children and adults with DBA has been brokered by and large through their efforts.

REFERENCES

1. Young NS. Inherited bone marrow failure syndromes: introduction. Philadelphia: WB Saunders Company; 1994.
2. Gripp KW, McDonald-McGinn DM, La Rossa D, et al. Bilateral microtia and cleft palate in cousins with Diamond-Blackfan anemia. Am J Med Genet 2001;101: 268–74.
3. Lipton JM, Federman N, Khabbaze Y, et al. Osteogenic sarcoma associated with Diamond-Blackfan anemia: a report from the Diamond-Blackfan Anemia Registry. J Pediatr Hematol Oncol 2001;23:39–44.
4. Dianzani I, Loreni F. Diamond-Blackfan anemia: a ribosomal puzzle. Haematologica 2008;93:1601–4.
5. Josephs H. Anemia of infancy and early childhood. Medicine 1936;15:307–451.
6. Diamond LK, Blackfan KD. Hypoplastic anemia. Am J Dis Child 1938;56:464–7.
7. Diamond LK, Wang WC, Alter BP. Congenital hypoplastic anemia. Adv Pediatr 1976;22:349–78.
8. Glader BE, Backer K, Diamond LK. Elevated erythrocyte adenosine deaminase activity in congenital hypoplastic anemia. N Engl J Med 1983;309:1486–90.
9. Vlachos A, Klein GW, Lipton JM. The Diamond Blackfan Anemia Registry: tool for investigating the epidemiology and biology of Diamond-Blackfan anemia. J Pediatr Hematol Oncol 2001;23:377–82.
10. Gustavsson P, Garelli E, Draptchinskaia N, et al. Identification of microdeletions spanning the Diamond-Blackfan anemia locus on 19q13 and evidence for genetic heterogeneity. Am J Hum Genet 1998;63:1388–95.
11. Draptchinskaia N, Gustavsson P, Andersson B, et al. The gene encoding ribosomal protein S19 is mutated in Diamond-Blackfan anaemia. Nat Genet 1999; 21:169–75.
12. Orfali KA, Ohene-Abuakwa Y, Ball SE. Diamond Blackfan anaemia in the UK: clinical and genetic heterogeneity. Br J Haematol 2004;125:243–52.
13. Vlachos A, Ball S, Dahl N, et al. Diagnosing and treating Diamond Blackfan anaemia: results of an international clinical consensus conference. Br J Haematol 2008;142:859–76.
14. Balaban EP, Buchanan GR, Graham M, et al. Diamond-Blackfan syndrome in adult patients. Am J Med 1985;78:533–8.
15. Willig TN, Niemeyer CM, Leblanc T, et al. Identification of new prognosis factors from the clinical and epidemiologic analysis of a registry of 229 Diamond-Blackfan anemia patients. DBA group of Societe d'Hematologie et d'Immunologie Pediatrique (SHIP), Gesellshaft fur Padiatrische Onkologie und Hamatologie

(GPOH), and the European Society for Pediatric Hematology and Immunology (ESPHI). Pediatr Res 1999;46:553–61.

16. Campagnoli MF, Garelli E, Quarello P, et al. Molecular basis of Diamond-Blackfan anemia: new findings from the Italian registry and a review of the literature. Haematologica 2004;89:480–9.

17. Ohga S, Mugishima H, Ohara A, et al. Diamond-Blackfan anemia in Japan: clinical outcomes of prednisolone therapy and hematopoietic stem cell transplantation. Int J Hematol 2004;79:22–30.

18. Freedman MH, Amato D, Saunders EF. Erythroid colony growth in congenital hypoplastic anemia. J Clin Invest 1976;57:673–7.

19. Nathan DG, Clarke BJ, Hillman DG, et al. Erythroid precursors in congenital hypoplastic (Diamond-Blackfan) anemia. J Clin Invest 1978;61:489–98.

20. Lipton JM, Kudisch M, Gross R, et al. Defective erythroid progenitor differentiation system in congenital hypoplastic (Diamond-Blackfan) anemia. Blood 1986; 67:962–8.

21. Chan HS, Saunders EF, Freedman MH. Diamond-Blackfan syndrome. II. In vitro corticosteroid effect on erythropoiesis. Pediatr Res 1982;16:477–8.

22. Matsson H, Davey EJ, Frojmark AS, et al. Erythropoiesis in the Rps19 disrupted mouse: analysis of erythropoietin response and biochemical markers for Diamond-Blackfan anemia. Blood Cells Mol Dis 2006;36:259–64.

23. Alter BP, Gaston T, Lipton JM. Lack of effect of corticosteroids in W/Wv and S1/S1d mice: these strains are not a model for steroid-responsive Diamond-Blackfan anemia. Eur J Haematol 1993;50:275–8.

24. Danilova N, Sakamoto KM, Lin S. Ribosomal protein S19 deficiency in zebrafish leads to developmental abnormalities and defective erythropoiesis through activation of p53 protein family. Blood 2008;112:5228–37.

25. Uechi T, Nakajima Y, Chakraborty A, et al. Deficiency of ribosomal protein S19 during early embryogenesis leads to reduction of erythrocytes in a zebrafish model of Diamond-Blackfan anemia. Hum Mol Genet 2008;17:3204–11.

26. Farrar JE, Nater M, Caywood E, et al. Abnormalities of the large ribosomal subunit protein, Rpl35a, in Diamond-Blackfan anemia. Blood 2008;112:1582–92.

27. McGowan KA, Li JZ, Park CY, et al. Ribosomal mutations cause p53-mediated dark skin and pleiotropic effects. Nat Genet 2008;40:963–70.

28. Ohene-Abuakwa Y, Orfali KA, Marius C, et al. Two-phase culture in Diamond Blackfan anemia: localization of erythroid defect. Blood 2005;105:838–46.

29. Perdahl EB, Naprstek BL, Wallace WC, et al. Erythroid failure in Diamond-Blackfan anemia is characterized by apoptosis. Blood 1994;83:645–50.

30. Tsai PH, Arkin S, Lipton JM. An intrinsic progenitor defect in Diamond-Blackfan anaemia. Br J Haematol 1989;73:112–20.

31. Ellis SR, Lipton JM. Diamond Blackfan anemia: a disorder of red blood cell development. Curr Top Dev Biol 2008;82:217–41.

32. Cmejla R, Cmejlova J, Handrkova H, et al. Ribosomal protein S17 gene (RPS17) is mutated in Diamond-Blackfan anemia. Hum Mutat 2007;28:1178–82.

33. Gazda HT, Grabowska A, Merida-Long LB, et al. Ribosomal protein S24 gene is mutated in Diamond-Blackfan anemia. Am J Hum Genet 2006;79:1110–8.

34. Gazda HT, Sheen MR, Vlachos A, et al. Ribosomal Protein L5 and L11 mutations are associated with cleft palate and abnormal thumbs in Diamond-Blackfan anemia patients. Am J Hum Genet 2008;83:769–80.

35. Idol RA, Robledo S, Du HY, et al. Cells depleted for RPS19, a protein associated with Diamond Blackfan Anemia, show defects in 18S ribosomal RNA synthesis and small ribosomal subunit production. Blood Cells Mol Dis 2007;39:35–43.

36. Flygare J, Aspesi A, Bailey JC, et al. Human RPS19, the gene mutated in Diamond-Blackfan anemia, encodes a ribosomal protein required for the maturation of 40S ribosomal subunits. Blood 2007;109:980–6.

37. Choesmel V, Bacqueville D, Rouquette J, et al. Impaired ribosome biogenesis in Diamond-Blackfan anemia. Blood 2007;109:1275–83.

38. Jin A, Itahana K, O'Keefe K, et al. Inhibition of HDM2 and activation of p53 by ribosomal protein L23. Mol Cell Biol 2004;24:7669–80.

39. Dai MS, Zeng SX, Jin Y, et al. Ribosomal protein L23 activates p53 by inhibiting MDM2 function in response to ribosomal perturbation but not to translation inhibition. Mol Cell Biol 2004;24:7654–68.

40. Marechal V, Elenbaas B, Piette J, et al. The ribosomal L5 protein is associated with mdm-2 and mdm-2-p53 complexes. Mol Cell Biol 1994;14:7414–20.

41. Lohrum MA, Ludwig RL, Kubbutat MH, et al. Regulation of HDM2 activity by the ribosomal protein L11. Cancer Cell 2003;3:577–87.

42. Zhang Y, Wolf GW, Bhat K, et al. Ribosomal protein L11 negatively regulates oncoprotein MDM2 and mediates a p53-dependent ribosomal-stress checkpoint pathway. Mol Cell Biol 2003;23:8902–12.

43. Held WA, Ballou B, Mizushima S, et al. Assembly mapping of 30 S ribosomal proteins from *Escherichia coli*: further studies. J Biol Chem 1974;249:3103–11.

44. Hage AE, Tollervey D. A surfeit of factors: why is ribosome assembly so much more complicated in eukaryotes than bacteria? RNA Biol 2004;1:10–5.

45. Lam YW, Lamond AI, Mann M, et al. Analysis of nucleolar protein dynamics reveals the nuclear degradation of ribosomal proteins. Curr Biol 2007;17:749–60.

46. Chen D, Zhang Z, Li M, et al. Ribosomal protein S7 as a novel modulator of p53-MDM2 interaction: binding to MDM2, stabilization of p53 protein, and activation of p53 function. Oncogene 2007;26:5029–37.

47. Horn HF, Vousden KH. Cooperation between the ribosomal proteins L5 and L11 in the p53 pathway. Oncogene 2008;27:5774–84.

48. Lindstrom MS, Deisenroth C, Zhang Y. Putting a finger on growth surveillance: insight into MDM2 zinc finger-ribosomal protein interactions. Cell Cycle 2007;6:434–7.

49. Maggi LB Jr, Kuchenruether M, Dadey DY, et al. Nucleophosmin serves as a rate-limiting nuclear export chaperone for the mammalian ribosome. Mol Cell Biol 2008;28:7050–65.

50. Brady SN, Yu Y, Maggi LB Jr, et al. ARF impedes NPM/B23 shuttling in an Mdm2-sensitive tumor suppressor pathway. Mol Cell Biol 2004;24:9327–38.

51. Cathie IAB. Erythrogenesis imperfecta. Arch Dis Child 1950;25:313–24.

52. Aase Jm SD. Congenital anemia and triphalangeal thumbs: a new syndrome. J Pediatr 1969;74:471–2.

53. Alter BP. Thumbs and anemia. Pediatrics 1978;62:613–4.

54. Lipton JM, Atsidaftos E, Zyskind I, et al. Improving clinical care and elucidating the pathophysiology of Diamond Blackfan anemia: an update from the Diamond Blackfan Anemia Registry. Pediatr Blood Cancer 2006;46:558–64.

55. Teber OA, Gillessen-Kaesbach G, Fischer S, et al. Genotyping in 46 patients with tentative diagnosis of Treacher Collins syndrome revealed unexpected phenotypic variation. Eur J Hum Genet 2004;12:879–90.

56. Fazen LE, Elmore J, Nadler HL. Mandibulo-facial dysostosis (Treacher-Collins syndrome). Am J Dis Child 1967;113:405–10.

57. Lipton JM. Diamond Blackfan anemia. Boca Raton (FL): CRC Press; 1993.

58. Wise CA, Chiang LC, Paznekas WA, et al. TCOF1 gene encodes a putative nucleolar phosphoprotein that exhibits mutations in Treacher Collins syndrome throughout its coding region. Proc Natl Acad Sci U S A 1997;94:3110–5.

59. So RB, Gonzales B, Henning D, et al. Another face of the Treacher Collins syndrome (TCOF1) gene: identification of additional exons. Gene 2004;328: 49–57.

60. Dixon J, Edwards SJ, Anderson I, et al. Identification of the complete coding sequence and genomic organization of the Treacher Collins syndrome gene. Genome Res 1997;7:223–34.

61. Dixon MJ. Treacher Collins syndrome. Hum Mol Genet 1996;5(Spec No):1391–6.

62. Valdez BC, Henning D, So RB, et al. The Treacher Collins syndrome (TCOF1) gene product is involved in ribosomal DNA gene transcription by interacting with upstream binding factor. Proc Natl Acad Sci U S A 2004;101:10709–14.

63. Gonzales B, Henning D, So RB, et al. The Treacher Collins syndrome (TCOF1) gene product is involved in pre-rRNA methylation. Hum Mol Genet 2005;14: 2035–43.

64. Dixon J, Brakebusch C, Fassler R, et al. Increased levels of apoptosis in the pre-fusion neural folds underlie the craniofacial disorder, Treacher Collins syndrome. Hum Mol Genet 2000;9:1473–80.

65. Jones NC, Lynn ML, Gaudenz K, et al. Prevention of the neurocristopathy Treacher Collins syndrome through inhibition of p53 function. Nat Med 2008;14:125–33.

66. Alter BP. Inherited bone marrow failure syndromes. Philadelphia: WB Saunders; 2003.

67. Yaris N, Erduran E, Cobanoglu U. Hodgkin lymphoma in a child with Diamond Blackfan anemia. J Pediatr Hematol Oncol 2006;28:234–6.

68. Janov AJ, Leong T, Nathan DG, et al. Diamond-Blackfan anemia: natural history and sequelae of treatment. Medicine (Baltimore) 1996;75:77–8.

69. Alter BP, Greene MH, Velazquez I, et al. Cancer in Fanconi anemia. Blood 2003; 101:2072.

70. Rosenberg PS, Alter BP, Link DC, et al. Neutrophil elastase mutations and risk of leukaemia in severe congenital neutropenia. Br J Haematol 2008;140:210–3.

71. Lensch MW, Rathbun RK, Olson SB, et al. Selective pressure as an essential force in molecular evolution of myeloid leukemic clones: a view from the window of Fanconi anemia. Leukemia 1999;13:1784–9.

72. Li J, Sejas DP, Zhang X, et al. TNF-alpha induces leukemic clonal evolution ex vivo in Fanconi anemia group C murine stem cells. J Clin Invest 2007;117: 3283–95.

73. Lindstrom MS, Jin A, Deisenroth C, et al. Cancer-associated mutations in the MDM2 zinc finger domain disrupt ribosomal protein interaction and attenuate MDM2-induced p53 degradation. Mol Cell Biol 2007;27:1056–68.

74. Pestov DG, Strezoska Z, Lau LF. Evidence of p53-dependent cross-talk between ribosome biogenesis and the cell cycle: effects of nucleolar protein Bop1 on G(1)/S transition. Mol Cell Biol 2001;21:4246–55.

75. Boon K, Caron HN, van Asperen R, et al. N-myc enhances the expression of a large set of genes functioning in ribosome biogenesis and protein synthesis. EMBO J 2001;20:1383–93.

76. Oskarsson T, Trumpp A. The myc trilogy: lord of RNA polymerases. Nat Cell Biol 2005;7:215–7.

77. Ruggero D, Pandolfi PP. Does the ribosome translate cancer? Nat Rev Cancer 2003;3:179–92.

78. Amsterdam A, Sadler KC, Lai K, et al. Many ribosomal protein genes are cancer genes in zebrafish. PLoS Biol 2004;2:E139.

79. Liu JM, Ellis SR. Ribosomes and marrow failure: coincidental association or molecular paradigm? Blood 2006;107:4583–8.

80. Morimoto K, Lin S, Sakamoto K. The functions of RPS19 and their relationship to Diamond-Blackfan anemia: a review. Mol Genet Metab 2007;90:358–62.
81. Palis J, Segel GB. Developmental biology of erythropoiesis. Blood Rev 1998;12: 106–14.
82. Weinberg RS, He LY, Alter BP. Erythropoiesis is distinct at each stage of ontogeny. Pediatr Res 1992;31:170–5.
83. Dessypris EN, Krantz SB, Roloff JS, et al. Mode of action of the IgG inhibitor of erythropoiesis in transient erythroblastopenia of children. Blood 1982;59:114–23.
84. Gasser C. Aplastische anämie (cronische erythroblastophthise) und cortison. Schweiz Med Wochenschr 1951;81:1241–2.
85. Olivieri NF, Brittenham GM. Iron-chelating therapy and the treatment of thalassemia. Blood 1997;89:739–61.
86. Nisbet-Brown E, Olivieri NF, Giardina PJ, et al. Effectiveness and safety of ICL670 in iron-loaded patients with thalassaemia: a randomised, double-blind, placebo-controlled, dose-escalation trial. Lancet 2003;361:1597–602.
87. Alter BP, Kumar M, Lockhart LL, et al. Pregnancy in bone marrow failure syndromes: Diamond-Blackfan anaemia and Shwachman-Diamond syndrome. Br J Haematol 1999;107:49–54.
88. Vlachos A, Federman N, Reyes-Haley C, et al. Hematopoietic stem cell transplantation for Diamond Blackfan anemia: a report from the Diamond Blackfan Anemia Registry. Bone Marrow Transplant 2001;27:381–6.
89. Roy V, Perez WS, Eapen M, et al. Bone marrow transplantation for Diamond-Blackfan anemia. Biol Blood Marrow Transplant 2005;11:600–8.
90. Kuliev A, Rechitsky S, Tur-Kaspa I, et al. Preimplantation genetics: improving access to stem cell therapy. Ann N Y Acad Sci 2005;1054:223–7.
91. Wagner JE, Kahn JP, Wolf SM, et al. Preimplantation testing to produce an HLA-matched donor infant. JAMA 2004;292:803–4, author reply 804.
92. Wynn RF, Grainger JD, Carr TF, et al. Failure of allogeneic bone marrow transplantation to correct Diamond-Blackfan anaemia despite haemopoietic stem cell engraftment. Bone Marrow Transplant 1999;24:803–5.
93. Flygare J, Olsson K, Richter J, et al. Gene therapy of Diamond Blackfan anemia CD34(+) cells leads to improved erythroid development and engraftment following transplantation. Exp Hematol 2008;36:1428–35.
94. Pospisilova D, Cmejlova J, Hak J, et al. Successful treatment of a Diamond-Blackfan anemia patient with amino acid leucine. Haematologica 2007;92:e66–7.
95. Anthony JC, Yoshizawa F, Anthony TG, et al. Leucine stimulates translation initiation in skeletal muscle of postabsorptive rats via a rapamycin-sensitive pathway. J Nutr 2000;130:2413–9.
96. Sakai D, Trainor PA. Treacher Collins syndrome: unmasking the role of Tcof1/treacle. Int J Biochem Cell Biol 2009;41:1229–32.
97. Ebert BL, Pretz J, Bosco J, et al. Identification of RPS14 as a 5q- syndrome gene by RNA interference screen. Nature 2008;451:335–9.

The Congenital Dyserythropoietic Anemias

Raffaele Renella, MD*, William G. Wood, PhD

KEYWORDS

- Anemia • Inherited • Erythropoiesis
- Dyserythropoiesis • Iron overload

The congenital dyserythropoietic anemias (CDAs) are a heterogeneous group of clinically challenging but biologically fascinating rare inborn disorders that principally affect erythropoiesis. They are distinct from other inherited bone marrow failure syndromes, being marked by morphologic abnormalities of the erythroblasts that lead to ineffective erythropoiesis. Other hematopoietic lineages seem to be unaffected. Therefore, CDAs have the potential to identify critical pathways and important players in the process of erythropoiesis. As with other rare disorders, the corpus of knowledge on CDA derives from an array of case reports or small series, which have been reviewed previously.[1,2] Registry-based data are only starting to emerge. This has limited our understanding of these syndromes and their management. Here, the authors aim to review the clinically relevant data available and focus on providing rational information to help with decision making.

The term *congenital dyserythropoietic anemia* was introduced by Crookston and colleagues,[3] and subsequently used by the German group of Heimpel and colleagues.[4] The recognition that the morphologic abnormalities in these and other cases had similarities but also significant differences led Heimpel and Wendt[5] to propose a working classification for a new category in the already extensive differential diagnosis list for dyserythropoiesis. Conceptually, CDAs were considered to be different because of their inborn and primary nature when compared with dyserythropoiesis associated with the thalassemias, vitamin B_{12} deficiency, acquired anemias, and certain infectious conditions (**Box 1**).[6]

Heimpel and Wendt[5] defined three major CDA subtypes (CDA-1, CDA-2, and CDA-3), and this still remains the basis of the classification today, although additional subgroups

R.R. is supported by the Lord Florey Scholarship (2005–2008) of the Berrow Foundation (Switzerland), the Lord Nathaniel Crewe Scholarship (2008–2009) of Lincoln College, University of Oxford (UK), and the "Eugenio Litta" Scholarship (2008–2009) of the Valeria Rossi di Montelera Trust (Switzerland).

Medical Research Council Molecular Haematology Unit, The Weatherall Institute of Molecular Medicine, University of Oxford, John Radcliffe Hospital, Oxford, OX3 9DS, UK

* Corresponding author.

E-mail address: raffaele.renella@imm.ox.ac.uk (R. Renella).

Box 1
Differential diagnosis and definition of dyserythropoiesis

Primary

  Homozygous β-thalassemia (hemoglobin [Hb] C or HbE), other unstable hemoglobins

  Sideroblastic anemia, thiamine-responsive anemia

  Acute myeloblastic leukemia, hairy cell leukemia, and preleukemic states[a]

  Myelodysplastic syndromes and chronic myeloproliferative disorders

  Aplastic anemia/paroxysmal nocturnal anemia

  GATA1/FOG1 X-linked thrombocytopenia/dyserythropoiesis/thalassemia syndrome

  Rare genetic conditions (hemophagocytic lymphohistiocytosis, Ellis-Van-Creveld syndrome, Majeed syndrome)

  CDA

Secondary

  Megaloblastic anemias (vitamin B_{12}, folate-deficient)

  Iron deficiency anemia

  Infection (HIV/AIDS, human herpesvirus-6, *Plasmodium falciparum* and *Plasmodium vivax* malaria, visceral leishmaniasis)

  Excess alcohol intake, liver disease

  Intoxication (benzene, arsenic, alternative medicine supplements)

  Drugs (linezolid, chloramphenicol, and probably many others)

  Autoimmune disorders

  After hematopoietic stem cell transplantation (HSCT) and cancer chemotherapy

Definition: Abnormal proportion of erythroid precursors in the bone marrow with morphologic features indicating aberrant proliferation or differentiation. The definition itself allows for some dyserythropoiesis to occur in normal bone marrow. In fact, anomalies, including nucleocytoplasmic maturation dissociation, karyorrhexis, and binucleation, can all be present but should not represent a dominant population. In a study of normal bone marrow, Nemec and Polak[131] (1947) stipulated that a maximum 4% of erythroblasts should be binucleate or multinucleate. A variable degree of chromatin bridging or basophilic stippling can be present in normal bone marrow but should not exceed 2%. These findings have been confirmed by independent investigators.

  [a] Particularly important differential diagnosis in children with nonclassic CDA-1, CDA-2, or CDA-3.

---

and variants have been added.[2] It ultimately made the systematic collection and analysis of cases possible, but the degree to which these disorders are related other than by morphologically abnormal erythroblasts is discussed later. After many years of mostly descriptive exploration, a molecular window on the pathogenesis of CDA was opened in 2002, when research by Tamary and colleagues[7,8] identified a gene linked to CDA-1. The discovery of the *CDAN1* gene and its protein, codanin-1, has opened new avenues in the field. The genes for CDA-2 and CDA-3 have also been localized to chromosomal segments, and their identification should go a long way toward determining how closely related these disorders are.[9,10]

DIAGNOSIS AND CLASSIFICATION OF THE CONGENITAL DYSERYTHROPOIETIC ANEMIAS

CDAs present a diagnostic challenge for the clinician, and the aim of this review is to provide the most recent knowledge for appropriate decision making. In fact, because

CDAs remain an exclusion diagnosis, a long time lapse from presentation of anemia to suspicion of CDA is a common problem. To think of CDA upfront in the workup of a patient displaying congenital anemia associated with suboptimal reticulocyte response and abnormal bone marrow red blood cell precursors is key to the correct diagnosis and further management. Many patients who have CDA have spent years with an incorrect diagnosis of hemolytic anemia, myelodysplastic syndrome, iron-deficient anemia, thalassemia, erythrocyte membrane abnormality, or hemochromatosis. Sometimes, this has exposed the patients to potentially harmful iron supplementation, aggressive transfusion, or steroids and cocktails of vitamins or has prevented screening for disorder-specific complications and therapy.[11,12] Copresentation of nonspecific and sometimes confounding features, such as mental retardation or congenital malformations (mostly cardiovascular and skeletal), which could be pleiotropic signs of the disease, coincidental findings, or byproducts of consanguinity, add to the diagnostic difficulty.[5,6,13–21] CDAs also present varied management challenges, because the ineffective erythropoiesis can be associated with severe iron overload (with secondary organ dysfunction), cholelithiasis, and hepatosplenomegaly.[11,12,22]

CDA is the association of hereditary or congenital ineffective erythropoiesis with morphologically abnormal bone marrow erythroid precursors as observed by light microscopy. This dyserythropoiesis is accompanied by increased phagocytosis of abnormal precursors by bone marrow macrophages and a suboptimal reticulocyte response.[23] Three major types of CDA can be distinguished, based on the classification proposed by Heimpel and Wendt[5] in 1968 (**Table 1**). All share the previously mentioned central features but are considered distinct because of their different bone marrow morphology and potentially different molecular causes. More importantly for the clinician, their presentation, evolution, and treatment are at least partly specific. Atypical cases have been reported as CDA variants, but without genetic identification of the loci involved, it is unclear whether these are distinct conditions or mutation-specific presentations of the known genes. Wickramasinghe has tentatively classified them into five groups (**Table 2**), but this needs to be reassessed when comprehensive molecular testing becomes available.[2,24]

Congenital Dyserythropoietic Anemia Type 1

In CDA-1, diagnosis may be made rarely in utero but also at any time between the neonatal period and late adulthood; the majority of cases come to attention during childhood and adolescence.[11,20,25,26] There is no gender preference, and the pattern of inheritance is autosomal recessive. Obligate heterozygotes have normal hematologic indices, peripheral blood, and bone marrow morphology.

The signs for neonatal presentation include intrauterine growth retardation, hepatomegaly, early jaundice with increased direct bilirubinemia (sometimes in association with Gilbert syndrome) and transaminases, and persistent pulmonary hypertension of the newborn. Most patients require transfusional therapy, although fewer than 10% remain dependent on transfusions.[20]

In childhood, the anemia is often diagnosed within episodes of erythropoietic stress (infection and, in young women, pregnancy). Symptoms can be highly variable, and mild cases may remain undetected. The management of women with CDA-1 through pregnancy has been described.[27] More severe presentations can include gallstones, cholecystitis from chronic hyperbilirubinemia, or extramedullary hemopoietic foci in the parietal and frontal bones of the skull (as observed in thalassemia).[28] Although iron overloading is rarely the primary symptom, it seems to be present in most patients after childhood.[11] Not surprisingly, this phenomenon is not limited to patients

Table 1
Summary of clinical and molecular features of congenital dyserythropoietic anemia

	Inheritance and Molecular	Epidemiology	Age at Presentation (Years)	Symptoms and Signs	Specific Therapy
CDA-1	Autosomal recessive Gene: CDAN1 (15q15) Other unknown locus[a]	Founder effects (Israel and Switzerland) Cases from central Europe, Arabic countries, India, Japan, China	In utero (hydrops foetalis), neonatal, childhood, or early adulthood	Anemia (most cases during neonatal period) Iron overload Splenomegaly and hepatomegaly Rare: extramedullary hemopoiesis (skull bones)	IFNα (HSCT)
CDA-2	Autosomal recessive Locus 20q11.2 Other unknown locus[a]	Most frequent Founder effect (southern Italy) Cases mostly European (including Eastern Europe and Mediterranean basin)	Most are diagnosed from age 5–30 (average 18–20)	Anemia and jaundice Gallstones (60%) Cholecystectomy (30%) Splenomegaly (usually by adulthood) Iron overload Rare: paravertebral hematopoiesis Aplastic crisis Parvovirus B19	Splenectomy (HSCT)
CDA-3	Autosomal dominant (familial cases) Locus 15q22 Autosomal recessive (sporadic cases)	Rarest form Founder effect (Sweden, Argentina, and United States)	N/A	Mild anemia No iron overload	N/A (HSCT?)

Abbreviations: HSCT, hematopoietic stem cell transplantation; IFNα, interferon-α; N/A, not available.
[a] Evidence for genetic heterogeneity in CDA-1/2.

Table 2
Wickramasinghe's congenital dyserythropoietic anemia variants group classification

	Features	Reference
Group CDA-IV	Severe transfusion-dependent normoblastic anemia with hypercellular marrow but absence of other features of CDA-1/2/3 If anemia is only moderate, then CDA-IVb Inheritance: not clear	112,113
Group CDA-V	Mild normomacrocytic anemia without medullary hyperplasia and erythroid dysplasia but with unconjugated hyperbilirubinemia Has been reported in the literature as "primary shunt hyperbilirubinemia" Inheritance: autosomal recessive/dominant	114–118
Group CDA-VI	Mild anemia with important macrocytosis (MCV: 120–130 fL) and marked megaloblastoid hypercellular erythropoiesis Orotic aciduria and thiamine-responsive anemia should be excluded Inheritance: not clear	119
Group CDA-VII	As CDA-IV, but marked irregular nuclear shapes and with cytoplasmic globin-like inclusions (not reactive to α- or β-antibodies) β-thalassemia has to be excluded Inheritance: not clear	120,121
Group CDA-VIII[a]	CDA with prominent postsplenectomy erythroblastemia ($10-40 \times 10^9$ erythroblasts/mL) but no resolution of a moderate anemia Marrow showed irregular nuclei (clover-leaf forms) and karyorrhexis Inheritance: not clear	107,122,123
Different variants	Case reports exist of unclear cases in which classification and further delineation was not possible Many of these may be classified within the spectrum of the major types when comprehensive molecular testing becomes available	124–130

For the sake of clarity, groups of variants are indicated with Roman numerals, whereas major types are indicated with Arabic numerals. To be considered a variant, at least three families were described with the features.

Abbreviation: MCV, mean corpuscular volume.

[a] Previously identified as CDA with prominent postsplenectomy erythroblastemia.

Data from Wickramasinghe SN. Congenital dyserythropoietic anemias. Curr Opin Hematol 2000;7:71.

receiving frequent transfusions, because the highly ineffective erythropoiesis results in decreased hepcidin levels, and thus increased iron absorbtion.[29] Levels of ferritin increase with age if chelation therapy is not initiated but tend to be in the range of 500 to 1500 µg/L in adulthood. Associations of CDA-1 with mutations in the HFE hemochromatosis gene have been described but do not seem to increase the severity of loading.[26,28,30] It is unclear whether mutations in the other genes associated with hemochromatosis (HJV, HAMP, TFR2, and TMPRSS6) may modulate this phenomenon. A recent study investigating the role of GDF15 (a member of the transforming growth factor-β superfamily that is highly increased in thalassemia intermedia) showed that it is also overexpressed in CDA-1.[31] This factor is believed to suppress hepcidin levels, thus contributing to increased iron absorption.

In certain rare cases, skeletal or other dysmorphic features can be identified, and the range of reported abnormalities is wide and includes short stature, distal limb and nail malformations, vertebral deformations or dysplasias, and skin pigmentation defects.[14–19,21,22,26,27] Although these signs are found in other bone marrow failure syndromes, it remains to be proved whether these are linked to genetic pleiotropism or if they are mere epiphenomena, especially in the highly consanguineous populations in which these signs have sometimes been described. Certain of the distal limb abnormalities could be secondary to undetected intrauterine anemia. These findings do not add value to the hematologic index of suspicion because they are nonspecific, but a complete examination with a suspicion-oriented radiologic and/or functional investigation is nonetheless warranted.

Hematologic and laboratory features of CDA-1/2/3 are shown in **Table 3**. In CDA-1, the anemia is macrocytic, with a mean corpuscular volume (MCV) up to 120 fL, and the blood smear shows anisopoikilocytosis with an inadequate reticulocyte response (when compared with hemolytic anemias). Macrocytes can be observed even in cases in which the MCV is within the normal range. In some cases, late normoblasts circulate in the periphery and basophilic stippling of red cells is common.

Light microscopy of the bone marrow demonstrates erythroid hyperplasia with abnormal precursors showing a megaloblastoid appearance. Dysplastic signs (**Table 4**) include markedly irregular nuclei with frequent (3.5%–7%) binucleate erythroblasts (particularly late cells) and occasional tri- and tetranucleate cells. None of these morphologic abnormalities are entirely specific for CDA-1 because they can be found in the other CDA types and in other acquired dyserythropoietic states. A particular diagnostic finding in CDA-1 is the presence in the marrow of intranuclear bridges between erythroblasts (**Fig. 1A**).[5] These require prolonged searching because they are only found in a small percentage of erythroblasts, with figures ranging from 0.5% to 8% among various studies and a mean of approximately 3%.[6]

Electron microscopy of the bone marrow erythroblast is the "gold standard" for the determination of CDA-1, wherein 40% to 60% of the intermediate and late erythroblasts show a characteristic heterochromatin pattern.[23,32–35] The heterochromatin is abnormally electron dense with a spongy appearance that has been described as Swiss cheese-like (**Fig. 2B**). The nuclear membrane is frequently invaginated into the nucleus and contains cytoplasmic organelles, a feature that is not limited to CDA-1 but is found in other dyserythropoietic states.

In some cases of CDA-1, there are increased amounts of HbA$_2$ and there may also be an increased α/non-α globin chain synthesis (1.2–1.8) ratio.[36] Foci of intracytoplasmic electron-dense deposits similar in appearance to precipitated globin chains may also be found.[37,38] These thalassemic-like features are most likely to be secondary to the dyserythropoiesis.

Table 3
Hematology and laboratory features of congenital dyserythropoietic anemia

	CDA-1	CDA-2	CDA-3
Blood smear	Anisopoikilocytosis with basophilic stippling Occasional circulating mature erythroblast	Anisopoikilocytosis with basophilic stippling Occasional circulating mature erythroblast	Anisopoikilocytosis with basophilic stippling
Hemoglobin (g/dL)	6.5–11.5 (mean = 9.5)	9–12 (mean = 11)	8–14 (mean = 12)
MCV	↑↑ (70% cases)	N/min ↑	N/min ↑
RDW	↑↑↑	↑↑	↑↑
Reticulocytes	Suboptimal response[a]		N/A
Bilirubin (total, mg/dL)	↑ (indirect)[b]	↑ (2–8)[b]	N/min ↑[b]
LDH	↑	↑	↑↑↑
Haptoglobin	N/A		↓/absent
Ferritin (μg/L)	↑ (in 60% = 1000–1500)	↑↑ (>50% >1000 by age 50 years)	N
Ham (acid sera lysis) test[c]	Negative	Positive	Negative
Anti-i antigen hemagglutination	N-strong	Strong	N-strong
Serum thymidine kinase	↑↑↑	↑↑	↑↑↑
SDS-PAGE	Normal	Abnormal migration of band-3	Normal
Hemosiderinuria	N/A	N/A	+++

Abbreviations: N, normal; EMP, erythrocyte membrane protein; LDH, lactate dehydrogenase; MCV, mean corpuscular volume; RDW, red cell distribution width; min, minimal; N/A, not available; SDS-PAGE, sodium dodecyl sulfate polyacrylamide gel electrophoresis.
[a] In comparison to anemia from intravascular hemolysis or blood loss (ie, trauma), indicating ineffective (suboptimal) stress erythropoiesis.
[b] Values might be modulated by coinheritance of Gilbert syndrome.
[c] See text for limitations of this test.

Table 4
Abnormalities observed in the bone marrow of patients who have CDA

	Light Microscopy	Electron Microscopy

CDA-1	Myeloid/erythroid ratio skewed <1
	Erythroblasts
	 Megaloblastic appearance
	 Binuclearity, mostly asymmetric
	  (3%–7%)
	 Internuclear chromatin bridges[a]
	  (1%–3%)
	 Cytoplasmic stippling (1%–15%)
	 Irregular or karyorrhectic nuclei
	  (1%–5%)
	 Howell-Jolly bodies (1%–2%)
		Most, but not all, erythroblasts display
		characteristic Swiss-cheese pattern
		of heterochromatin (see **Fig. 1**).
		There can be marked invagination
		of the nuclear membrane with
		intranuclearization of cytoplasmic
		organelles
		In certain cases, electron-dense
		cytoplasmic precipitates
		(eg, α-globin in thalassemia)

CDA-2	Myeloid/erythroid ratio skewed <1
	Erythroblasts
	 Binuclearity, usually symmetric
	  (10%–35%)
	 Multinuclearity (rare)
	 Late orthochromatic cytoplasm,
	  highly condensed nuclei
	Pseudo-Gaucher cells
	 (lipid-laden bone marrow
	 macrophages, visible under
	 birefringent light)
		Double membranes (possibly
		peripheral cisternae of smooth
		endoplasmic reticulum) running
		parallel (40–60-nm interval) to
		cytoplasmic membrane of
		erythroblasts

CDA-3	Myeloid/erythroid ratio skewed <1
	Erythroblasts (basophilic and
	 polychromatophilic)
	 Multinuclearity (up to 12 nuclei
	  per cell)
	 Nuclear lobulation and
	  karyorrhexis
		Multiple intranuclear clefts in
		erythroblasts
		Intracytoplasmic β-globin chain
		precipitates

[a] To be distinguished from erythroblast cytoplasmic bridges, which can be found in normal bone marrow at a rate of 1% to 5%.

Congenital Dyserythropoietic Anemia Type 2

Diagnosis of CDA-2 is usually made later in life compared with CDA-1, because symptoms can be mild.[12,39] Patients may come to attention because of the anemia but also with jaundice (present in 90% of cases), splenomegaly (70%), or hepatomegaly (45%).[40] In older patients, signs of iron overload (eg, liver cirrhosis, cardiac or endocrine dysfunction) can lead to the diagnosis, whereas in certain cases, the presence of posterior mediastinal or paravertebral masses consisting of extramedullary hemopoietic tissue has led to correction of an erroneous diagnosis.[41–47] Patients remain susceptible to decreased hemoglobin levels during intercurrent infections, or to severe aplastic phenomena in the case of parvovirus B19 infection (as in CDA-1).[48,49] Mental retardation has been described in a subset of patients but is not a recurrent feature of the disease.[50]

The anemia of CDA-2 is normocytic, and the peripheral smear shows anisopoikilocytosis with variable anisochromasia. Occasional basophilic stippling of red blood cells and circulating erythroid precursors can be found. The bone marrow is hypercellular with erythroid hyperplasia but, in contrast to CDA-1, is of normoblastic

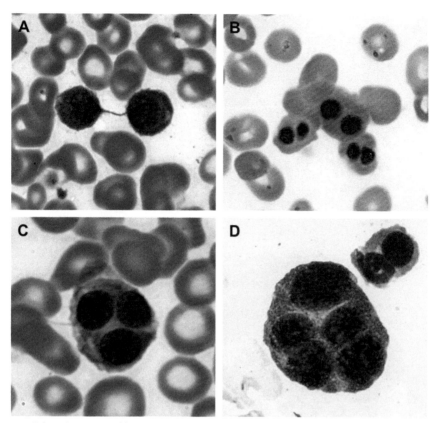

Fig. 1. Light microscopy of bone marrow erythroblasts obtained by aspiration, indicating the spectrum of nuclear abnormalities. (*A*) Internuclear chromatin bridging in CDA-1. (*B*) Binuclearity in CDA-2. (*C*) Trinuclearity, as observed in all CDA types. (*D*) Multinuclearity in CDA-3. (*Courtesy of* H. Heimpel, Ulm, Germany.)

appearance with a large number of binuclear erythroblasts (10%–35%).[50] A striking difference between the binuclearity of CDA-1 and CDA-2 is that the nuclei are of similar size and development in the latter, whereas they are often asymmetric in the former. In certain cases, bone marrow macrophages can be loaded with lipids mimicking cells observed in storage disorders (referred to as pseudo-Gaucher cells), which can best be visualized with birefringent light.[51] Again, none of these features is specific for the disorder.

On electron microscopic examination, CDA-2 erythroblasts lack the "Swiss cheese" chromatin appearance characteristic of CDA-1, but they are marked by stretches of double membranes approximately 50 nm from the outer membrane. These are peripheral cisternae of excess smooth endoplasmic reticulum and contain normal components of this organelle, such as calreticulin and protein disulfide isomerase.[33,52–54]

Early cases of CDA-2 were initially reported by Crookston and colleagues[55] as "hereditary erythroblastic multinuclearity with a positive acidified serum lysis test" syndrome before being reclassified by Heimpel and Wendt.[5] In fact, erythrocytes of patients with CDA-2 lyse in acidified serum (Ham test) because of an IgM class antibody that recognizes an antigen present on CDA-2 cells but absent on normal cells. The technical difficulty of this test, and the fact that cross-testing of more than 30 normal sera is

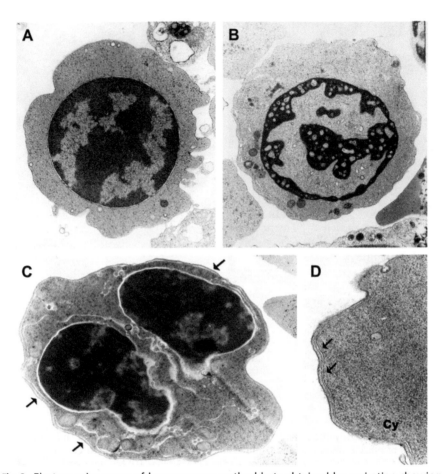

Fig. 2. Electron microscopy of bone marrow erythroblasts obtained by aspiration showing the specific abnormalities observed in CDA-1 and CDA-2. (*A*) Normal erythroblast. The nucleus is composed of heterochromatin (high electron density) and euchromatin (low electron density). (*B*) CDA-1 erythroblast with characteristic "Swiss-cheese" (spongy) heterochromatin. (*C*) CDA-2 binucleate erythroblast. Arrows show characteristic "double membrane." (*D*) CDA-2 erythroblast cytoplasmic membrane (detail). Arrows show double membrane (possibly peripheral cisternae of smooth endoplasmic reticulum) running parallel (40–60-nm interval) to cytoplasmic membrane of erythroblasts. Cy, cytoplasm.

needed to obtain a reliable result, has undermined its usefulness.[1] The test is highly specific for CDA-2, but it has become difficult to find accredited laboratories that can perform it with adequate quality controls, and there is general agreement that it should no longer be used as the standard confirmation. Cases in which the results of properly performed Ham tests were negative in patients with all other findings and investigations pointing to CDA-2 have been reclassified as variants in the literature (CDA-IV).[56] Other variants have presented with macrocytosis, gout, Kpb-negative Kell phenotype, and abnormal electron microscopic abnormalities not limited to the erythroid compartment but showing peripheral cisternae in granulocytes and thrombocytes.[57]

In addition to the tendency to lyze in acidified sera, red blood cells of patients who have CDA-2 agglutinate in sera containing anti-i antigens. This test is sensitive but not specific, and results cannot be compared among different institutions because of the different anti-i sera used. It is useful to note that red blood cells of patients who have CDA-2 are sucrose-lysis test-negative, which helps to discriminate it from cases of paroxysmal nocturnal hemoglobinuria.

Analysis of erythrocyte membrane proteins by sodium dodecyl sulfate polyacryl-amide gel electrophoresis (SDS-PAGE) has proved its value in all patients who have CDA-2 in identifying the narrower band size and faster migration of the band-3 and band-4.5 proteins.[58–61] Samples have to be taken outside of transfusional windows and tested within 48 hours, ideally in a laboratory with experience in red blood cell membrane disorders. Exceptional cases that do not show the characteristic SDS-PAGE pattern have been reported, but it is recommended that these should be considered CDA-2–like conditions. It is now clear that biosynthesis of N-linked oligo-saccharides is perturbed, although it remains to be determined whether this is the primary disturbance or a secondary effect, because a certain degree of glycosylation abnormalities can also be found in CDA-1 and CDA-3.[62]

Research on the abnormalities found in CDA-2 red blood cells has yielded several additional tests (eg, Western blotting of endoplasmic reticulum proteins of red blood cells, tomato-lectin binding Western blotting), and their diagnostic value still needs to be confirmed.[63]

Congenital Dyserythropoietic Anemia Type 3

CDA-3 constitutes a rare subtype. Familial cases have been described in Sweden, Argentina, and the United States.[10,64–67] The largest is a five-generation family from the Västerbotten district of Sweden, whose ancestry can be traced back since the 19th century. It contains more than 30 cases inherited in an autosomal dominant manner. CDA-3 does not seem to be as severe as the other types, and the anemia is mild. Patients present with ocular abnormalities (angioid streaks with macular degeneration), do not have iron overload (probably attributable to predominant intra-vascular hemolysis with hemosiderinuria), and do not have splenomegaly (except the Argentinean family). In the Swedish family, there is an increased tendency to develop monoclonal gammopathy and multiple myeloma, although sporadic cases have demonstrated lymphoma.[64,68,69] Sporadic cases do not have autosomal dominant inheritance, because parents and relatives were entirely normal; they may represent de novo mutations or demonstrate genetic heterogeneity. The clinical features of the sporadic cases are also extremely variable.[69–76]

The only identifying features of CDA-3 are those displayed by the bone marrow. The blood smear of patients who have CDA-3 shows moderate to marked anisopoikilocy-tosis with occasional basophilic stippling and macrocytes. In the bone marrow, there are abundant "giant" erythroid precursors of all developmental stages. These are frequently multinucleated (up to 12 nuclei per cell), whereas other nuclei are highly polyploid with a DNA content up to 48 times normal. Ultrastructural analysis showed intranuclear clefts, abnormal nuclear membrane, cytoplasmic autophagosomes, myelin deposits, hemoglobin precipitates, or abnormal mitochondria. It is important to note that multinucleated erythroblasts are not specific to CDA-3 because they can be seen in myelodysplasia and erythroleukemia.

MOLECULAR PATHOGENESIS OF CONGENITAL DYSERYTHROPOIETIC ANEMIAS
Congenital Dyserythropoietic Anemia Type 1

A breakthrough in the molecular basis of the CDAs came with the landmark discovery of the gene responsible for CDA-1 in a consanguineous family of Israeli Bedouins presenting with classic CDA-1 features.[8] It was localized to chromosome 15q15 using a genome-wide scan to identify regions of homozygosity by descent. The gene was identified by linkage analysis and designated *CDAN1*. This large 15-kb gene has 28 exons and encodes the protein codanin-1. This 134-kd protein does not contain any known motif or domain that would allow its inclusion in any of the known protein families or might give clues to its function. It is highly conserved evolutionarily and has no orthologs within the human genome, suggesting a nonredundant function. The expression of *CDAN1* is ubiquitous, which is intriguing when one thinks of the restriction of the phenotype to the erythroid lineage. The regulation of this gene seems to depend on the cell cycle, and it has an upstream promoter containing multiple transcription factor binding sites, including several E2F sites that may be important in its expression.[77] The function of codanin-1 remains elusive, but its localization is mainly nuclear, allowing speculation about its role in the abnormal chromatin structure observed on electron microscopy.[77,78]

To date, approximately 30 mutations have been found in the *CDAN1* gene in cases of CDA-1, which are spread throughout the gene (**Fig. 3**). Most of these are missense mutations resulting in amino acid substitutions, but frameshift and premature stop codons are also observed. So far, no homozygotes or compound heterozygotes for null mutations have been observed, which may indicate that such a condition would be lethal.

The continued study and investigation of human mutants should lead to a better understanding of the genotype-phenotype relation in CDA-1 cases with codanin-1 alterations. Ideally, one or more of the human mutations could be knocked in to the highly conserved mouse *CDAN1* locus to provide an animal model that recapitulates the phenotypic features of the human patients who have CDA-1. In the absence of a knock-in transgenic model, a gene-trap knockout mouse model has shown that homozygotes are embryonically lethal at a stage of development before the onset of erythropoiesis.[78] This demonstrates that mouse codanin-1 has essential functions in nonerythroid tissues, consistent with the suggestion that a total lack of this protein might be lethal in people.

It is important to note that not all cases with the classic features of CDA-1 segregate with the *CDAN1* locus and that at least one other locus unlinked to chromosome 15q15 must exist.[79,80] Genetic heterogeneity may explain some of the CDA-1 cases reported in the literature, in which thorough analysis of the *CDAN1* gene has failed

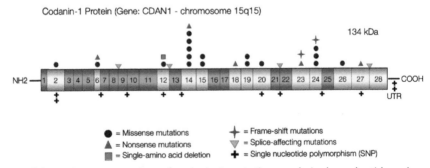

Fig. 3. Schematic representation of codanin-1 mutations and single-nucleotide polymorphisms (SNPs). Blocks represent exons on CDAN1 gene in relative size. Yellow blocks represent exons with mutations, and green blocks represent exons without mutations. SNPs depicted at the junctions of blocks (exons) indicate SNPs in intronic sequence.

to identify any mutations. More extensive sequencing of the promoter region and the introns of *CDAN1* is also likely to uncover previously missed mutations. This emphasizes the importance of building up a comprehensive collection of cases to identify new mutations and the identity of other genes involved. This again highlights the important role of clinicians in recognizing the condition to find not only sporadic cases, but also to identify families sufficiently large for further genetic studies.

Congenital Dyserythropoietic Anemia Type 2

Genome-wide linkage of families from France and Italy pointed to a 5-cm region of chromosome 20q11.2 as bearing a potential *CDAN2* gene. The region contains more than 90 transcripts, and seven of the most likely candidate genes (including integrin β4-binding protein, oligosaccharide α-1,2-mannosidase–like protein, and erythrocyte band 4.1-like protein) have been screened in 17 unrelated patients who had CDA-2. This failed to identify the gene responsible.[81] Techniques for genome-wide linkage analysis continue to improve, and its identity is likely to emerge soon. As with CDA-1, there are cases of CDA-2 that are unlinked to genetic markers around the chromosome 20q11.2 region, suggesting that there is likely to be genetic heterogeneity in this condition also.[82]

Speculation on the pathogenesis of CDA-2 has been based on the comprehensive analysis of red blood cell membrane protein glycosylation defects.[83] In fact, as described previously, erythrocyte-specific protein band-3 and band-4.5, in addition to glycophorin-A, are underglycosylated, whereas lipids seem to be overglycosylated in patients who have CDA-2.[84,85] Biochemical analysis has suggested that there is disturbed processing of asparagine and N-linked oligosaccharides associated with modified activities of enzymes involved. In fact, reduced *N*-acetyl-glucosaminyltransferase II and α-mannosidase II have been reported in patients who have CDA-2.[57,86–89] Intriguingly, the sequencing of these genes has failed to reveal potential pathogenic mutations.[90] Recent work has shown that glycosylation abnormalities can also be found in CDA-1 and CDA-3 and may indicate that these could be secondary phenomena.[62,91,92]

A zebrafish mutant, called retsina, mimics the phenotype of CDA-2 in that it has an erythroid-specific defect in cell division and binucleate cells containing double membranes.[93] The mutation was mapped to the fish homolog of the band-3 anion exchanger 1 gene. The human band 3 gene has been excluded as a cause of CDA-2.

Congenital Dyserythropoietic Anemia Type 3

For CDA-3, the value of a single large family for linkage analysis was demonstrated by the Swedish "Västerbotten" family, in which a 4.5-cM region of chromosome 15q22 was identified as harboring the *CDAN3* gene.[10] This region lies some distance telomeric to the *CDAN1* gene.

Dyserythropoiesis with multinucleated erythroblasts is not specific to CDA-3, and one case with these features (but with additional platelet abnormalities) was shown to be attributable to a *GATA1* mutation that abrogated the interaction between Gata-1 and Fog-1, indicating that defects in certain erythroid-specific pathways can mimic some phenotypic features of CDA-3.[94]

WHAT MIGHT THE MOLECULAR BASIS OF CONGENITAL DYSERYTHROPOIETIC ANEMIAS TEACH US ABOUT THE DISEASE(S)?

CDAs are hereditary lineage-restricted disorders characterized by ineffective erythropoiesis that does not progress to multilineage bone marrow failure or neoplastic transformation. The phenotypes of the various subtypes are distinct, but the common presence of nuclear abnormalities in erythroblasts has allowed the cases to be grouped together. It is possible that they represent defects in different genes of a shared metabolic pathway that lead to the common dyserythropoietic and karyorrhectic abnormalities. Subtle differences in the maturation process might then produce the distinguishing features of the various subtypes.

Alternatively, there may be no common pathway; the various CDA lesions may be unrelated to each other, and, instead, the constraints of the erythropoietic process result in a limited number of morphologic outcomes. Erythroid cells proliferate rapidly in the marrow and are highly specialized to maximize the production of a single protein (hemoglobin) inside a membrane that combines stability and flexibility to survive the rigors of an extended life in the circulation. As such, the control of erythroblast maturation divisions in the marrow may follow a specialized pathway in which perturbations of several unrelated systems may result in the morphologic similarities of karyorrhexis but with unrelated underlying causality. Arguing against this idea of constrained erythroid morphologies, other marrow failure disorders that have a marked erythroid component (eg, Diamond-Blackfan anemia) do not show dyserythropoiesis in the marrow; equally, these disorders seem to act at a much earlier stage in the erythroid differentiation process than the CDA defects.

Only genetic and functional molecular understanding can clarify whether these three types of CDA are indeed related conditions, or at least a pathologic cluster based on a novel pathway crucial for erythropoiesis. Why is the phenotype restricted to erythroid cells? It is intriguing that in CDA-1, as is the case for RPS19 mutations in Diamond-Blackfan anemia, for example, the gene is ubiquitously expressed, whereas the manifesting phenotype is limited to the erythroid lineage. One might argue that the signs and symptoms in the patient are merely the tip of the iceberg. Analysis of other tissues with rapidly proliferating cell types might reveal clinically silent but clearly abnormal "cryptophenotypes."

HOW FREQUENT ARE CONGENITAL DYSERYTHROPOIETIC ANEMIAS?

The literature and registry-based analyses (from Italy, France, Israel, Spain, Poland, Germany, United Kingdom, and Sweden) have allowed the collection of more than 400 families and more than 500 cases of CDA in Europe. Many cases are sporadic, lacking direct evidence of a genetic basis. Although efforts have been made to centralize reporting of cases, at best, we have only rather crude measures of the relative prevalence of these disorders. As with many other rare diseases, misdiagnosis and underreporting remain major issues even for the more advanced population-based registries. Thus, the incidence of CDAs and their subtypes remains speculative.

Nonetheless, some information is available to suggest that CDA-2 is the most frequent subtype, whereas CDA-3 seems to be isolated to familial clusters in Sweden, Argentina, and the United States. Founder events have been described for southern Italy (CDA-2), Switzerland and Israel (CDA-1), and Sweden (CDA-3); therefore, the prevalence and incidence of CDA subtypes might seem skewed in these geographic positions.

In CDA-1, several European cases have *CDAN1* mutations, which are also found in normal controls at a frequency of 0.5% to 1.0%. Although there are no functional assays to confirm that such mutations are the direct cause of the disease (rather than a neutral polymorphism), these carrier frequencies, if confirmed, would suggest that the disease might not be as rare as currently believed.

The observation and experience of many rare genetic conditions hold true in CDA; although rare, this entity needs to be thought of whenever the major clinical criteria fit, without any epidemiologic discrimination.

DIAGNOSTIC STRATEGY

Diagnosis of cases should follow the general guideline shown in **Fig. 4** and rely on the analysis of the bone marrow by light and electron microscopy. Because of the rarity of the condition, confirmation by an expert is recommended. In the case of CDA-1, genetic testing should be undertaken, although not all patients have mutations within the CDAN1 gene.[79,80] In fact, it is sometimes difficult to come to a diagnosis with certainty. Sharing cases, with their history, presentation, and clinical evolution, is vital in this field, and clinicians should participate in research efforts whenever possible.

TREATMENT OPTIONS

CDAs are rare conditions, and treatment recommendations are therefore based on case- or small series-based evidence. Clinicians should remember to tailor the therapeutic options to fit the patient's specific needs and consider seeking an expert opinion whenever possible. Treatment for CDA is mostly supportive and targeted to prevent the consequences of anemia and iron overload. The progressive accumulation of iron has

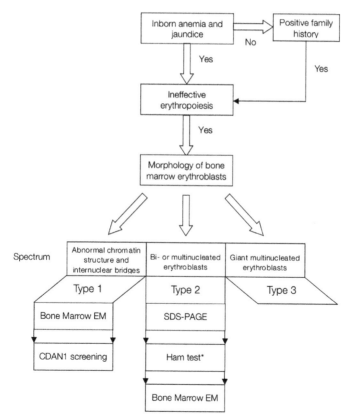

Fig. 4. Diagnostic algorithm for CDA. See text for diagnostic limitations of Ham (acid serum lysis) test. EM, electron microscopy.

been particularly well studied in CDA-2 and resembles that of untreated hemochromatosis. Most patients suffer from clinical consequences as early as the third decade of life. In patients whose anemia is relatively mild but demonstrates evidence of iron loading, phlebotomy may be considered. Expert-based consensus suggests that iron chelation should be introduced, or at least considered, when repeated ferritin levels are greater than 1000 μg/L. Desferrioxamine has been the standard chelation therapy, but it is anticipated that newer oral chelation drugs, when approved for iron overload conditions, can greatly contribute to the care of patients who have CDA.

During the treatment of hepatitis C infection with interferon-α (IFNα) in a patient who had CDA-1, Lavabre-Bertrand and colleagues[95] observed a progressive and impressive correction of the hemoglobin levels. Furthermore, most bone marrow erythroblasts became morphologically normal even by electron microscopy analysis. This finding led to the successful administration of IFNα to many other patients who had confirmed CDA-1 and has proved to be safe and effective in the long term.[11,25,96] The schedule of IFN-α2b used was 10^6 U three times a week or 2×10^6 U twice a week administered subcutaneously. Pegylated forms at a dosage of 30 μg/wk have been given with success. In infants, IFNα might be off limits because of reports of toxicity and tolerance should modulate application.[97] Nonresponders clustered where a diagnosis of CDA-1 could not be entirely confirmed;[98] other subtypes of CDA do not respond to IFNα. Patients who have CDA-1, CDA-2, or CDA-IV do not respond to erythropoietin stimulation.[99]

For CDA-2, splenectomy can lead to a sustained increase in hemoglobin values, although it does not have a beneficial effect on iron overload.[12,50,100] Strategies in place for hereditary red blood cell membrane disorders are a good guide for patients who have CDA.[101,102] Potential candidates who could benefit from the procedure might be identified when peripheral hemolysis is severe.[103] Postsplenectomy thrombotic consequences should be looked for in all patients.[1,34] In certain cases, splenectomy can be effective in CDA-1, CDA-3 (sporadic), and CDA-IV, although the effect is unpredictable.[18,72,104–107] Age and severity of the condition must be balanced against the risks and detrimental effects of the procedure.

The only available curative treatment for genetic conditions of hematopoiesis is HSCT, and it has been used with some success in patients who have CDA-1 or CDA-2 and in one variant case. It has been limited to severe cases in which splenectomy was ineffective, transfusion needs exceeded tolerance levels for iron overload, and a human leukocyte antigen-identical donor was available.[108–111]

SUMMARY

The CDAs are a fascinating but heterogeneous group of hereditary, lineage-restricted, inherited bone marrow disorders characterized by ineffective erythropoiesis with abnormal erythroblast morphology, with at least three definable subtypes. Progress is being made in determining the defective genes responsible for the condition, and that should determine the degree to which the CDAs may be considered a homogeneous group rather than unrelated diseases. Although CDA is rare, the clinician should include this disorder in his/her list of differential diagnosis of dyserythropoiesis and use expert resources, which can help with the management of cases.

ACKNOWLEDGMENTS

We thank Professor David Ferguson, Nuffield Department of Clinical Laboratory Sciences, The John Radcliffe Hospital, Oxford, UK, for the electron microscopy analysis.

APPENDIX
Useful Resources and Contacts

Oxford congenital dyserythropoietic anaemia research initiative
Dr. Raffaele Renella and Prof. Bill Wood, Medical Research Council Molecular Haematology Unit, The Weatherall Institute of Molecular Medicine, Oxford (see author information for contact details). Available at: www.imm.ox.ac.uk/mhu/cda. This resource offers clinical and diagnostic advice and a comprehensive array of tests, including *CDAN1* analysis.

German registry on congenital dyserythropoietic anemias
Prof. Emerit. Dr. med. Hermann Heimpel, FRCPath, Medizinische Universitätsklinik, KFA 210, Albert Einstein Allee 23, D-89081 Ulm, Germany; telephone: +49(0)731-500- 69413; fax, +49(0)731-500-69412; e-mail: hermann.heimpel@uniklinik-ulm.de; or contact Rosi Leichtle via e-mail: rosi.leichtle@uniklinik-ulm.de. Available at: www.bone-marrow-failure-syndromes.de/erkrankungen/arztinfo_cda.htm (in German). This resource offers clinical and diagnostic advice and a comprehensive array of tests, including *CDAN1* analysis.

International registry of congenital dyserythropoietic anemia type 2
Prof. Achille Iolascon, CEINGE, Via C. Margherita, 80131 Naples, Italy; telephone: 081 3737897; fax: 081 3737804/821; e-mail: iolascondbbm.unina.it. This resource offers clinical and diagnostic advice and testing for CDA-2.

National institutes of health/national cancer institute expert on inherited bone marrow failure
Blanche P. Alter, MD, MPH, 6120 Executive Boulevard, EPS Room 7020, MSC 7242, Bethesda, Maryland 20892–7335, USA; telephone: 301-594-7642; fax: 301-496-1854; e-mail: alterb@mail.nih.gov. This resource offers clinical and diagnostic advice and links to test-providing institutions.

Online hematopathological atlas of congenital dyserythropoietic anemia
Prof. Hermann Heimpel, Ulm, Germany. Available at: http://bildatlas.onkodin.de/bildatlas/content/e1352/e1775/e1872/e2500/index_ger.html (in German).

REFERENCES

1. Heimpel H. Congenital dyserythropoietic anemias: epidemiology, clinical significance, and progress in understanding their pathogenesis. Ann Hematol 2004; 83:613.
2. Wickramasinghe SN, Wood WG. Advances in the understanding of the congenital dyserythropoietic anaemias. Br J Haematol 2005;131:431.
3. Crookston JH, Godwin TF, R Wkj, et al. Congenital dyserythropoietic anaemia. Abstracts from the XIth Congress of the International Society of Haematology, Sydney:18, 1966.
4. Heimpel H, Wendt F, Klemm D, et al. [Congenital dyserythropoietic anemia]. Arch Klin Med 1968;215:174 [in German].
5. Heimpel H, Wendt F. Congenital dyserythropoietic anemia with karyorrhexis and multinuclearity of erythroblasts. Helv Med Acta 1968;34:103.
6. Wickramasinghe SN. Dyserythropoiesis and congenital dyserythropoietic anaemias. Br J Haematol 1997;98:785.
7. Tamary H, Shalmon L, Shalev H, et al. Localization of the gene for congenital dyserythropoietic anemia type I to a <1-cM interval on chromosome 15q15.1-15.3. Am J Hum Genet 1998;62:1062.

8. Dgany O, Avidan N, Delaunay J, et al. Congenital dyserythropoietic anemia type I is caused by mutations in codanin-1. Am J Hum Genet 2002;71:1467.

9. Gasparini P, Miraglia del Giudice E, Delaunay J, et al. Localization of the congenital dyserythropoietic anemia II locus to chromosome 20q11.2 by genomewide search. Am J Hum Genet 1997;61:1112.

10. Lind L, Sandstrom H, Wahlin A, et al. Localization of the gene for congenital dyserythropoietic anemia type III, CDAN3, to chromosome 15q21-q25. Hum Mol Genet 1995;4:109.

11. Heimpel H, Schwarz K, Ebnother M, et al. Congenital dyserythropoietic anemia type I (CDA I): molecular genetics, clinical appearance, and prognosis based on long-term observation. Blood 2006;107:334.

12. Heimpel H, Anselstetter V, Chrobak L, et al. Congenital dyserythropoietic anemia type II: epidemiology, clinical appearance, and prognosis based on long-term observation. Blood 2003;102:4576.

13. Jean R, Dossa D, Navarro M, et al. [Congenital aplastic anemia, type I]. Arch Fr Pediatr 1975;32:337 [in French].

14. Holmberg L, Jansson L, Rausing A, et al. Type I congenital dyserythropoietic anaemia with myelopoietic abnormalities and hand malformations. Scand J Haematol 1978;21:72.

15. Brichard B, Vermylen C, Scheiff JM, et al. Two cases of congenital dyserythropoietic anaemia type I associated with unusual skeletal abnormalities of the limbs. Br J Haematol 1994;86:201.

16. Le Merrer M, Girot R, Parent P, et al. Acral dysostosis dyserythropoiesis syndrome. Eur J Pediatr 1995;154:384.

17. Sabry MA, Zaki M, al Awadi SA, et al. Non-haematological traits associated with congenital dyserythropoietic anaemia type 1: a new entity emerging. Clin Dysmorphol 1997;6:205.

18. Tamary H, Dgany O, Proust A, et al. Clinical and molecular variability in congenital dyserythropoietic anaemia type I. Br J Haematol 2005;130:628.

19. Tamary H, Offret H, Dgany O, et al. Congenital dyserythropoietic anaemia, type I, in a Caucasian patient with retinal angioid streaks (homozygous arg1042trp mutation in codanin-1). Eur J Haematol 2008.

20. Shalev H, Kapelushnik J, Moser A, et al. A comprehensive study of the neonatal manifestations of congenital dyserythropoietic anemia type I. J Pediatr Hematol Oncol 2004;26:746.

21. Goede JS, Benz R, Fehr J, et al. Congenital dyserythropoietic anemia type I with bone abnormalities, mutations of the CDAN I gene, and significant responsiveness to alpha-interferon therapy. Ann Hematol 2006;85:591.

22. Tamary H, Shalev H, Luria D, et al. Clinical features and studies of erythropoiesis in Israeli Bedouins with congenital dyserythropoietic anemia type I. Blood 1996; 87:1763.

23. Heimpel H, Forteza-Vila J, Queisser W, et al. Electron and light microscopic study of the erythroblasts of patients with congenital dyserythropoietic anemia. Blood 1971;37:299.

24. Wickramasinghe SN. Congenital dyserythropoietic anemias. Curr Opin Hematol 2000;7:71.

25. Parez N, Dommergues M, Zupan V, et al. Severe congenital dyserythropoietic anaemia type I: prenatal management, transfusion support and alpha-interferon therapy. Br J Haematol 2000;110:420.

26. Shalev H, Kapleushnik Y, Haeskelzon L, et al. Clinical and laboratory manifestations of congenital dyserythropoietic anemia type I in young adults. Eur J Haematol 2002;68:170.

27. Shalev H, Perez Avraham G, Hershkovitz R, et al. Pregnancy outcome in congenital dyserythropoietic anemia type I. Eur J Haematol 2008;81:317.

28. Wickramasinghe SN, Thein SL, Srichairatanakool S, et al. Determinants of iron status and bilirubin levels in congenital dyserythropoietic anaemia type I. Br J Haematol 1999;107:522.

29. Papanikolaou G, Tzilianos M, Christakis JI, et al. Hepcidin in iron overload disorders. Blood 2005;105:4103.

30. Chrobak L, Hulek P, Nozicka J. [Congenital dyserythropoietic anemia—type II (CDA-II) in 3 siblings with long-term follow up and iron overload]. Acta Medica (Hradec Kralove) Suppl 2004;47:29.

31. Tamary H, Shalev H, Perez-Avraham G, et al. Elevated growth differentiation factor 15 expression in patients with congenital dyserythropoietic anemia type I. Blood 2008.

32. Lewis SM, Nelson DA, Pitcher CS. Clinical and ultrastructural aspects of congenital dyserythropoietic anaemia type I. Br J Haematol 1972;23:113.

33. Breton-Gorius J, Daniel MT, Clauvel JP, et al. [Ultrastructural abnormalities of erythroblasts and erythrocytes in 6 cases of congenital dyserythropoietic anemia]. Nouv Rev Fr Hematol 1973;13:23.

34. Wickramasinghe SN. Congenital dyserythropoietic anaemias: clinical features, haematological morphology and new biochemical data. Blood Rev 1998;12:178.

35. Wickramasinghe SN, Pippard MJ. Studies of erythroblast function in congenital dyserythropoietic anaemia, type I: evidence of impaired DNA, RNA, and protein synthesis and unbalanced globin chain synthesis in ultrastructurally abnormal cells. J Clin Pathol 1986;39:881.

36. Alloisio N, Jaccoud P, Dorleac E, et al. Alterations of globin chain synthesis and of red cell membrane proteins in congenital dyserythropoietic anemia I and II. Pediatr Res 1982;16:1016.

37. Antonelou M, Papassideri IS, Karababa F, et al. A novel case of haemoglobin H disease associated with clinical and morphological characteristics of congenital dyserythropoietic anaemia type I. Eur J Haematol 2002;68:247.

38. Antonelou MH, Papassideri IS, Karababa FJ, et al. Ultrastructural characterization of the erythroid cells in a novel case of congenital anemia. Blood Cells Mol Dis 2003;30:30.

39. Iolascon A, D'Agostaro G, Perrotta S, et al. Congenital dyserythropoietic anemia type II: molecular basis and clinical aspects. Haematologica 1996;81:543.

40. Perrotta S, del Giudice EM, Carbone R, et al. Gilbert's syndrome accounts for the phenotypic variability of congenital dyserythropoietic anemia type II (CDA-II). J Pediatr 2000;136:556.

41. Bird AR, Jacobs P, Moores P. Congenital dyserythropoietic anaemia (type II) presenting with haemosiderosis. Acta Haematol 1987;78:33.

42. Lugassy G, Michaeli J, Harats N, et al. Paravertebral extramedullary hematopoiesis associated with improvement of anemia in congenital dyserythropoietic anemia type II. Am J Hematol 1986;22:295.

43. Hines GL. Paravertebral extramedullary hematopoiesis (as a posterior mediastinal tumor) associated with congenital dyserythropoietic anemia. J Thorac Cardiovasc Surg 1993;106:760.

44. Imran A, Mawhinney R, Swirsky D, et al. Paravertebral extramedullary haemopoiesis occurring in a case of congenital dyserythropoietic anaemia type II. Br J Haematol 2008;140:1.

45. Steiner W, Denzlinger C, Weiss M. [Paravertebral extramedullary hematopoiesis in congenital dyserythropoietic anemia type II (CDA II)]. Rontgenpraxis 1995;48: 110.

46. Halpern Z, Rahmani R, Levo Y. Severe hemochromatosis: the predominant clinical manifestation of congenital dyserythropoietic anemia type 2. Acta Haematol 1985;74:178.

47. Tamura H, Matsumoto G, Itakura Y, et al. A case of congenital dyserythropoietic anemia type II associated with hemochromatosis. Intern Med 1992;31:380.

48. West NC, Meigh RE, Mackie M, et al. Parvovirus infection associated with aplastic crisis in a patient with HEMPAS. J Clin Pathol 1986;39:1019.

49. Heimpel H, Wilts H, Hirschmann WD, et al. Aplastic crisis as a complication of congenital dyserythropoietic anemia type II. Acta Haematol 2007;117:115.

50. Verwilghen RL, Lewis SM, Dacie JV, et al. HEMPAS: congenital dyserythropoietic anaemia (type II). Q J Med 1973;42:257.

51. Van Dorpe A, Broeckaert-van O, Desmet V, et al. Gaucher-like cells and congenital dyserythropoietic anaemia, type II (HEMPAS). Br J Haematol 1973;25:165.

52. Verwilghen RL, Tan P, De Wolf-Peeters C, et al. Cell membrane anomaly impeding cell division. Experientia 1971;27:1467.

53. Wong KY, Hug G, Lampkin BC. Congenital dyserythropoietic anemia type II: ultrastructural and radioautographic studies of blood and bone marrow. Blood 1972;39:23.

54. Alloisio N, Texier P, Denoroy L, et al. The cisternae decorating the red blood cell membrane in congenital dyserythropoietic anemia (type II) originate from the endoplasmic reticulum. Blood 1996;87:4433.

55. Crookston JH, Crookston MC, Burnie KL, et al. Hereditary erythroblastic multinuclearity associated with a positive acidified-serum test: a type of congenital dyserythropoietic anaemia. Br J Haematol 1969;17:11.

56. Benjamin JT, Rosse WF, Daldorf FG, et al. Congential dyserythropoietic anemia—type IV. J Pediatr 1975;87:210.

57. Lowenthal RM, Marsden KA, Dewar CL, et al. Congenital dyserythropoietic anaemia (CDA) with severe gout, rare Kell phenotype and erythrocyte, granulocyte and platelet membrane reduplication: a new variant of CDA type II. Br J Haematol 1980;44:211.

58. Mawby WJ, Tanner MJ, Anstee DJ, et al. Incomplete glycosylation of erythrocyte membrane proteins in congenital dyserythropoietic anaemia type II (CDA II). Br J Haematol 1983;55:357.

59. Baines AJ, Banga JP, Gratzer WB, et al. Red cell membrane protein anomalies in congenital dyserythropoietic anaemia, type II (HEMPAS). Br J Haematol 1982; 50:563.

60. Scartezzini P, Forni GL, Baldi M, et al. Decreased glycosylation of band 3 and band 4.5 glycoproteins of erythrocyte membrane in congenital dyserythropoietic anaemia type II. Br J Haematol 1982;51:569.

61. Tomita A, Parker CJ. Aberrant regulation of complement by the erythrocytes of hereditary erythroblastic multinuclearity with a positive acidified serum lysis test (HEMPAS). Blood 1994;83:250.

62. Zdebska E, Golaszewska E, Fabijanska-Mitek J, et al. Glycoconjugate abnormalities in patients with congenital dyserythropoietic anaemia type I, II and III. Br J Haematol 2001;114:907.

63. Denecke J, Kranz C, Nimtz M, et al. Characterization of the N-glycosylation phenotype of erythrocyte membrane proteins in congenital dyserythropoietic anemia type II (CDA II/HEMPAS). Glycoconj J 2008;25:375.
64. Sandstrom H, Wahlin A. Congenital dyserythropoietic anemia type III. Haematologica 2000;85:753.
65. Wolff JA, Von Hofe FH. Familial erythroid multinuclearity. Blood 1951;6:1274.
66. Bergstrom I, Jacobsson L. Hereditary benign erythroreticulosis. Blood 1962;19:296.
67. Accame EA, de Tezanos Pinto M. [Congenital dyserythropoiesis with erythroblastic polyploidy. Report of a variety found in Argentinian Mesopotamia (author's translation)]. Sangre (Barc) 1981;26:545.
68. Byrnes RK, Dhru R, Brady AM, et al. Congenital dyserythropoietic anemia in treated Hodgkin's disease. Hum Pathol 1980;11:485.
69. McCluggage WG, Hull D, Mayne E, et al. Malignant lymphoma in congenital dyserythropoietic anaemia type III. J Clin Pathol 1996;49:599.
70. Goudsmit R, Beckers D, De Bruijne JI, et al. Congenital dyserythropoietic anaemia, type 3. Br J Haematol 1972;23:97.
71. Wickramasinghe SN, Parry TE, Williams C, et al. A new case of congenital dyserythropoietic anaemia, type III: studies of the cell cycle distribution and ultrastructure of erythroblasts and of nucleic acid synthesis in marrow cells. J Clin Pathol 1982;35:1103.
72. Jijina F, Ghosh K, Yavagal D, et al. A patient with congenital dyserythropoietic anaemia type III presenting with stillbirths. Acta Haematol 1998;99:31.
73. Rohrig G, Kilter H, Beuckelmann D, et al. Congenital dyserythropoietic anemia type III associated with congenital atrioseptal defect has led to severe cardiac problems in a 32-year-old patient. Am J Hematol 2000;64:314.
74. Sigler E, Shaft D, Shtalrid M, et al. New sporadic case of congenital dyserythropoietic anemia type III in an aged woman: detailed description of ultrastructural findings. Am J Hematol 2002;70:72.
75. Krouwels FH, Bresser P, von dem Borne AE. Extramedullary hematopoiesis: breathtaking and hair-raising. N Engl J Med 1999;341:1702.
76. Clauvel JP, Cosson A, Breton-Gorius J, et al. [Congenital dyserythropoiesis (study of 6 cases)]. Nouv Rev Fr Hematol 1972;12:653.
77. Noy-Lotan S, Dgany O, Lahmi R, et al. Codanin-1, the protein encoded by the gene mutated in CDA-1 (CDAN1), is cell-cycle regulated. In: 50th Annual Meeting of the American Society of Hematology. San Francisco, USA, 2008.
78. Renella R, Roberts NA, Sharpe J, et al. A transgenic mouse model for congenital dyserythropoietic anemia type 1. In: 50th Annual Meeting of the American Society of Hematology. San Francisco, USA, 2008.
79. Ahmed MR, Chehal A, Zahed L, et al. Linkage and mutational analysis of the CDAN1 gene reveals genetic heterogeneity in congenital dyserythropoietic anemia type I. Blood 2006;107:4968.
80. Ahmed MR, Zaki M, Sabry MA, et al. Evidence of genetic heterogeneity in congenital dyserythropoietic anaemia type I. Br J Haematol 2006;133:444.
81. Lanzara C, Ficarella R, Totaro A, et al. Congenital dyserythropoietic anemia type II: exclusion of seven candidate genes. Blood Cells Mol Dis 2003;30:22.
82. Iolascon A, De Mattia D, Perrotta S, et al. Genetic heterogeneity of congenital dyserythropoietic anemia type II. Blood 1998;92:2593.
83. Fukuda MN. Congenital dyserythropoietic anaemia type II (HEMPAS) and its molecular basis. Baillieres Clin Haematol 1993;6:493.

84. Bouhours JF, Bouhours D, Delaunay J. Abnormal fatty acid composition of erythrocyte glycosphingolipids in congenital dyserythropoietic anemia type II. J Lipid Res 1985;26:435.

85. Zdebska E, Anselstetter V, Pacuszka T, et al. Glycolipids and glycopeptides of red cell membranes in congenital dyserythropoietic anaemia type II (CDA II). Br J Haematol 1987;66:385.

86. Fukuda MN, Dell A, Scartezzini P. Primary defect of congenital dyserythropoietic anemia type II. Failure in glycosylation of erythrocyte lactosaminoglycan proteins caused by lowered N-acetylglucosaminyltransferase II. J Biol Chem 1987;262:7195.

87. Fukuda MN, Gaetani GF, Izzo P, et al. Incompletely processed N-glycans of serum glycoproteins in congenital dyserythropoietic anaemia type II (HEMPAS). Br J Haematol 1992;82:745.

88. Fukuda MN, Klier G, Yu J, et al. Anomalous clustering of underglycosylated band 3 in erythrocytes and their precursor cells in congenital dyserythropoietic anemia type II. Blood 1986;68:521.

89. Fukuda MN, Masri KA, Dell A, et al. Defective glycosylation of erythrocyte membrane glycoconjugates in a variant of congenital dyserythropoietic anemia type II: association of low level of membrane-bound form of galactosyltransferase. Blood 1989;73:1331.

90. Iolascon A, Miraglia del Giudice E, Perrotta S, et al. Exclusion of three candidate genes as determinants of congenital dyserythropoietic anemia type II (CDA-II). Blood 1997;90:4197.

91. Zdebska E, Mendek-Czajkowska E, Ploski R, et al. Heterozygosity of CDAN II (HEMPAS) gene may be detected by the analysis of erythrocyte membrane glycoconjugates from healthy carriers. Haematologica 2002;87:126.

92. Zdebska E, Wozniewicz B, Adamowicz-Salach A, et al. Short report: erythrocyte membranes from a patient with congenital dyserythropoietic anaemia type I (CDA-I) show identical, although less pronounced, glycoconjugate abnormalities to those from patients with CDA-II (HEMPAS). Br J Haematol 2000;110:998.

93. Paw BH, Davidson AJ, Zhou Y, et al. Cell-specific mitotic defect and dyserythropoiesis associated with erythroid band 3 deficiency. Nat Genet 2003;34:59.

94. Nichols KE, Crispino JD, Poncz M, et al. Familial dyserythropoietic anaemia and thrombocytopenia due to an inherited mutation in GATA1. Nat Genet 2000;24:266.

95. Lavabre-Bertrand T, Blanc P, Navarro R, et al. Alpha-interferon therapy for congenital dyserythropoiesis type I. Br J Haematol 1995;89:929.

96. Lavabre-Bertrand T, Ramos J, Delfour C, et al. Long-term alpha interferon treatment is effective on anaemia and significantly reduces iron overload in congenital dyserythropoiesis type I. Eur J Haematol 2004;73:380.

97. Dubois J, Hershon L, Carmant L, et al. Toxicity profile of interferon alfa-2b in children: a prospective evaluation. J Pediatr 1999;135:782.

98. Marwaha RK, Bansal D, Trehan A, et al. Interferon therapy in congenital dyserythropoietic anemia type I/II. Pediatr Hematol Oncol 2005;22:133.

99. Tamary H, Shalev H, Pinsk V, et al. No response to recombinant human erythropoietin therapy in patients with congenital dyserythropoietic anemia type I. Pediatr Hematol Oncol 1999;16:165.

100. Iolascon A, Delaunay J, Wickramasinghe SN, et al. Natural history of congenital dyserythropoietic anemia type II. Blood 2001;98:1258.

101. Bolton-Maggs P, Stevens R, Dodd N, et al. Guidelines for the diagnosis and management of hereditary spherocytosis. Br J Haematol 2004;126:455.

102. Perrotta S, Gallagher PG, Mohandas N. Hereditary spherocytosis. Lancet 2008; 372:1411.
103. Barosi G, Cazzola M, Stefanelli M, et al. Studies of ineffective erythropoiesis and peripheral haemolysis in congenital dyserythropoietic anaemia type II. Br J Haematol 1979;43:243.
104. Choudhry VP, Saraya AK, Kasturi J, et al. Congenital dyserythropoietic anaemias: splenectomy as a mode of therapy. Acta Haematol 1981;66:195.
105. Maeda K, Saeed SM, Rebuck JW, et al. Type I dyserythropoietic anemia. A 30-year follow-up. Am J Clin Pathol 1980;73:433.
106. Samson D, Halliday D, Chanarin I. Congenital dyserythropoietic anaemia: response to splenectomy and quantitation of ineffective erythropoiesis. J Clin Pathol 1977;30:184.
107. Bird AR, Karabus CD, Hartley PS. Type IV congenital dyserythropoietic anemia with an unusual response to splenectomy. Am J Pediatr Hematol Oncol 1985;7: 196.
108. Ayas M, al-Jefri A, Baothman A, et al. Transfusion-dependent congenital dyserythropoietic anemia type I successfully treated with allogeneic stem cell transplantation. Bone Marrow Transplant 2002;29:681.
109. Iolascon A, Sabato V, de Mattia D, et al. Bone marrow transplantation in a case of severe, type II congenital dyserythropoietic anaemia (CDA II). Bone Marrow Transplant 2001;27:213.
110. Remacha AF, Badell I, Pujol-Moix N, et al. Hydrops fetalis-associated congenital dyserythropoietic anemia treated with intrauterine transfusions and bone marrow transplantation. Blood 2002;100:356.
111. Ariffin WA, Karnaneedi S, Choo KE, et al. Congenital dyserythropoietic anaemia: report of three cases. J Paediatr Child Health 1996;32:191.
112. Carter C, Darbyshire PJ, Wickramasinghe SN. A congenital dyserythropoietic anaemia variant presenting as hydrops fetalis. Br J Haematol 1989;72:289.
113. Wickramasinghe SN, Vora AJ, Will A, et al. Transfusion-dependent congenital dyserythropoietic anaemia with non-specific dysplastic changes in erythroblasts. Eur J Haematol 1998;60:140.
114. Israel LG. The bilirubin shunt and shunt hyperbilirubinemia. In: Popper H, Schaffner F, editors. Progress in liver disease III. New York & London: Grune and Stratton, Inc; 1970. p. 1.
115. Bird AR, Knottenbelt E, Jacobs P, et al. Primary shunt hyperbilirubinaemia: a variant of the congenital dyserythropoietic anaemias. Postgrad Med J 1991; 67:396.
116. Frank DJ, Dusol M, Schiff ER. Primary shunt hyperbilirubinemia with secondary iron overload: a case report. Gastroenterology 1979;77:754.
117. Ohisalo JJ, Viitala J, Lintula R, et al. A new congenital dyserythropoietic anaemia. Br J Haematol 1988;68:111.
118. Hamer JW, Fitzgerald PH. Disturbed bone marrow cell proliferation in primary shunt hyperbilirubinemia. Blood 1973;41:539.
119. Wickramasinghe SN, Andrews VE, O'Hea AM. Congenital dyserythropoiesis characterized by marked macrocytosis, vitamin B12- and folate-independent megaloblastic change and absence of the defining features of congenital dyserythropoietic anaemia types I or III. Br J Haematol 1996;95:73.
120. Iolascon A, Martire B, Lee MJ, et al. Transfusion-dependent congenital dyserythropoietic anaemia with intraerythroblastic inclusions of a non-globin protein. Eur J Haematol 2000;65:140.

121. Wickramasinghe SN, Lee MJ, Furukawa T, et al. Composition of the intra-erythroblastic precipitates in thalassaemia and congenital dyserythropoietic anaemia (CDA): identification of a new type of CDA with intra-erythroblastic precipitates not reacting with monoclonal antibodies to alpha- and beta-globin chains. Br J Haematol 1996;93:576.
122. Bethlenfalvay NC, Hadnagy C, Heimpel H. Unclassified type of congenital dyserythropoietic anaemia (CDA) with prominent peripheral erythroblastosis. Br J Haematol 1985;60:541.
123. Adams CD, Kessler JF. Circulating nucleated red blood cells following splenectomy in a patient with congenital dyserythropoietic anemia. Am J Hematol 1991; 38:120.
124. Agre P, Smith BL, Baumgarten R, et al. Human red cell Aquaporin CHIP. II. Expression during normal fetal development and in a novel form of congenital dyserythropoietic anemia. J Clin Invest 1994;94:1050.
125. Parsons SF, Jones J, Anstee DJ, et al. A novel form of congenital dyserythropoietic anemia associated with deficiency of erythroid CD44 and a unique blood group phenotype [In(a-b-), Co(a-b-)]. Blood 1994;83:860.
126. Wickramasinghe SN, Illum N, Wimberley PD. Congenital dyserythropoietic anaemia with novel intra-erythroblastic and intra-erythrocytic inclusions. Br J Haematol 1991;79:322.
127. Wickramasinghe SN, Spearing RL, Hill GR. Congenital dyserythropoiesis with intererythroblastic chromatin bridges and ultrastructurally-normal erythroblast heterochromatin: a new disorder. Br J Haematol 1998;103:831.
128. Kenny MW, Ibbotson RM, Hand MJ, et al. Congenital dyserythropoietic anaemia with unusual cytoplasmic inclusions. J Clin Pathol 1978;31:1228.
129. Woessner S, Trujillo M, Florensa L, et al. Congenital dyserthropoietic anaemia other than type I to III with a peculiar erythroblastic morphology. Eur J Haematol 2003;71:211.
130. Heimpel H, Kohne E, Schrod L, et al. A new type of transfusion-dependent congenital dyserythropoietic anemia. Haematologica 2007;92:1427.
131. Němec J, Polák. Erythropoietic polyploidy. I. The morphology of polyploid erythroid elements and their incidence in healthy subjects. Folia Haematol Int Mag Klin Morphol Blutforsch 1965;84(1):24–40.

Severe Congenital Neutropenia

Karl Welte, MD[a],*, Cornelia Zeidler, MD[b]

KEYWORDS

- G-CSFR mutations • ELA2 • HAX1
- Severe congenital neutropenia
- Acute myelogenous leukemia

The current knowledge of the pathophysiologic mechanisms of severe congenital neutropenia (CN) suggests that CN is a heterogeneous disorder with a common hematologic and clinical phenotype characterized by a maturation arrest of myelopoiesis at the level of the promyelocyte/myelocyte stage with peripheral blood absolute neutrophil counts (ANCs) below $0.5 \times 10^9/L$ and early onset of bacterial infections. CN follows an autosomal dominant or autosomal recessive pattern of inheritance. During the last 10 years, marked progress has been made in identifying the genetic defects causing CN. CN was first described in 1956 by Rolf Kostmann[1] as an autosomal recessive hematologic disorder with severe neutropenia with an ANC below $0.5 \times 10^9/L$ and early onset of severe bacterial infections,[1] later termed "Kostmann syndrome." The underlying genetic defect of Kostmann syndrome has been identified recently as mutations in the *HAX1* gene.[2,3] Genetic analyses in autosomal dominant and sporadic cases of CN indicate that most of these cases are attributable to mutations in the elastase 2 (*ELA2*) gene encoding neutrophil elastase.[4,5] In addition, other less frequent mutations have been identified, such as *p14*, *G6PC3*, *TAZ*, and *WASP* in recessive CN and *GFI-1* in dominant CN. CN needs to be differentiated from secondary causes of neutropenia such as autoimmune neutropenia, infection, and drug-induced neutropenia.

Both the prognosis and the quality of life of patients who have CN improved dramatically following the introduction of granulocyte colony-stimulating factor (G-CSF) therapy in 1987.[6] Since the establishment of the Severe Chronic Neutropenia International Registry (SCNIR) in 1994, data on more than 700 patients who had or have CN have been collected worldwide to monitor the clinical course, treatment, and disease outcomes in these patients. More than 90% of patients who have CN respond to

This work was supported by the German Network on Congenital Bone Marrow Failure Syndromes, Deutsche Forschungsgemeinschaft, and Deutsche Jose Carreras Leukämie-Stiftung e.V.

[a] Department of Molecular Hematopoiesis, Kinderklinik, Medizinische Hochschule Hannover, Carl-Neuberg-Str.1, D-30625 Hannover, Germany
[b] Department of Molecular Hematopoiesis, Severe Chronic Neutropenia Registry, Kinderklinik, Medizinische Hochschule Hannover, Carl-Neuberg-Str.1, D-30625 Hannover, Germany
* Corresponding author.
E-mail address: welte.karl.h@mh-hannover.de (K. Welte).

Hematol Oncol Clin N Am 23 (2009) 307–320
doi:10.1016/j.hoc.2009.01.013
0889-8588/09/$ – see front matter © 2009 Elsevier Inc. All rights reserved.

G-CSF treatment with an increase in ANC to more than 1.0×10^9/L. Importantly, all responding patients require significantly fewer antibiotics and days of hospitalization.[7-11] G-CSF clearly is the treatment of choice in patients who have this disorder. Hematopoietic stem cell transplantation (HSCT) remains the only currently available treatment for patients who have disease refractory to G-CSF and for patients in whom CN has transformed into myelodysplastic syndrome and leukemia.[12]

DIAGNOSIS

CN usually is detected in infancy or during the first months of life because of recurrent severe infections (eg, pneumonitis, abscesses). Diagnosis requires repeated differential blood counts indicating persistent neutropenia with an ANC range of 0 to 0.5×10^9/L. Blood monocytes and blood eosinophil counts usually are elevated. Intriguingly, the level of serum immunoglobulins often is elevated.[11] Anti-neutrophil–specific antibodies are absent.[13] The bone marrow usually shows a maturation arrest of neutrophil precursors at the promyelocyte/myelocyte stage independent of the genetic subtypes. Promyelocytes often reveal morphologic atypical nuclei and vacuolization of the cytoplasm. The number of promyelocytes is increased slightly.[10] Bone marrow cellularity usually is normal or slightly decreased. Current data suggest that CN is a multigene disorder.

PATHOPHYSIOLOGY
ELA2 Congenital Neutropenia

Heterozygous mutations in the ELA2 gene are the most common genetic abnormality, found in approximately 50% to 60% of patients who have CN, suggesting a dominant mechanism of action.[4,5] Some cases of CN with ELA2 mutations arise sporadically, however, consistent with its transmission as an autosomal dominant disorder.[5] More than 50 ELA2 mutations in all five exons have been described in patients who have CN, resulting in proteins with a wide range of enzyme activities. No obvious connection could be made linking the abnormalities of the mutant proteins and neutropenia. Two case reports of paternal mosaicism for an ELA2 mutation also provide evidence for autosomal dominant inheritance and suggest that mutant neutrophil elastase (NE) protein has no effect on wild-type neutrophils.[14,15] Evidence for the causative role of ELA2 mutations is derived from a recently published study of five unrelated children from healthy mothers who had been impregnated with the semen from the same sperm donor.[16] Furthermore, mutations in the ELA2 gene are responsible for the clinical phenotype of cyclic neutropenia, another autosomal dominant inherited disorder with regular neutropenic phases caused by the cycling of blood cells but less severe infections. Genetic analysis has shown that ELA2 mutations can occur at the same site of the gene in patients who have congenital and cyclic neutropenia. The pathophysiologic mechanisms responsible for the development of the different phenotypes—congenital or cyclic neutropenia—are not yet understood. The diversity of mutations within the ELA2 gene in CN and the lack of any consistent effect of the mutated NE protein on its enzymatic properties[5] led the authors and others to hypothesize that structural rather than functional enzymatic properties of the mutated NE protein may be responsible for the neutropenia.[17,18] Three studies hypothesize that mutations in the ELA2 gene result in the production of misfolded NE protein in the endoplasmatic reticulum (ER) that induces an unfolded protein response (UPR) and the subsequent UPR-dependent apoptosis.[17-19] Indeed, the chaperone family member HsP70 protein BiP, which is associated with misfolded protein–induced ER stress, was up-regulated in CN.[17] Interestingly, neither targeting of CN-associated mutations into murine ELA2[18] nor complete deletion of ELA2[20] has an effect on murine hematopoiesis, a finding that supports the notion that enzymatic NE activities are not required for granulopoiesis. An as yet unexplained finding is that the expression of NE protein is severely down-regulated in CN, independent of the presence of ELA2 mutations.[21,22] In summary, further studies regarding the role of ELA2 mutations in CN are required to explain the pathophysiologic mechanism leading to a maturation arrest of promyelocytes in these patients.

HAX1 Congenital Neutropenia

Biallelic HAX1 mutations were detected in patients belonging to the original pedigree described by Kostmann[1] and were found in patients who had CN who were born of consanguineous parents.[2] HAX1-CN is an autosomal recessive form of CN. Patients who have HAX1 mutations did not have mutations in the ELA2 gene. HAX1 protein is a mitochondrial molecule with distant structural similarity to the anti-apoptotic members of the Bcl2 family, but the pathophysiologic mechanisms of neutropenia are not completely resolved. Mitochondrial inner membrane permeabilization, manifested as a dissipation of $\Delta\Psi_m$, compromises the vital function of mitochondria and leads to cell death associated with release of proteins such as cytochrome c, Smac/DIABLO, and Omi/HtrA2 from the intermembrane space into the cytosol. Studies in a murine Hax1-knockout model suggest that suppression of apoptosis by HAX1 is dependent on the mitochondrial proteases Parl (presenilin-associated, rhomboid-like) and HtrA2/Omi (high-temperature regulated A2).[23] The biochemical interaction of Parl, HtrA2/Omi, and Hax1 allows Hax1 to present HtrA2 to Parl, thereby facilitating the proteolytic cleavage of HtrA2 to the active protease. Processed HtrA2 prevents Bax-mediated mitochondrial apoptosis. Although these studies shed light on mechanisms of HAX1 in controlling apoptosis, it remains unclear why in human patients premature cell death of neutrophils is the most obvious and consistent finding in HAX1 deficiency. Whether HAX1 may have additional functions is under active investigation. Central nervous system involvement seems to be restricted to patients in whom the HAX1 mutation affects both alternatively spliced isoforms of HAX1.[3]

G6PC3 Congenital Neutropenia

The authors recently have identified a previously unrecognized syndrome associated with CN and variable extra-hematopoietic features caused by biallelic mutations in the gene encoding the glucose-6-phosphate catalytic subunit 3 (G6PC3).[24] Eleven of the 12 patients also had additional organ involvement, including structural heart defects or urogenital defects, and increased visibility of superficial veins. The role of G6PC3 in granulopoiesis is supported by the finding that $g6pc3^{-/-}$ knockout mice also reveal neutropenia and increased myeloid cell apoptosis.[25] In contrast to glycogen storage disease, type Ib, which also is associated with severe neutropenia, patients who have G6PC3-CN do not reveal glycogen storage symptoms. Because in glycogen storage disease, type Ib, the glucose-6-phosphate transporter (G6PT) is defective and because G6PT forms a complex with G6PC3, it is very likely that the G6PT/G6PC3 complex is needed to maintain myeloid cell viability, including neutrophil homeostasis. The underlying pathway leading to neutropenia in the absence of G6PC3 involves increased ER stress and increased apoptosis.[24]

OTHER RARE CAUSES OF CONGENITAL NEUTROPENIA

Neutropenia caused by mutations in other genes such as GFI-1,[26] WASP,[27,28] p14,[29] TAZ,[30] and others is very rare and has been reported in only a few patients or families.

COMMON PATHOPHYSIOLOGIC MECHANISMS

Patients who have ELA2-, HAX1-, or G6PC3 mutations reveal a similar morphologic and similar clinical phenotype in terms of myelopoiesis, suggesting these mutations cause common downstream molecular events. Both misfolded elastase protein and G6PC3 protein cause ER stress and an UPR. The UPR induces a general decrease of protein synthesis by inhibiting translation initiation, increasing chaperone protein expression, and activating ER-associated protein degradation.[31] If these responses are inadequate to compensate for the quantity of misfolded proteins, they induce apoptosis through increased caspase expression.[31] HAX1 mutation leading to lack of a functional HAX1 protein compromises a vital function of mitochondria, also leading to increased apoptosis. The link between mitochondrial dysfunction, ER stress, and cell death is well known.[31] Downstream signals secondary to these events include lack of expression of the transcription factor LEF-1 and subsequent C/EBP-alpha down-regulation, reducing survival and differentiation of granulocytic progenitors and leading to the maturation arrest of granulopoiesis in bone marrow and decreased blood neutrophils.[32] C/EBP-alpha, however, is the transcription factor required for steady-state neutrophilic granulopoiesis. Therefore, the question arises, which transcription factor(s) are responsible for the in vivo response of patients who have CN to pharmacologic doses of G-CSF? In a recent study, the authors were able to document that G-CSF acts through Nampt/PEBF to increase intracellular NAD^+, which in combination with SIRT1 binds and activates C/EBP-beta and leads to the so-called "emergency" neutrophil granulopoiesis.[33]

ACQUIRED GRANULOCYTE COLONY-STIMULATING FACTORS RECEPTOR MUTATIONS

Mutations in a region of the CSF3R gene coding for the intra-cytoplasmic domain of the G-CSF receptor (G-CSFR) were discovered in 1994[34] and initially were suggested as the cause of CN. In the following years it became obvious that these mutations were acquired somatic mutations arising during the lifetime of patients who had CN.[35,36] All mutations introduce a stop codon predicted to lead to the truncation of the intracellular part of the G-CSFR protein with the loss of the C-terminal–negative regulatory domain and leading to a loss of one or more tyrosines.[35] In most patients, however, only one allele of CSF3R is affected. Expression of these mutations in myeloid cell lines leads to enhanced proliferation, resistance to apoptosis, and increased cell survival.[37–39] Knock-in mice bearing receptor mutants equivalent to those found in patients who have CN revealed a hyperproliferative response to exogenous G-CSF, but, despite prolonged G-CSF administration, no patient developed leukemia.[39] In the authors' recent study,[40] CSF3R mutation analysis could be performed in 148 patients who had CN, of whom 61 (41%) harbored CSF3R mutations. Even 5 of 30 patients tested before G-CSF treatment revealed CSF3R mutations, suggesting that G-CSF administration is not responsible for these mutations. Interestingly, no mutations were detected in patients who had cyclic neutropenia or other types of chronic neutropenia. The incidence of CSF3R mutations in patients who had CN but who thus far had not developed leukemia was 34% (43 of 125 patients) and was 78% in patients whose disease had progressed to acute myelogenous leukemia (AML) or acute lymphoid leukemia (18 of 23 patients). CSF3R mutations were detected at 17 different nucleotide positions.[40] Some patients displayed a CSF3R mutation at one nucleotide position only, whereas other patients were found to harbor mutations at two or more nucleotide positions. In many cases increasing numbers of different mutations developed during the patient's lifetime. Low percentages of clones were detected at initial analysis, with the frequency of mutation (both the number of different nucleotides and the number of positive clones) increasing over several years,[40,41] suggesting genetic instability of at least the *CSF3R* gene.

The percentage of patients who have CN and who harbor *CSF3R* mutations reported by the authors (40%) is higher than that in studies reported by other investigators. For instance Ancliff and colleagues[42] reported a frequency of only 7% in a cohort of 29 patients who had CN and argued against the inevitability of leukemic progression in the presence of these mutations. Most of the published data on *CSF3R* mutations in CN cannot be compared with the authors' data because they are biased by the restriction of the analysis only to patients who had CN and who developed leukemia. There are a number of possible explanations for the apparent discrepancy between the different reports. Most of the studies used direct sequencing of cDNA or restriction analysis, which might be inappropriate to detect low levels of heterozygously mutated cells, and screened only for the five mutations previously described. In addition, one could assume a higher cumulative effect in the authors' study compared with others, because the authors survey a large cohort of patients over a period of several years, including patients older than 20 years. This difference also is reflected in the higher percentage of patients who progress to leukemia. From their investigations of the clonal succession of various *CSF3R* mutations, the authors can conclude that the acquisition of a *CSF3R* mutation is an event that does occur before malignant transformation.[40] The highly elevated risk for leukemic progression in patients who have acquired a *CSF3R* mutation argues that these mutations contribute significantly to leukemogenesis.

The way *CSF3R* mutations are acquired in the course of a lifetime and the way these cells contribute to the progression to leukemia still are not understood. One possible explanation is that the truncated G-CSFR protein affects G-CSFR endocytosis and G-CSFR signaling.[43–46] Indeed, cells harboring mutated G-CSFR protein reveal activated (phosphorylated) STAT5 protein, most likely by defective endocytosis of G-CSFR, thereby prolonging the G-CSFR signaling. Touw and colleagues[44] suggested that SOCS3 efficiently suppresses STAT3 and STAT5 activation by G-CSFR in wild-type cells, whereas in cells harboring truncated G-CSFR SOCS3 still inhibits STAT3, but the inhibition of STAT5 activation is completely lost.[44–46] SOCS3-induced inhibition of STAT5 requires mechanisms controlled by the G-CSFR C-terminus, which is missing in the G-CSFR (*CSF3R*) mutated protein. The increased STAT5/STAT3 activation ratio results in signaling abnormalities of truncated G-CSFR (*CSF3R*) that might be leukemogenic.[44] The authors and others have shown that constitutive activation of STAT5 alters myelopoiesis by down-regulation of myeloid-associated differentiation factors such as C/EBP-alpha[47,48] and LEF-1.[32] Recently the authors found that G-CSF–treated myeloid progenitor cells from patients who have CN express high levels of activated phospho-STAT5 protein.[49] These data were confirmed further by findings in a recently published mouse model.[50] These investigators have shown that G-CSFR (*CSF3R*) mutations confer a strong clonal advantage of hematopoietic stem cells via activation of STAT5 that is dependent on exogenous G-CSF.[50,51] Activated STAT5 multimerizes and then translocates to the nucleus to function as a transcription factor. Defining promoter binding sites unique to stem cells bearing the G-CSFR (*CSF3R*) mutation may help identify gene products that are directly involved in clonal expansion of hematopoietic stem cells and/or leukemic clones.[51] A possible mechanism of leukemogenesis could be the prolonged activation of STAT5 in G-CSFR (*CSF3R*) mutation-bearing cells, rendering them susceptible to additional molecular aberrations. Intriguingly, levels of another protein reported to be involved in leukemogenesis, the proto-oncogene β-catenin,[52] were found to be two to three times higher and were nuclear translocated in CD33$^+$ cells from patients who had CN, as compared with healthy individuals (authors' observation). It is very likely, however, that in addition to these two leukemogenic pathways, other molecules might contribute to the development of overt leukemia.

In a recent study the authors were able to demonstrate that *CSF3R* mutations are not restricted to the myeloid compartment but also are detectable in lymphoid cells, although in lower percentages.[53] In this study the authors also showed that the mutated G-CSFR–bearing cells have an growth advantage in vivo over cells without mutation. The altered signaling in *CSF3R*-mutated cells that confers a G-CSF–dependent competitive advantage over hematopoietic progenitors may provide a background for the acquisition of additional mutations or chromosomal aberrations that ultimately lead to overt leukemia.

CLINICAL PRESENTATION

At diagnosis ANCs, site of infections, and bone marrow morphology (**Fig. 1**) do not distinguish among patients harboring *ELA2*, *HAX1*, or *G6PC3* mutations. A family history of consanguineous parenthood is indicative for the recessive subtypes with *HAX1* or *G6PC3* mutations, however. In the course of the disease, all patient groups, independent of the underlying genetic defect, respond well to treatment with the hematopoietic growth factor G-CSF but do not respond to granulocyte macrophage-colony stimulating factor.[54] The course of ANCs in patients receiving G-CSF treatment for up to 17 years is shown in **Fig. 2**. In *HAX1*-deficient patients, the onset of neurologic symptoms during childhood (cognitive defects, mental retardation, epilepsy) may be associated with congenital neutropenia.[3,55–57] Recent findings suggest a genotype–phenotype correlation, because central nervous system involvement seems to be restricted to those patients in whom the *HAX1* mutation affects both alternatively spliced isoforms of *HAX1*.[3,55]

The genetic distribution in 122 patients who had CN from the European Branch of the SCNIR (SCNER) tested for *ELA2*, *HAX1*, *G6PC3*, or *p14* mutations is shown in **Fig. 3**. Of the 122 patients who were tested and registered by the SCHER, 65 patients harbored *ELA2* mutations, 16 had *HAX1* mutations, 7 had *G6PC3* mutations, and 4 had *p14* mutations. Thirty patients were negative for all mutations tested. Currently a comprehensive genetic analysis of all registered patients within the SCNIR is ongoing to determine the prevalence of *HAX1/ELA2* and other mutations. The authors

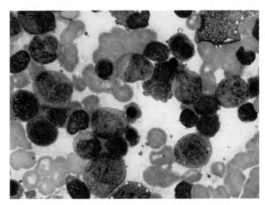

Fig. 1. Bone marrow morphology at diagnosis. Primitive myeloid precursors are abundant, but there is a complete maturation arrest at the promyelocyte/myelocyte stage.

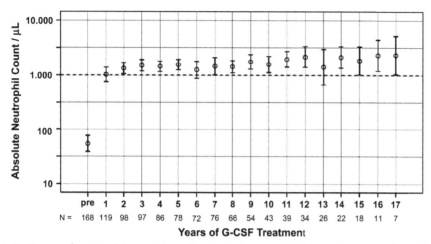

Fig. 2. Course of neutrophil counts in patients who have received G-CSF treatment for CN for up to 17 years.

anticipate that the frequency of mutations in various neutropenia-related genes will be associated with ethnic background and consanguinity. Patients in both *HAX1*-CN and *ELA2*-CN groups have an increased risk of leukemic transformation, whereas no leukemias have been reported so far in any of the other groups of patients with known mutations (eg, *G6PC3*, *WASP*, *p14*, *GFI1*). Under cytokine treatment, the most important parameter for the risk of bacterial infections is the neutrophil count, not the genetic subtype. Therefore maintenance of sufficient neutrophil counts (> 1000/μL) is essential to minimize the risk of severe infections. Patients who have these blood counts still may suffer from gingivitis, however, and may develop early periodontitis even during childhood. A current study evaluates the correlation between genetic subtype, ANC response, and dental care. Preliminary results suggest no difference by genetic subtype but a lower risk with sufficient mean ANCs and continuous good dental hygiene.[58,59] The development of early-onset osteopenia and osteoporosis has been reported in approximately 40% of patients,[60] but the underlying pathomechansims in patients who have CN still are unclear. The development of osteopenia also seems to be independent of the underlying genetic defect, but further genotype–phenotype correlation analysis is required.

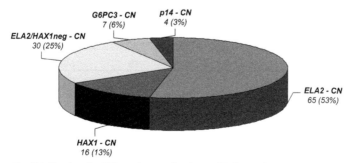

Fig. 3. Genetic distribution in 122 patients who have CN from the European Branch of the Severe Chronic Neutropenia International Registry tested for *ELA2*, *HAX1*, *G6PC3*, or *p14*.

Besides the hematopoietic manifestation, genetic subtypes may present with additional clinical features, such as organ anomalies of the heart and urogenital tract in *G6PC3*-CN and neurologic abnormalities (eg, seizures and delayed mental development) in a percentage of patients who have *HAX1*-CN. It is known from other bone marrow failure syndromes associated with neutropenia, such as Shwachman-Diamond syndrome and Barth syndrome, that the clinical presentation may be extremely heterogenous. In the CN subtypes described here, however, the clinical presentation is yet not fully clear, and further clinical features may be described as new patients are identified.

TREATMENT

Since 1987, recombinant human G-CSF has been available for treatment of CN.[6] An extensive study of the first 374 patients demonstrated that the median pretreatment ANC was 129/μL and that ANC increased with G-CSF treatment to a median of 2125/μL.[61] The G-CSF dose to achieve and maintain an ANC above 1000/μL varied between 1 and 120 μg/kg/d, with most patients responding to G-CSF dosages below 25 μg/kg/d.[11,61] Discrimination of G-CSF dosages by genotype (**Table 1**) shows that patients who have *HAX1*-CN require a median dose (5.5 μg/kg/d) similar to the median dose required by patients who have *ELA2*-CN (5 μg/kg/d), suggesting an equivalent severity of the underlying defect of granulocyte differentiation. Patients who have *G6PC3* mutations require a median dose of 4 μg/kg/d. (The statistical significance of these findings is not given because of the limited number of patients in the subgroups.)

For patients who do not respond to G-CSF treatment, HSCT is the only currently available treatment.[12] Following successful transplantation, peripheral blood counts normalize, and patients do not require further G-CSF treatment.

LEUKEMIA SECONDARY TO CONGENITAL NEUTROPENIA

It now is well accepted that CN is a preleukemic syndrome and that a significant proportion of CN patients develop leukemia.[8,9,40,42,62,63]

To identify the risk of leukemic transformation, the SCNIR recently reported in more detail on the first 374 patients who had CN (enrolled from 1987–2000) and who received long-term G-CSF therapy.[61] The cumulative incidence of leukemia was 21% after 10 years.[61] Intriguingly, the risk of leukemia increased with the dose of G-CSF. The cumulative incidence of leukemia was 40% after 20 years in less responsive patients, who require more than 8 μg/kg/d of G-CSF, compared with 11% in more

Table 1
G-CSF dose (μg/kg/d) required according to genetic subtype

Gene Mutation	N	Median	Mean	SD	Minimum	Maximum
ELA2-CN	61	5.00	17.271	35.81	0.17	240.00
HAX1-CN	16	5.50	8.535	8.977	0.70	48.00
ELA2-/HAX1-CN	27	10.00	18.847	30.309	0.7	231.00
G6PC3-CN	7	4.00	4.894	2.999	1.00	15.00
P14-CN	4	5.00	5.043	0.743	3.59	6.00
Total	115	5.39	11.9067	19.41784	0.24	180.00

responsive patients.[61] The data were interpreted as indicating that a poor response to G-CSF defines an at-risk CN population and predicts an adverse outcome.

Within the SCNER, data are available up to 2008. The cumulative incidence of leukemia is approximately 23% (crude rate, 15.4%) for all patients who have CN followed for up to 25 years. The leukemic transformation occurred in the groups of patients who had autosomal dominant CN (with *ELA2* mutations)[64] or autosomal recessive CN (Kostmann syndrome with *HAX1* mutations)[2] but also occurred in patients negative for these mutations, as shown in **Fig. 4**. The subtypes of leukemia were predominantly AML, but acute lymphoid leukemia, chronic myelomonocytic leukemia,[65,66] and bi-phenotypic leukemia[67] also have been reported.

Independent of the genetic subtype, conversion to leukemia in patients who had CN was associated with one or more cellular genetic abnormalities (eg, monosomy 7, *RAS* mutations, trisomy 21, or *G-CSFR* mutations), which may be diagnostically useful to identify subgroups of patients at high risk of developing leukemia. Interestingly, marrow cells from nearly 80% of the patients who had CN who transformed to leukemia showed point mutations in the *G-CSFR* (*CSF3R*) gene, suggesting that these mutations play an important role in leukemogenesis. The frequency of *CSF3R* mutations is much lower (approximately 30%) in patients who have not yet developed leukemia.[40] Both in patients who have *ELA2* mutations and in patients who have *HAX1* mutations, crucial mutations occurred during the course of the disease. The time course between acquisition of a *CSF3R* mutation and development of leukemia varies considerably. In some patients *CSF3R* gene mutations are present only in the leukemic cells. Other patients show single or multiple mutations of the *CSF3R* gene for several years before leukemic transformation.[40,41] Interestingly, *G-CSFR* (*CSF3R*) mutations can be detected in patients transforming not only into AMLs but also acute lymphoid leukemia and chronic myelomonocytic leukemia.[40,65,66] G-CSFR (*CSF3R*) analyses cannot be used for diagnostic purposes in the underlying disease but may be helpful to screen for the risk of malignant transformation, that is, for the growth of preleukemic cell clones and for overt leukemia. The presence of acquired mutations in the *CSF3R* gene is a strong predictor of later leukemic development and therefore should result in more intensive diagnostic monitoring. In contrast

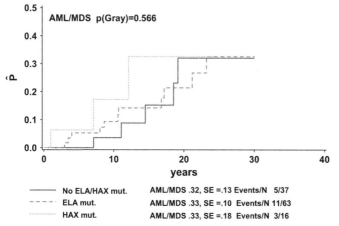

Fig. 4. Thirty-year incidence of leukemia in patients who had CN by subdiagnosis up to June 2008.

to expectations arising from the mouse models, the occurrence of *CSF3R* mutations is not accompanied by a change in response to G-CSF treatment.

Interestingly, in the small group of patients who have *G6PC3* mutations, none of the patients acquired *CSF3R* mutations, and none of the patients has developed leukemia thus far.

Intriguingly, genetic aberrations seen in de novo AML, such as *NPM1* or *FLT3* mutations, were not detected in AML secondary to CN.[68] A recent report hypothesized a link between G-CSF administration and the development of monosomy 7 in patients who have CN,[69] documenting that monosomy 7 cells are abnormally sensitive to high concentrations of G-CSF and that G-CSF leads to an expansion of a pre-existing monosomy 7 clone.

The development of leukemia is a multistep process characterized by a series of cellular genetic changes, suggesting a genetic predisposition to malignant transformation. If and how G-CSF affects this predisposition remains unclear; furthermore, there are no historical controls for comparison to resolve the issue. Long-term therapy with pharmacologic doses of G-CSF may cause genomic instability because of the increased pressure on cell division and DNA replication. Moreover, G-CSF may lead to a preferential secondary outgrowth of a pre-existing cell clone with mutations, for example in the *G-CSFR* (*CSF3R*) gene.[53]

SUMMARY

Gene mutations involved in the pathophysiology of CN include *ELA2* mutations in autosomal dominant CN and *HAX1* mutations in autosomal recessive CN. Clinical presentation and bone marrow morphology do not discriminate between genetic subtypes in early childhood, but additional symptoms such as epilepsy, which are typical for a subgroup of patients who have *HAX1* mutations, may occur later in childhood. Patients who have *G6PC3* or *TAZ* mutations present with additional heart anomalies. The use of G-CSF remains the first-line treatment for all patients who have CN. Maintenance of ANC above 1000/μL is important to prevent severe infections. Independent of the genetic subtype, patients who have CN are at risk of leukemic transformation. The acquisition of *G-CSFR* (*CSF3R*) mutations occurs irrespective of the underlying genetic defect and identifies patients at risk of leukemic transformation. Patients who develop monosomy 7, other significant chromosomal abnormalities, or myelodysplastic syndrome/leukemia should proceed urgently to HSCT. Further analysis of genotype–phenotype correlation is required to identify subgroup-specific risks.

ACKNOWLEDGMENTS

Tha authors are indebted to all patients and their families who agreed to participate in these studies. They also are grateful to the many physicians worldwide who faithfully and generously submitted data on their patients. They thank all colleagues of the Severe Chronic Neutropenia International Registry at the University of Washington, Seattle, Washington (Dr. David Dale, Director) and the European Branch of the Severe Chronic Neutropenia International Registry at the Medizinische Hochschule Hannover, Hannover, Germany.

REFERENCES

1. Kostmann R. Infantile genetic agranulocytosis. Acta Paediatr Scand 1956;45: 1–78.

2. Klein C, Grudzien M, Appaswamy G, et al. HAX1 deficiency causes autosomal recessive severe CN (Kostmann disease). Nat Genet 2007;39:86–92.

3. Germeshausen M, Grudzien M, Zeidler C, et al. Novel HAX1 mutations in patients with severe congenital neutropenia reveal isoform-dependent genotype-phenotype associations. Blood 2008;111:4954–7.

4. Dale DC, Person DE, Bolyard AA, et al. Mutations in the gene encoding neutrophil elastase. Paternal mosaicism proves the pathogenic nature of mutations in neutrophil elastase in severe congenital neutropenia. Blood 2000;100:707–9.

5. Horwitz MS, Duan Z, Korkmaz B, et al. Neutrophil elastase in cyclic and severe congenital neutropenia. Blood 2007;109:1817–24.

6. Bonilla MA, Gillio AP, Ruggeiro, et al. Effects of recombinant human granulocyte colony-stimulating factor on neutropenia in patients with congenital agranulocytosis. N Engl J Med 1989;320:1574–80.

7. Dale DC, Bonilla MA, Davis MW, et al. A randomized controlled phase III trial of recombinant human granulocyte colony-stimulating factor (filgrastim) for treatment of severe chronic neutropenia. Blood 1993;81:2496–502.

8. Freedman MH. Safety of long-term administration of granulocyte colony-stimulating factor for severe chronic neutropenia. Curr Opin Hematol 1997;4:217–24.

9. Welte K, Dale D. Pathophysiology and treatment of severe chronic neutropenia. Ann Hematol 1996;72:158–65.

10. Welte K, Boxer L. Severe chronic neutropenia: pathophysiology and therapy. Semin Hematol 1997;34:267–78.

11. Welte K, Zeidler C, Dale DC. Severe congenital neutropenia. Semin Hematol 2006;43:189–95.

12. Zeidler C, Welte K, Barak Y, et al. Stem cell transplantation in patients with severe CN without evidence of leukemic transformation. Blood 2000;95:1195–8.

13. Bux J, Behrens G, Jaeger G, et al. Diagnosis and clinical course of autoimmune neutropenia in infancy: analysis of 240 cases. Blood 1998;91:181–6.

14. Ancliff PJ, Gale RE, Watts MJ, et al. Paternal mosaicism proves the pathogenic nature of mutations in neutrophil elastase in severe congenital neutropenia. Blood 2002;100:707–9.

15. Germeshausen M, Schulze H, Ballmaier M, et al. Mutations in the gene encoding neutrophil elastase (ELA2) are not sufficient to cause the phenotype of congenital neutropenia. Br J Haematol 2001;115:222–4.

16. Boxer LA, Stein S, Buckley D, et al. Strong evidence for autosomal dominant inheritance of severe congenital neutropenia associated with ELA2 mutations. J Pediatr 2006;148:633–6.

17. Köllner I, Sodeik B, Schreek S, et al. Mutations in neutrophil elastase causing congenital neutropenia lead to cytoplasmic protein accumulation and induction of the unfolded protein response. Blood 2006;108:493–500.

18. Grenda DS, Murakami M, Ghatak J, et al. Mutations of the ELA2 gene found in patients with severe congenital neutropenia induce the unfolded protein response and cellular apoptosis. Blood 2007;110:4179–87.

19. Xia J, Link DC. Severe congenital neutropenia and the unfolded protein response. Curr Opin Hematol 2008;15:1–7 [Review].

20. Belaaouaj A, McCarthy R, Baumann M, et al. Mice lacking neutrophil elastase reveal impaired host defense against gram negative bacterial sepsis. Nat Med 1998;4:615–8.

21. Kawaguchi H, Kobayashi M, Nakamura K, et al. Dysregulation of transcriptions in primary granule constituents during myeloid proliferation and differentiation in patients with severe congenital neutropenia. J Leukoc Biol 2003;73(2):225–34.

22. Skokowa J, Germeshausen M, Zeidler C, et al. Severe congenital neutropenia: inheritance and pathophysiology. Curr Opin Hematol 2007;14:22–8.

23. Chao JR, Parganas E, Boyd K, et al. Hax1-mediated processing of HtrA2 by Parl allows survival of lymphocytes and neurons. Nature 2008;452:98–102.

24. Boztug K, Appaswamy G, Ashikov A, et al. A novel syndrome with severe congenital neutropenia is caused by mutations in G6PC3. N Engl J Med 2009; 360:32–43.

25. Cheung YY, Kim SY, Yiu WH, et al. Impaired neutrophil activity and increased susceptibility to bacterial infections in mice lacking glucose-6-phosphate-beta. J Clin Invest 2007;117:784–93 b.

26. Person RE, Li FQ, Duan Z, et al. Mutations in proto-oncogene GFI1 causes human neutropenia and target ELA2. Nat Genet 2003;34:308–12.

27. Devriendt K, Kim AS, Mathijs G, et al. Constitutive activating mutations in WASP causes X-linked severe congenital neutropenia. Nat Genet 2001;27:313–7.

28. Ancliff PJ, Blundell MP, Cory G, et al. Two novel activating mutations in the Wiskott-Aldrich syndrome protein result in congenital neutropenia. Blood 2006; 108:2182–9.

29. Bohn G, Allroth A, Brandes G, et al. A novel human primary immunodeficiency syndrome caused by deficiency of the endosomal adaptor protein p14. Nat Med 2007;13:38–45.

30. Barth PG, Scholte HR, Berden JA, et al. An X-linked mitochondrial disease affecting cardiac muscle, skeletal muscle and neutrophil leucocytes. J Neurol Sci 1983;62:327–55.

31. Ron D, Walter P. Signal integration in the endoplasmic reticulum unfolded protein response. Natl Rev 2007;8:519–29.

32. Skokowa J, Cario G, Uenalan M, et al. LEF-1 is crucial for neutrophil granulocy-topoiesis and its expression is severely reduced in CN. Nat Med 2006;12:1191–7.

33. Skokowa J, Lan D, Thakur BK, et al. Nampt is essential for the G-CSF induced myeloid differentiation via a novel NAD+/SIRT1-dependent pathway. Nat Med 2009;15:151–8.

34. Dong F, Hoefsloot LH, Schelen AM, et al. Identification of a nonsense mutation in the granulocyte-colony-stimulating factor receptor in severe congenital neutrope-nia. Proc Natl Acad Sci U S A 1994;91(10):4480–4.

35. Dong F, Brynes RK, Tidow N, et al. Mutations in the gene for the granulocyte-colony stimulating factor receptor in patients with acute myeloid leukemia preceded by severe CN. N Engl J Med 1995;333:487–93.

36. Tidow N, Pilz C, Teichmann B, et al. Clinical relevance of point mutations in the cytoplasmatic domain of the granulocyte-colony stimulating factor gene in patients with severe CN. Blood 1997;88:2369–75.

37. McLemore ML, Poursine-Laurent J, Link DC. Increased granulocyte colony-stimulating factor responsiveness but normal resting granulopoiesis in mice carrying a targeted granulocyte colony-stimulating factor receptor mutation derived from a patient with severe congenital neutropenia. J Clin Invest 1998;102:483–92.

38. Hunter MG, Avalos BR. Granulocyte colony-stimulating factor receptor mutations in severe congenital neutropenia transforming to acute myelogenous leukemia confer resistance to apoptosis and enhance cell survival. Blood 2000;95:2132–7.

39. Hermans MH, Antonissen C, Ward AC, et al. Sustained receptor activation and hyperproliferation in response to granulocyte colony-stimulating factor (G-CSF) in mice with a severe congenital neutropenia/acute myeloid leukemia-derived mutation in the G-CSF receptor gene. J Exp Med 1999;189:683–92.

40. Germeshausen M, Ballmaier M, Welte K. Incidence of CSF3R mutations in severe CN and relevance for leukemogenesis: results of a long-term survey. Blood 2007; 109:93–9.
41. Tschan CA, Pilz C, Zeidler C, et al. Time course of increasing numbers of mutations in the granulocyte colony-stimulating factor receptor gene in a patient with CN who developed leukemia. Blood 2001;97:1882–4.
42. Ancliff PJ, Gale RE, Liesner R, et al. Long-term follow-up of granulocyte colony-stimulating factor receptor mutations in patients with severe congenital neutropenia: implications for leukaemogenesis and therapy. Br J Haematol 2003;120: 685–90.
43. Hermans MH, van de Geijn GJ, Antonissen C, et al. Signaling mechanisms coupled to tyrosines in the granulocyte colony-stimulating factor receptor orchestrate G-CSF-induced expansion of myeloid progenitor cells. Blood 2003;101: 2584–90.
44. Touw IP, van de Geijn GJ. Granulocyte colony-stimulating factor and its receptor in normal myeloid cell development, leukemia and related blood cell disorders. Front Biosci 2007;12:800–15 [Review].
45. van de Geijn GJ, Gits J, Aarts LH, et al. G-CSF receptor truncations found in SCN/AML relieve SOCS3-controlled inhibition of STAT5 but leave suppression of STAT3 intact. Blood 2004;104:667–74.
46. Irandoust MI, Aarts LH, Roovers O, et al. Suppressor of cytokine signaling 3 controls lysosomal routing of G-CSF receptor. EMBO J 2007;26:1782–93.
47. Moore MA, Dorn DC, Schuringa JJ, et al. Constitutive activation of Flt3 and STAT5A enhances self-renewal and alters differentiation of hematopoietic stem cells. Exp Hematol 2007;35(Suppl 1):105–16.
48. Wierenga AT, Schepers H, Moore MA, et al. STAT5-induced self-renewal and impaired myelopoiesis of human hematopoietic stem/progenitor cells involves down-modulation of C/EBPalpha. Blood 2006;107:4326–33.
49. Gupta K, Skokowa J, Müller Brechlin A, et al. The effects of STAT5 activation on the proliferation and differentiation of myeloid hematopoietic progenitors in healthy individuals and in patients with severe congenital neutropenia (CN). Blood 2008;112:122 [abstract 316].
50. Liu F, Kunter G, Krem MM, et al. Csf3r mutations in mice confers a strong clonal HSC advantage via activation of Stat5. J Clin Invest 2008;118:946–55.
51. Bagby GC. Discovering early molecular determinants of leukemogenesis. J Clin Invest 2008;118:847–50.
52. Jamieson CH, Ailles LE, Dylla SJ, et al. Granulocyte-macrophage progenitors as candidate leukemic stem cells in blast-crisis CML. N Engl J Med 2004;351: 657–67.
53. Germeshausen M, Welte K, Ballmaier M. In vivo expansion of cells expressing acquired CSF3R mutations in patients with severe congenital neutropenia. Blood 2009;113:668–70.
54. Welte K, Zeidler C, Reiter A, et al. Differential effects of granulocyte-macrophage colony-stimulating factor and granulocyte colony-stimulating factor in children with severe congenital neutropenia. Blood 1990;75:1056–63.
55. Carlsson G, van't Hooft I, Melin M, et al. Central nervous system involvement in severe congenital neutropenia: neurological and neuropsychological abnormalities associated with specific HAX1 mutations. J Intern Med 2008;264(4):388–400.
56. Matsubara K, Imai K, Okada S, et al. Severe developmental delay and epilepsy in a Japanese patient with severe congenital neutropenia due to HAX1 deficiency. Haematologica 2007;92:123–5.

57. Rezaei N, Chavoshzadeh Z, Alaei OR, et al. Association of HAX1-deficiency with neurological disorder. Neuropediatrics 2007;38:261–3.
58. Carlsson G, Wahlin YB, Johansson A, et al. Periodontal disease in patients from the original Kostmann family with severe congenital neutropenia. J Periodontol 2006;77(4):744–51.
59. Schilke R, Stanulla M, Finke CH, et al. Influence of periodontitis co-factors in patients with severe chronic neutropenia. J Dent Res 2006;85:1138.
60. Yakisan E, Schirg E, Zeidler C, et al. High incidence of significant bone loss in patients with severe congenital neutropenia (Kostmann's syndrome). J Pediatr 1997;131:592–7.
61. Rosenberg PS, Alter BP, Bolyard AA, et al. Severe Chronic Neutropenia International Registry. The incidence of leukemia and mortality from sepsis in patients with severe CN receiving long-term G-CSF therapy. Blood 2006;107:4628–35.
62. Donadieu J, Leblanc T, Meunier Bader, et al. Analysis of risk factors for myelodysplasia/leukemia and infectious death among patients with CN: experience of the French Severe Chronic Neutropenia Study Group. Haematologica 2005;90: 45–53.
63. Carlsson G, Aprikyan AA, Ericson KG, et al. Neutrophil elastase and granulocyte colony-stimulating factor receptor mutation analyses and leukemia evolution in severe congenital neutropenia patients belonging to the original Kostmann family in northern Sweden. Hematologica 2006;91:589–95.
64. Bellanné-Chantelot C, Clauin S, Leblanc T, et al. Mutations in the ELA2 gene correlate with more severe expression of neutropenia: a study of 81 patients from the French Neutropenia Register. Blood 2004;103:4119–25.
65. Germeshausen M, Ballmaier M, Schulze H, et al. Granulocyte colony-stimulating factor receptor mutations in a patient with acute lymphoblastic leukemia secondary to severe CN. Blood 2001;97:829–30.
66. Germeshausen M, Schulze H, Kratz C, et al. An acquired G-CSF receptor mutation results in increased proliferation of CMML cells from a patient with severe CN. Leukemia 2005;19:611–7.
67. Göhring G, Karow A, Steinemann D, et al. Chromosomal aberrations in congenital bone marrow failure disorders—an early indicator for leukemogenesis? Ann Hematol 2007;86:733–9.
68. Link DC, Kunter G, Kasai Y, et al. Distinct patterns of mutations occurring in de novo AML versus AML arising in the setting of severe CN. Blood 2007;110: 1648–55.
69. Sloand EM, Yong AS, Ramkissoon S, et al. Granulocyte colony-stimulating factor preferentially stimulates proliferation of monosomy 7 cells bearing the isoform IV receptor. Proc Natl Acad Sci U S A 2007;103:14483–8.

Congenital Amegakaryocytic Thrombocytopenia and Thrombocytopenia with Absent Radii

Amy E. Geddis, MD, PhD

KEYWORDS

- Neonatal thrombocytopenia • c-Mpl
- Inherited thrombocytopenia • Thrombopoietin
- Thrombocytopenia with absent radii

Thrombocytopenia is a relatively common clinical problem in hospitalized neonates, and it is critical to distinguish infants who have rare congenital thrombocytopenias from those who have acquired disorders. Two well-described inherited thrombocytopenia syndromes that present in the newborn period are congenital amegakaryocytic thrombocytopenia (CAMT) and thrombocytopenia with absent radii (TAR). Although both are characterized by severe (< 50,000/μL) thrombocytopenia at birth, the molecular mechanisms underlying these disorders and their clinical presentations and courses are distinct. CAMT is an autosomal recessive disorder caused by mutations in the thrombopoietin (TPO) receptor c-Mpl. TAR is a syndrome of variable inheritance and unclear genetic etiology consisting of thrombocytopenia in association with bilateral absent radii and frequently additional congenital abnormalities. This article summarizes the current understanding of the pathophysiology and clinical course of CAMT and TAR.

CONGENITAL AMEGAKARYOCYTIC THROMBOCYTOPENIA: PRESENTATION AND DIFFERENTIAL DIAGNOSIS

CAMT is an autosomal recessive disorder that presents at birth with severe thrombocytopenia. Mean platelet counts at diagnosis are 21,000/μL, and platelets are of normal size and morphology.[1] Importantly, phenotypic findings in CAMT usually are limited to those related to thrombocytopenia, such as cutaneous and intracranial

The author receives research support from National Institutes of Health grant R01DK049858 and Amgen.
Department of Pediatrics, University of California San Diego, Rady Children's Hospital, 9500 Gilman Dr., Mailcode 0671, San Diego, CA 92093, USA
E-mail address: ageddis@ucsd.edu

Hematol Oncol Clin N Am 23 (2009) 321–331
doi:10.1016/j.hoc.2009.01.012
0889-8588/09/$ – see front matter © 2009 Elsevier Inc. All rights reserved.

hemorrhages. An increased incidence of psychomotor retardation has been described in patients who have CAMT, although some neurologic abnormalities may be sequelae of intracranial bleeding.[1] Because no specific congenital malformations are characteristic of CAMT, consideration should be given to an alternative syndrome if such malformations are present.

Bone marrow evaluation in newborns who have CAMT typically demonstrates normal overall cellularity with an isolated reduction or absence of megakaryocytes,[1] although in some cases marrow studied early in the course of the disease can have misleadingly minimal findings and serial evaluations may be required to clarify the diagnosis.[2,3] Although originally a clinical diagnosis, CAMT now can be defined molecularly by mutations involving the TPO receptor *c-Mpl*.[4,5] Mutations have been identified throughout *c-Mpl* and include nonsense, missense, and splicing mutations (Fox and colleagues, unpublished data, and [2,5–12]), although in severely affected patients mutations frequently are located in exons 2 and 3, which encode the first cytokine receptor homology domain (**Fig. 1**). Some patients who have CAMT have inherited two different mutations of *c-Mpl*, resulting in a compound heterozygous state, whereas in families with consanguinity the inheritance of homozygous mutations is more common. Clinically certified mutation analysis of *c-Mpl* now can be obtained at GeneDx (Gaithersburg, MD) and Prevention Genetics (Marshfield, Wisconsin).

Another diagnostic evaluation that is useful in establishing the diagnosis of CAMT is determination of the plasma TPO level. In CAMT, plasma levels of TPO are high, consistent with severely reduced platelet production and the absence of c-Mpl.[4] The relationship between TPO and thrombopoiesis reflects the normal metabolism of TPO, which is produced at a constant rate by the liver and removed from the circulation by receptor-mediated uptake and destruction.[13–15] c-Mpl receptors expressed on megakaryocytes and platelets are responsible for most TPO uptake.[16] In CAMT, impaired expression of c-Mpl means that there is little, if any, receptor-mediated destruction of TPO, and therefore circulating levels of the cytokine increase to as high as 10-fold above those seen in normal controls. By comparison, in disorders such as immune thrombocytopenia, in which c-Mpl is normal and thrombocytopenia is caused by platelet destruction, TPO levels are normal or are elevated only modestly.[17,18] Elevated TPO levels are not specific for CAMT and can occur in other conditions in which the production of megakaryocytes and platelets is severely impaired (eg, acquired aplastic anemia); however, in the appropriate clinical setting a highly elevated TPO level supports a diagnosis of CAMT and justifies further confirmation by specific gene sequencing.

CAMT is a rare cause of thrombocytopenia in the newborn period; much more common causes of thrombocytopenia include prenatal factors (such as pre-eclampsia, placental insufficiency, and intrauterine growth retardation), anoxic insult, infection, or maternal transfer of platelet allo- or autoantibodies. The timing of onset, severity of thrombocytopenia, clinical history, and maternal platelet counts often are often helpful in identifying underlying factors contributing to neonatal thrombocytopenia.[19] Neonatal alloimmune thrombocytopenia (NAIT) is an especially important cause of severe thrombocytopenia that must be differentiated from CAMT. Like CAMT, NAIT typically presents as severe thrombocytopenia in an otherwise normal newborn whose mother's platelets are normal. NAIT is more common (1:1000–1:2000 live births)[20,21] than CAMT (< 100 cases reported). DNA-based platelet phenotyping can establish whether there is incompatibility between maternal and paternal platelet antigens that would predispose the neonate to alloimmunization, and serologic assays using patient or maternal serum may detect platelet-specific alloantibodies.[22–24] Bone marrow aspiration usually is not required to diagnose NAIT but, if performed, typically shows normal to

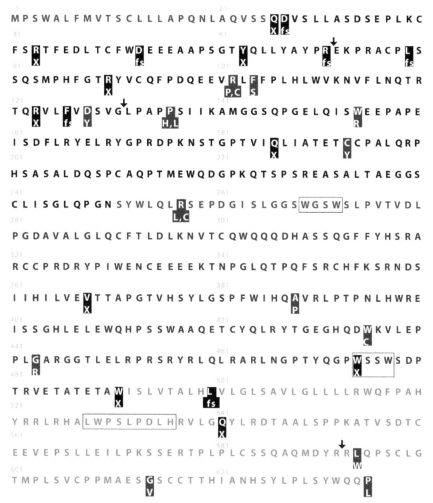

Fig.1. Summary of reported *c-Mpl* mutations in CAMT. Amino acids are represented by single letters. The signal peptide (residues 1–25) is shown in dark gray, the extracellular domain of the receptor (residues 26–491) in black, and the intracellular domain of the receptor (residues 492–635) in light gray. The WSXW motifs and Box 1 are indicated by open boxes. Identified mutations are highlighted, and the resulting changes are listed below. Changes resulting in stop codons (X) and frameshifts (fs) are highlighted with black. Substitutions are highlighted in gray. Arrows indicate the positions of splicing mutations.

increased megakaryocytes. After birth the maternally derived platelet alloantibody diminishes, and platelet counts are expected to improve after the first month of life. Even when antigen incompatibility is consistent with the possibility of NAIT, alternative diagnoses such as CAMT should be explored when thrombocytopenia does not resolve after 3 months (Fox and colleagues, unpublished data).

CONGENITAL AMEGAKARYOCYTIC THROMBOCYTOPENIA: PATHOPHYSIOLOGY

Platelets are produced by bone marrow megakaryocytes, which, like all blood cells, are derived from the hematopoietic stem cell. Although many cytokines and factors contribute to the growth and maturation of megakaryocytes, TPO is required for normal thrombopoiesis.[25–28] Consistent with the critical role of TPO signaling in megakaryocyte and platelet development, deletion of TPO or c-Mpl in mouse models results in severe thrombocytopenia with reduction of platelet counts to 10% of normal values.[28,29] In *c-Mpl–* and *TPO*-null mice, however, hematopoietic progenitors and stem cells also are reduced to approximately 10% of normal values.[28,30,31] Thus, TPO is critical both for thrombopoiesis and for the maintenance of the hematopoietic stem cell compartment. Clinical confirmation of this experimental finding came in 1999 when mutations in *c-Mpl* were discovered in children who had CAMT,[5] a disease characterized by thrombocytopenia and also by the development of bone marrow failure. It now is well established that the lack of TPO signaling in CAMT caused by absent or defective c-Mpl expression leads to impaired megakaryocyte and platelet production and ultimately to aplastic anemia in affected patients.[4,5]

Further studies of patients who have CAMT have described two classes of *c-Mpl* mutation, type I and type II.[1,6] Type I mutations completely eliminate receptor signaling through disruption of all or most of the intracellular domain, often through the creation of a stop codon or frameshift. Type II mutations typically create amino acid substitutions or altered splice sites that result in a small degree of residual receptor signaling. One of the most frequently identified mutations in CAMT involves the substitution of proline for arginine at position 102 in the extracellular domain, a nonconservative change that is predicted to alter receptor conformation significantly. In contrast, another common amino acid substitution has been described (methionine for valine at residue 114) that is not associated with disease.[9] The mechanisms by which some substitutions interfere with signaling are not obvious, and further study using structural or cell line models may lead to new insights into interactions between c-Mpl and its ligand or other signaling molecules.

Although *c-Mpl* mutations cause thrombocytopenia in CAMT, other mutations that alter c-Mpl and TPO signaling are associated with thrombocytosis. Constitutional mutations in the transmembrane domain of *c-Mpl* that lead to persistent receptor activation have been described in familial thrombocytosis,[32] and acquired mutations in c-Mpl or its associated kinase Jak2 that promote chronic activation of signaling are found in approximately 50% of patients who have essential thrombocythemia and almost all patients who have polycythemia vera.[33–38] A receptor variant called "c-Mpl Baltimore" has been described in which a substitution in the extracellular domain of the receptor leads to reduced expression of c-Mpl and paradoxically increased platelet counts,[39] possibly because of the relatively increased availability of circulating TPO. Thus, alterations of c-Mpl signaling may contribute both to thrombocytopenia and to thrombocytosis.

Not all children who have thrombocytopenia and a clinical picture resembling CAMT can be shown to have *c-Mpl* mutations, and therefore it is possible that other genetic loci for this disease exist. For example, because TPO is the only known ligand for c-Mpl, mutations that eliminate or severely reduce circulating TPO would be predicted to cause a clinical picture identical to CAMT. In fact, *TPO*-null mice phenocopy *c-Mpl*–null mice,[31] but mutations leading to the absence of TPO have not been described in humans. Whether there is active selection against *TPO* mutations in humans or whether they simply have not yet been discovered is not known. Children who have CAMT who do not have demonstrable mutations in *c-Mpl* may have novel mutations affecting *c-Mpl* transcription or other components of the TPO signaling pathway. Further research is needed to understand the etiology of thrombocytopenia in such patients.

CONGENITAL AMEGAKARYOCYTIC THROMBOCYTOPENIA: CLINICAL COURSE AND MANAGEMENT

Thrombocytopenia in patients who have CAMT can have a variable clinical course.[1] Although infants who have type I receptor mutations generally remain thrombocytopenic and have a rapid progression to trilineage bone marrow failure (mean age of onset, 1 year 11 months), infants who have type II mutations may show transient modest improvement of platelet counts during the first year of life and have a delayed onset of marrow failure (mean age of onset, 5 years).[1] Nevertheless, with rare exceptions, most patients who have CAMT go on to develop bone marrow failure. Importantly, patients who have CAMT also are at increased risk for the development of myelodysplasia and acute myeloid leukemia.[40] The mechanism by which the absence of c-Mpl predisposes a person to malignancy is not understood, but it is possible that the environment of impaired hematopoiesis selects for the outgrowth of abnormal clones.[41]

Supportive care in patients who have CAMT consists primarily of platelet transfusion, adjunctive therapies such as fibrinolytic inhibitors to manage bleeding symptoms, and red cell transfusions and antibiotics if needed. The use of alternative cytokines to stimulate thrombopoiesis has shown some efficacy in mouse models,[42] but clinical use has been limited by toxicity. Given the lack of functional c-Mpl in hematopoietic stem cells and megakaryocytic progenitors, it is unlikely that currently available TPO mimetics will be therapeutically useful in this disease (Fox and colleagues, unpublished data, and [43]). Gene therapy, although an attractive strategy for correction of the stem cell defect,[44,45] has not been studied clinically in CAMT, and concerns regarding its potential leukemogenicity remain.

Currently, the only definitive treatment for the long-term management of patients who have CAMT is hematopoietic stem cell transplantation. HLA typing for the patient and siblings should be obtained at the time of diagnosis to direct management decisions. Transplantation with a matched sibling donor is the treatment of choice.[1,46,47] Siblings who are heterozygous carriers of the c-Mpl mutation have been used successfully as stem cell donors.[10] Outcomes are less favorable for patients who do not have a matched sibling donor; failures caused by delayed engraftment, rejection, graft-versus-host disease, and regimen-related toxicity have been reported.[1,48,49] Although the numbers of patients are very small, haploidentical donors have been used with some success as an alternative to unrelated donors.[1,46] The optimal timing for transplantation is not known but has been suggested to be before pancytopenia develops, thus limiting transfusion exposures and risk for infections that could compromise transplant outcomes. In the review by King and colleagues,[1] 15 of 20 patients received transplants at a median age of 38 months (range, 7–89 months). Further studies are needed to optimize donor selection and conditioning regimens for patients who have CAMT, particularly those who lack a matched sibling donor.

THROMBOCYTOPENIA WITH ABSENT RADII: PRESENTATION AND DIAGNOSIS

TAR is a clinically defined syndrome characterized by thrombocytopenia and bilateral radial aplasia with thumbs present.[50,51] At birth thrombocytopenia may be of variable severity, with platelet counts ranging from 10 to 100,000/μL; platelets are normal in size and granularity. Bone marrow examination typically demonstrates a reduction in the size and number of bone marrow megakaryocytes, and plasma TPO levels, if obtained, usually are elevated.[52,53] Although bilateral radial aplasia is the defining skeletal feature in TAR, additional skeletal abnormalities frequently are observed, including more extensive upper limb malformations, phocomelia, and lower limb malformations in as many as 50% of the patients.[54] Nonskeletal abnormalities also are common, including gastroenteritis and cow's milk intolerance in 47%, renal malformations in 23%, cardiac defects in 15%, facial dysmorphism in 53%, short stature in 95%, macrocephaly in 76%, and capillary hemangiomata in 24% of patients.[54] Thus, when a child is born with absent radii, a multisystem evaluation with genetics and orthopedics consultations should be initiated to detect and manage associated congenital malformations.

Although TAR is distinctive, several syndromes have interesting phenotypic similarities to TAR. Amegakaryocytic thrombocytopenia with radioulnar synostosis (ATRUS) is a rare disorder characterized by neonatal thrombocytopenia in association with proximal fusion of the radius and ulna.[55] This skeletal finding may be identified by limited supination of the wrist or detected by radiographic evaluation. In two unrelated families with autosomal dominant transmission of ATRUS, genetic analysis revealed heterozygous inheritance of a point mutation in the homeobox gene *HoxA11*, which leads to truncation of this transcription factor within its DNA binding domain.[56] Studies using a cell line model demonstrated that overexpression of this truncated *HoxA11* impairs megakaryocytic differentiation,[57] whereas in mouse models deletion of *HoxA11* is associated with forelimb abnormalities.[58] Further studies are needed to define the role of HoxA11 in hematopoiesis. Despite their association with ATRUS, *Hox* gene mutations have not been identified in TAR.[59] Radial abnormalities and thrombocytopenia also may be found in Fanconi's anemia, a chromosomal instability syndrome with a constellation of findings that may include bone marrow failure, predisposition to malignancy, skeletal malformations, abnormal pigmentation, and growth failure.[60] Although Fanconi's anemia may present with thrombocytopenia, hematopoietic findings usually are not present at birth, and therefore the timing of onset of thrombocytopenia should distinguish Fanconi's anemia from TAR or ATRUS. Also, upper limb abnormalities in patients who have Fanconi's anemia often involve the thumbs, whereas in TAR thumbs characteristically are normal. The diagnosis of Fanconi's anemia can be confirmed by examining peripheral blood lymphocytes for the increased chromosomal breakage in the presence of clastogenic agents such as diepoxybutane or mitomycin C.

THROMBOCYTOPENIA WITH ABSENT RADII: PATHOPHYSIOLOGY

Despite significant interest, the molecular basis of TAR is not yet known. The inheritance pattern of TAR is complex, and autosomal recessive as well as autosomal dominant with variable penetrance inheritance patterns have been reported. Females are over-represented (27:7).[54] As with CAMT, plasma TPO levels in patients who have TAR are elevated, and studies of patients who have TAR reveal that megakaryocyte maturation is blocked and signaling in response to TPO is abnormal.[61–63] Nevertheless, no mutations in *c-Mpl* or its associated kinase *Jak2* have been identified,[62,64] and the underlying reason for this signaling defect is not understood. Recently an interstitial microdeletion involving chromosome 1q was identified in a cohort of 30 individuals who had TAR.[65] Although all affected patients carried the microdeletion, in approximately 75% of the cases the microdeletion was identified in an unaffected parent, suggesting that co-inheritance of an additional, unknown modifier is required for the expression of the disease. Nevertheless, there are 11 genes within this critical region, including a negative regulator of STAT3, an integrin subunit, and a ribosomal binding protein, and these genes now provide novel candidates for proteins that could be involved in the pathogenesis of TAR. These proteins also may have previously unsuspected and important functions in megakaryopoiesis.

Any mechanism proposed for impaired megakaryopoiesis in TAR must account for the observation that platelet counts typically recover spontaneously to nearly normal levels after the first year of life. This pattern has led some to postulate that the defect underlying TAR is relatively specific for fetal megakaryocytes. Although the differences between fetal and adult megakaryopoiesis remain poorly understood, it is clear that fetal and adult megakaryocytes respond differently to cytokine stimulation and have different potentials for proliferation and maturation.[66] Insights into the basis of TAR could have implications for the understanding of megakaryopoiesis during fetal development.

THROMBOCYTOPENIA WITH ABSENT RADII: CLINICAL COURSE AND MANAGEMENT

Although CAMT and TAR both involve abnormal TPO signaling, the clinical course of the two disorders is very different. Although patients who have CAMT nearly always develop bone marrow failure, platelet counts in TAR generally improve over the first year of life and eventually can approach normal adult levels. Marrow failure generally is not seen. As with CAMT, however, patients who have TAR have been reported to develop both acute myeloid and lymphoid leukemias,[67–69] suggesting that this disorder also is associated with a predisposition to malignancy. Nevertheless, lymphocytes from patients who have TAR do not exhibit abnormal chromosomal instability,[54] and an explanation of this tendency to develop cancer will require a better molecular understanding of the disorder.

Because thrombocytopenia tends to remit, the treatment of TAR is largely supportive with platelet transfusions in the first year of life as needed to control bleeding symptoms and facilitate orthopedic or other procedures. Much of the clinical management following the first year of life is directed toward the nonhematologic manifestations of this disorder. Hematopoietic stem cell transplantation generally is not indicated, although matched related-donor transplantation has been performed successfully in a child who had TAR and unusually persistent thrombocytopenia.[70] The advent of TPO agonists for the stimulation of platelet production offers an exciting new possibility for a targeted therapy in TAR, but this approach may be of limited efficacy if plasma levels of endogenous TPO are high and megakaryocytes have a downstream signaling defect. There are case reports of patients in whom thrombocytopenia has responded to alternative cytokines such as erythropoietin and interleukin-6.[71,72] Following resolution of the thrombocytopenia, long-term monitoring of patients for late recurrence of thrombocytopenia or leukemia is recommended.

SUMMARY

Thrombocytopenia in the newborn period can have diverse etiologies, but among them it is important to consider congenital disorders such as CAMT and TAR. Making the correct diagnosis is critical for optimal patient management, although not all patients who have inherited thrombocytopenia will fulfill criteria for a known disorder. Few physicians outside large referral centers will encounter more than one or a few patients who have these rare diseases, and therefore participation in national or international registries may be helpful in gaining access to specialized testing. Widespread participation in registries also will facilitate additional studies of the molecular basis and long-term outcomes and will support the development of novel therapies for inherited thrombocytoptenias. The discovery of new mutations may provide insights into TPO signaling and thrombopoiesis.

ACKNOWLEDGMENTS

The author thanks Norma E. Fox for ongoing essential research contributions, Kenneth Kaushansky for critical review of the manuscript, and Monica Gudea for valuable administrative assistance.

REFERENCES

1. King S, Germeshausen M, Strauss G, et al. Congenital amegakaryocytic thrombocytopenia: a retrospective clinical analysis of 20 patients. Br J Haematol 2005;131(5):636–44.
2. Rose MJ, Nicol KK, Skeens MA, et al. Congenital amegakaryocytic thrombocytopenia: the diagnostic importance of combining pathology with molecular genetics. Pediatr Blood Cancer 2008;50:1263–5.
3. Fox NE, Chen R, Hitchcock I, et al. Compound heterozygous c-Mpl mutations in a child with congenital amegakaryocytic thrombocytopenia: functional characterization and review of the literature. Experimental Hematology 2009; in press.
4. Ballmaier M, Germeshausen M, Schulze H, et al. c-Mpl mutations are the cause of congenital amegakaryocytic thrombocytopenia. Blood 2001;97(1):139–46.
5. Ihara K, Ishii E, Eguchi M, et al. Identification of mutations in the c-Mpl gene in congenital amegakaryocytic thrombocytopenia. Proc Natl Acad Sci U S A 1999;96(6):3132–6.
6. Germeshausen M, Ballmaier M, Welte K. Mpl mutations in 23 patients suffering from congenital amegakaryocytic thrombocytopenia: the type of mutation predicts the course of the disease. Hum Mutat 2006;27(3):296.
7. Steinberg O, Gilad G, Dgany O, et al. Congenital amegakaryocytic thrombocytopenia-3 novel c-Mpl mutations and their phenotypic correlations. J Pediatr Hematol Oncol 2007;29(12):822–5.
8. Passos-Coelho JL, Sebastiao M, Gameiro P, et al. Congenital amegakaryocytic thrombocytopenia—report of a new c-Mpl gene missense mutation. Am J Hematol 2007;82(3):240–1.
9. Gandhi MJ, Pendergrass TW, Cummings CC, et al. Congenital amegakaryocytic thrombocytopenia in three siblings: molecular analysis of atypical clinical presentation. Exp Hematol 2005;33(10):1215–21.
10. Muraoka K, Ishii E, Ihara K, et al. Successful bone marrow transplantation in a patient with c-Mpl-mutated congenital amegakaryocytic thrombocytopenia from a carrier donor. Pediatr Transplant 2005;9(1):101–3.
11. van den Oudenrijn S, Bruin M, Folman CC, et al. Mutations in the thrombopoietin receptor, Mpl, in children with congenital amegakaryocytic thrombocytopenia. Br J Haematol 2000;110(2):441–8.
12. Savoia A, Balduini CL, Savino M, et al. Autosomal dominant macrothrombocytopenia in Italy is most frequently a type of heterozygous Bernard-Soulier syndrome. Blood 2001;97(5):1330–5.
13. Kuter DJ, Rosenberg RD. The reciprocal relationship of thrombopoietin (c-Mpl ligand) to changes in the platelet mass during busulfan-induced thrombocytopenia in the rabbit. Blood 1995;85(10):2720–30.
14. Nagata Y, Shozaki Y, Nagahisa H, et al. Serum thrombopoietin level is not regulated by transcription but by the total counts of both megakaryocytes and platelets during thrombocytopenia and thrombocytosis. Thromb Haemost 1997;77(5):808–14.
15. Yang C, Li YC, Kuter DJ. The physiological response of thrombopoietin (c-Mpl ligand) to thrombocytopenia in the rat. Br J Haematol 1999;105(2):478–85.

16. Geddis AE, Fox NE, Kaushansky K. The Mpl receptor expressed on endothelial cells does not contribute significantly to the regulation of circulating thrombopoietin levels. Exp Hematol 2006;34(1):82–6.

17. Kunishima S, Tahara T, Kato T, et al. Serum thrombopoietin and plasma glycocalicin concentrations as useful diagnostic markers in thrombocytopenic disorders. Eur J Haematol 1996;57(1):68–71.

18. Mukai HY, Kojima H, Todokoro K, et al. Serum thrombopoietin (TPO) levels in patients with amegakaryocytic thrombocytopenia are much higher than those with immune thrombocytopenic purpura. Thromb Haemost 1996;76(5):675–8.

19. Roberts I, Stanworth S, Murray NA. Thrombocytopenia in the neonate. Blood Rev 2008;22(4):173–86.

20. Williamson LM, Hackett G, Rennie J, et al. The natural history of fetomaternal alloimmunization to the platelet-specific antigen HPA-1a (PIA1, Zwa) as determined by antenatal screening. Blood 1998;92(7):2280–7.

21. Panzer S, Auerbach L, Cechova E, et al. Maternal alloimmunization against fetal platelet antigens: a prospective study. Br J Haematol 1995;90(3):655–60.

22. Bussel JB. Alloimmune thrombocytopenia in the fetus and newborn. Semin Thromb Hemost 2001;27(3):245–52.

23. McFarland JG. Detection and identification of platelet antibodies in clinical disorders. Transfus Apheresis Sci 2003;28(3):297–305.

24. Arnold DM, Smith JW, Kelton JG. Diagnosis and management of neonatal alloimmune thrombocytopenia. Transfus Med Rev 2008;22(4):255–67.

25. Kaushansky K. The Mpl ligand: molecular and cellular biology of the critical regulator of megakaryocyte development. Stem Cells 1994;12(Suppl 1):91–6 [discussion: 96–7].

26. Kaushansky K, Lok S, Holly RD, et al. Promotion of megakaryocyte progenitor expansion and differentiation by the c-Mpl ligand thrombopoietin. Nature 1994; 369(6481):568–71.

27. Bartley TD, Bogenberger J, Hunt P, et al. Identification and cloning of a megakaryocyte growth and development factor that is a ligand for the cytokine receptor Mpl. Cell 1994;77(7):1117–24.

28. Alexander WS, Roberts AW, Maurer AB, et al. Studies of the c-Mpl thrombopoietin receptor through gene disruption and activation. Stem Cells 1996;14(Suppl 1):124–32.

29. Gurney AL, Carver-Moore K, de Sauvage FJ, et al. Thrombocytopenia in c-Mpl-deficient mice. Science 1994;265(5177):1445–7.

30. Alexander WS, Roberts AW, Nicola NA, et al. Deficiencies in progenitor cells of multiple hematopoietic lineages and defective megakaryocytopoiesis in mice lacking the thrombopoietic receptor c-Mpl. Blood 1996;87(6):2162–70.

31. Carver-Moore K, Broxmeyer HE, Luoh SM, et al. Low levels of erythroid and myeloid progenitors in thrombopoietin-and c-Mpl-deficient mice. Blood 1996; 88(3):803–8.

32. Ding J, Komatsu H, Wakita A, et al. Familial essential thrombocythemia associated with a dominant-positive activating mutation of the c-Mpl gene, which encodes for the receptor for thrombopoietin. Blood 2004;103(11):4198–200.

33. Levine RL, Wadleigh M, Cools J, et al. Activating mutation in the tyrosine kinase JAK2 in polycythemia vera, essential thrombocythemia, and myeloid metaplasia with myelofibrosis. Cancer Cell 2005;7(4):387–97.

34. Vainchenker W, Constantinescu SN. A unique activating mutation in JAK2 (V617F) is at the origin of polycythemia vera and allows a new classification of myeloproliferative diseases. Hematology Am Soc Hematol Educ Program 2005;195–200.

35. Baxter EJ, Scott LM, Campbell PJ, et al. Acquired mutation of the tyrosine kinase JAK2 in human myeloproliferative disorders. Lancet 2005;365(9464):1054–61.
36. James C, Ugo V, Le Couedic JP, et al. A unique clonal JAK2 mutation leading to constitutive signalling causes polycythaemia vera. Nature 2005;434(7037): 1144–8.
37. Kralovics R, Passamonti F, Buser AS, et al. A gain-of-function mutation of JAK2 in myeloproliferative disorders. N Engl J Med 2005;352(17):1779–90.
38. Pikman Y, Lee BH, Mercher T, et al. MPLW515L is a novel somatic activating mutation in myelofibrosis with myeloid metaplasia. PLoS Med 2006;3(7):e270.
39. Moliterno AR, Williams DM, Gutierrez-Alamillo LI, et al. Mpl Baltimore: a thrombopoietin receptor polymorphism associated with thrombocytosis. Proc Natl Acad Sci U S A 2004;101(31):11444–7.
40. Alter BP. Bone marrow failure syndromes in children. Pediatr Clin North Am 2002; 49(5):973–88.
41. Bagby GC, Meyers G. Bone marrow failure as a risk factor for clonal evolution: prospects for leukemia prevention. Hematology Am Soc Hematol Educ Program 2007;2007:40–6.
42. Gainsford T, Roberts AW, Kimura S, et al. Cytokine production and function in c-Mpl-deficient mice: no physiologic role for interleukin-3 in residual megakaryocyte and platelet production. Blood 1998;91(8):2745–52.
43. Tijssen MR, di Summa F, van den Oudenrijn S, et al. Functional analysis of single amino-acid mutations in the thrombopoietin-receptor Mpl underlying congenital amegakaryocytic thrombocytopenia. Br J Haematol 2008;141(6):808–13.
44. Jin L, Siritanaratkul N, Emery DW, et al. Targeted expansion of genetically modified bone marrow cells. Proc Natl Acad Sci U S A 1998;95(14):8093–7.
45. Richard RE, Blau CA. Small-molecule-directed Mpl signaling can complement growth factors to selectively expand genetically modified cord blood cells. Stem Cells 2003;21(1):71–8.
46. Lackner A, Basu O, Bierings M, et al. Haematopoietic stem cell transplantation for amegakaryocytic thrombocytopenia. Br J Haematol 2000;109(4):773–5.
47. Al-Ahmari A, Ayas M, Al-Jefri A, et al. Allogeneic stem cell transplantation for patients with congenital amegakaryocytic thrombocytopenia (CAT). Bone Marrow Transplant 2004;33(8):829–31.
48. MacMillan ML, Davies SM, Wagner JE, et al. Engraftment of unrelated donor stem cells in children with familial amegakaryocytic thrombocytopenia. Bone Marrow Transplant 1998;21(7):735–7.
49. Gluckman E, Wagner JE. Hematopoietic stem cell transplantation in childhood inherited bone marrow failure syndrome. Bone Marrow Transplant 2008;41(2): 127–32.
50. Hall JG, Levin J, Kuhn JP, et al. Thrombocytopenia with absent radius (TAR). Medicine (Baltimore) 1969;48(6):411–39.
51. Hedberg VA, Lipton JM. Thrombocytopenia with absent radii. A review of 100 cases. Am J Pediatr Hematol Oncol 1988;10(1):51–64.
52. Ballmaier M, Schulze H, Strauss G, et al. Thrombopoietin in patients with congenital thrombocytopenia and absent radii: elevated serum levels, normal receptor expression, but defective reactivity to thrombopoietin. Blood 1997;90(2):612–9.
53. Homans AC, Cohen JL, Mazur EM. Defective megakaryocytopoiesis in the syndrome of thrombocytopenia with absent radii. Br J Haematol 1988;70(2):205–10.
54. Greenhalgh KL, Howell RT, Bottani A, et al. Thrombocytopenia-absent radius syndrome: a clinical genetic study. J Med Genet 2002;39(12):876–81.

55. Thompson AA, Woodruff K, Feig SA, et al. Congenital thrombocytopenia and radio-ulnar synostosis: a new familial syndrome. Br J Haematol 2001;113(4): 866–70.
56. Thompson AA, Nguyen LT. Amegakaryocytic thrombocytopenia and radio-ulnar synostosis are associated with HOXA11 mutation. Nat Genet 2000;26(4):397–8.
57. Horvat-Switzer RD, Thompson AA. HOXA11 mutation in amegakaryocytic thrombocytopenia with radio-ulnar synostosis syndrome inhibits megakaryocytic differentiation in vitro. Blood Cells Mol Dis 2006;37(1):55–63.
58. Boulet AM, Capecchi MR. Multiple roles of Hoxa11 and Hoxd11 in the formation of the mammalian forelimb zeugopod. Development 2004;131(2):299–309.
59. Fleischman RA, Letestu R, Mi X, et al. Absence of mutations in the HoxA10, HoxA11 and HoxD11 nucleotide coding sequences in thrombocytopenia with absent radius syndrome. Br J Haematol 2002;116(2):367–75.
60. Alter BP. Bone marrow failure: a child is not just a small adult (but an adult can have a childhood disease). Hematology Am Soc Hematol Educ Program 2005;96–103.
61. Letestu R, Vitrat N, Masse A, et al. Existence of a differentiation blockage at the stage of a megakaryocyte precursor in the thrombocytopenia and absent radii (TAR) syndrome. Blood 2000;95(5):1633–41.
62. Ballmaier M, Schulze H, Cremer M, et al. Defective c-Mpl signaling in the syndrome of thrombocytopenia with absent radii. Stem Cells 1998;16(Suppl 2): 177–84.
63. al-Jefri AH, Dror Y, Bussel JB, et al. Thrombocytopenia with absent radii: frequency of marrow megakaryocyte progenitors, proliferative characteristics, and megakaryocyte growth and development factor responsiveness. Pediatr Hematol Oncol 2000;17(4):299–306.
64. Strippoli P, Savoia A, Iolascon A, et al. Mutational screening of thrombopoietin receptor gene (c-Mpl) in patients with congenital thrombocytopenia and absent radii (TAR). Br J Haematol 1998;103(2):311–4.
65. Klopocki E, Schulze H, Strauss G, et al. Complex inheritance pattern resembling autosomal recessive inheritance involving a microdeletion in thrombocytopenia-absent radius syndrome. Am J Hum Genet 2007;80(2):232–40.
66. Pastos KM, Slayton WB, Rimsza LM, et al. Differential effects of recombinant thrombopoietin and bone marrow stromal-conditioned media on neonatal versus adult megakaryocytes. Blood 2006;108(10):3360–2.
67. Fadoo Z, Naqvi SM. Acute myeloid leukemia in a patient with thrombocytopenia with absent radii syndrome. J Pediatr Hematol Oncol 2002;24(2):134–5.
68. Go RS, Johnston KL. Acute myelogenous leukemia in an adult with thrombocytopenia with absent radii syndrome. Eur J Haematol 2003;70(4):246–8.
69. Camitta BM, Rock A. Acute lymphoidic leukemia in a patient with thrombocytopenia/absent radii (Tar) syndrome. Am J Pediatr Hematol Oncol 1993;15(3):335–7.
70. Brochstein JA, Shank B, Kernan NA, et al. Marrow transplantation for thrombocytopenia-absent radii syndrome. J Pediatr 1992;121(4):587–9.
71. Dempfle CE, Burck C, Grutzmacher T, et al. Increase in platelet count in response to rHuEpo in a patient with thrombocytopenia and absent radii syndrome. Blood 2001;97(7):2189–90.
72. Aquino VM, Mustafa MM, Vaickus L, et al. Recombinant interleukin-6 in the treatment of congenital thrombocytopenia associated with absent radii. J Pediatr Hematol Oncol 1998;20(5):474–6.

Bone Marrow Failure Syndromes: Paroxysmal Nocturnal Hemoglobinuria

Charles J. Parker, MD

KEYWORDS

- Hemolysis • Aplastic anemia • Myelodysplasia
- Bone marrow failure • Bone marrow transplant
- Eculizumab

Speaking in London as President of the Section of Pathology of the Royal Society in March 1963, Professor John V. Dacie (1912–2005) gave a prescient review of paroxysmal nocturnal hemoglobinuria (PNH), which he regarded as *the* blood disease.[1] Dacie's review focused on the following five central problems connected with PNH that were unresolved at the time:

1. The nature of the red cell defect
2. The nature of the factors in normal plasma that bring about hemolysis of the PNH red cell
3. Whether the patient's leukocytes and platelets are abnormal
4. The relationship between PNH and thrombosis
5. The ultimate problem—the etiology of the disease and its relationship to marrow hypoplasia

In the ensuing 45 years, Dacie's first,[2,3] second,[4] and third[5–7] central problems have been solved. The fourth central problem, the basis of the thrombophilia of PNH, remains largely speculative.[8] Dacie's ultimate problem, the etiology of the disease and its relationship to marrow hypoplasia, is the subject of this article.

AN OVERVIEW OF PAROXYSMAL NOCTURNAL HEMOGLOBINURIA

PNH is an acquired disease that results from nonmalignant clonal expansion of one or more hematopoietic stem cells[9] that have undergone somatic mutation of the X-chromosome gene *PIGA*.[6,7,10] The protein encoded by *PIGA* is essential for synthesis of the glycosyl phosphatidylinositol (GPI) moiety that serves as the membrane anchor

Division of Hematology and Bone Marrow Transplantation, Department of Medicine, University of Utah School of Medicine, 50 North Medical Drive, Salt Lake City, UT 84132, USA
E-mail address: charles.parker@hsc.utah.edu

Hematol Oncol Clin N Am 23 (2009) 333–346
doi:10.1016/j.hoc.2009.01.014
0889-8588/09/$ – see front matter © 2009 Elsevier Inc. All rights reserved.

for a functionally diverse group of cellular proteins.[3] As a consequence of mutant *PIGA*, all GPI-anchored proteins (GPI-APs) are deficient on affected stem cells and their progeny. Two proteins, CD55 (decay accelerating factor, DAF)[11–13] and CD59 (membrane inhibitor of reactive lysis, MIRL)[14,15] that inhibit the activation and cytolytic functions of complement are among the GPI-APs normally expressed by hematopoietic cells. The Coombs-negative intravascular hemolysis (and the resultant hemoglobinuria) that are the clinical hallmarks of classic PNH are a direct consequence of the deficiency of CD55 and CD59, because peripheral blood erythrocytes derived from the mutant clone lack the capacity to restrict cell-surface activation of the alternative pathway of complement and to block formation of the cytolytic membrane attack complex.[4]

Thromboembolism is the leading cause of morbidity and mortality in PNH.[8,16–19] Unusual sites of involvement, including hepatic vein thrombosis (Budd-Chiari syndrome) and thrombosis of mesenteric, cerebral, and dermal veins, characterize the thrombophilia of PNH.[20] In contrast to the present thorough understanding of the complement-mediated hemolytic anemia of PNH,[4] however, the pathobiology of the thrombosis of PNH is largely speculative.[8]

An association between PNH and acquired aplastic anemia has been recognized for more than 50 years,[1,21–23] and all patients who have PNH have evidence of bone marrow dysfunction.[24] Understanding the association between PNH and aplastic anemia seems to be a key to unlocking the complex pathophysiology of this eccentric disease. The close association of PNH with an immune-mediated bone marrow failure syndrome (ie, aplastic anemia) suggests that hematopoietic stem cells with mutant *PIGA* have a conditional growth or survival advantage in the setting of a specific type of bone marrow injury with subsequent independent, nonmalignant expansion of the *PIGA*-mutant clone in some (but not all) cases. In this view of PNH, acquired deficiency of one or more GPI-APs in hematopoietic stem cells through somatic mutation of *PIGA* is seen as nature's approach (by way of natural selection) to treatment of immune-mediated bone marrow injury.

THE CLINICAL PROBLEM

The peripheral blood of patients who have PNH is a mosaic of normal and abnormal cells (**Fig. 1**), and the percentage of abnormal cells varies widely among patients. For example, hypothetical patient A may have 90% abnormal, GPI-AP–deficient cells with 10% of the cells showing normal expression of GPI-APs (based on flow cytometric analysis of peripheral blood neutrophils or erythrocytes), whereas hypothetical patient B may have 10% abnormal cells and 90% phenotypically normal cells. The degree of mosaicism among different patients is determined by the extent to which the *PIGA*-mutant clone expands, but the factors that determine clonal expansion in an individual patient are largely speculative.[25] *PIGA*-mutant stem cells seem to have no intrinsic growth or survival advantage,[26,27] suggesting that clonal expansion is driven by factors that are distinct from but that work in concert with mutant *PIGA*.[3] Although the clinical manifestations of PNH depend in large part on the size of the clone, the extent of the associated bone marrow failure also contributes significantly to disease manifestations. Thus, PNH is not a binary process; based on the clinical features, bone marrow characteristics, and the size of the mutant clone (based on the percentage of GPI-AP–deficient PMNs), the International PNH Interest Group recognizes three disease subcategories (**Table 1**).

Although the bone marrow of patients who have classic PNH appears fairly normal morphologically (**Table 1**), numerous in vitro studies have shown that the growth characteristics of marrow-derived stem cells are aberrant.[24] Moreover, when stem cells

High-Resolution Flow Cytometry for Diagnosis of PNH

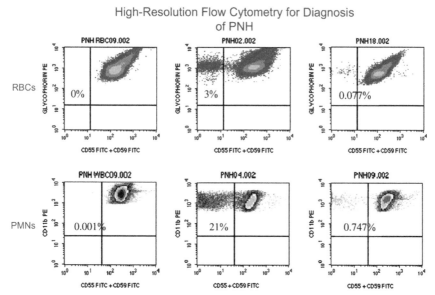

Fig. 1. High-sensitivity flow cytometry of peripheral blood cells for diagnosis of PNH. Peripheral blood erythrocytes (RBCs) and neutrophils (PMNs) from a healthy volunteer and two patients who had bone marrow failure were analyzed by flow cytometry using anti-glycophorin A (*top row, vertical axis*) to identify RBCs and anti-CD11b (*bottom row, vertical axis*) to identify PMNs. GPI-AP expression was detected using a combination of anti-CD55 and anti-CD59 (*top and bottom rows, horizontal axis*). PNH cells are deficient in both CD55 and CD59 (*upper left quadrant* of each histogram). The percentage of GPI-AP–deficient (PNH) cells is shown for each sample. These results demonstrate variability in the size of the PNH clone among patients and phenotypic mosaicism, both characteristic of PNH. The *left panels*, normal control; *middle panels*, a patient who has PNH/anaplastic anemia; *right panels*, a patient with subclinical PNH.

are sorted into GPI-AP$^-$ and GPI-AP$^+$ populations, the growth characteristics of the GPI-AP$^-$ population approach those of normal control cells more closely than do those of the GPI-AP$^+$ population.[28,29] One plausible explanation for this observation is that the GPI-AP$^-$ cells are relatively protected from the pathophysiologic process that mediates the bone marrow injury, thereby providing a basis for natural selection of the *PIGA*-mutant clone. In this view of PNH, outgrowth of the *PIGA*-mutant clone is seen as an example of Darwinian evolution occurring within the microenvironment of the bone marrow. Although this interpretation is hypothetically appealing, rigorous experimental support is lacking.

Although anecdotal reports of an association of PNH with bone marrow failure syndromes had appeared sporadically, Dacie[22] and Lewis[23] were the first to study the relationship systematically, and Dacie[1] emphasized the significance of marrow hypoplasia in PNH in his 1963 address to the Royal Society. In that address, he stated that of his 48 patients who had PNH, 7 (16%) had been diagnosed initially with aplastic anemia. He also noted that screening of 32 patients who had aplastic anemia produced four (13%) positive acidified serum lysis tests, revealing the presence of PNH erythrocytes in patients who had aplastic anemia but in whom PNH had not been suspected clinically.

In 1995, Hillmen and colleagues[18] reported on 80 patients originally diagnosed by Professor Dacie, noting that 23 (29%) had an antecedent history of aplastic anemia.

Table 1
Classification of PNH[a]

Category	Rate of Intravascular Hemolysis[b]	Bone Marrow	Analysis of Glycosyl Phosphatidylinositol– Anchored Protein Expression by Flow Cytometry
Classic	Florid (macroscopic hemoglobinuria is frequent or persistent)	Cellular marrow with erythroid hyperplasia and normal or near-normal morphology[c]	Large population (> 50%) of GPI-AP–deficient PMNs[e]
PNH in the setting of another bone marrow failure syndrome[d]	Mild to moderate (macroscopic hemoglobinuria is intermittent or absent)	Evidence of a concomitant bone marrow failure syndrome[d]	Although variable, the percentage of GPI-AP–deficient PMNs[e] usually is relatively small (< 30%)
Subclinical	No clinical or biochemical evidence of intravascular hemolysis	Evidence of a concomitant bone marrow failure syndrome[d]	Small (< 1%) population of GPI-AP–deficient PMNs detected by high-resolution flow cytometry

[a] Based on recommendations of the International PNH Interest Group.[20]
[b] Based on macroscopic hemoglobinuria, serum lactate dehydrogenase concentration, and reticulocyte count.
[c] Karyotypic abnormalities are uncommon.
[d] Aplastic anemia and refractory anemia/MDS are the most commonly associated marrow failure syndromes.
[e] Analysis of PMNs is more informative than analysis of RBCs because of selective destruction GPI-AP–deficient RBCs.

In a series of 220 French patients who had PNH, Socié and colleagues[19] identified 65 (30%) in whom the diagnosis of aplastic anemia preceded that of PNH. This group of investigators also found that 10% of patients who had PNH but no antecedent history of aplastic anemia developed evidence of bone marrow failure during the period of observation covered by the study (median follow-up of 2 years). The estimated cumulative incidence of pancytopenia in the French study was 8.2% (± 2.4% SE) at 2 year and 14.2% (± 3.3% SE) at 4 years.[19] This incidence of bone marrow failure developing in the setting of classic PNH seems to be somewhat higher than that observed in the British study in which 5 of 80 patients (6%) who had classic PNH subsequently developed aplasia.[18] The disparity in outcome between the two studies may be the result of differences in the criteria used to define bone marrow failure.

The French natural history study that was expanded and updated in 2008 reported that 106 of 460 patients who had PNH (23%) had an antecedent diagnosis of aplastic anemia, and of 176 patients who had PNH diagnosed at Duke University, 51 (29%) had a prior history of aplastic anemia; of 209 Japanese patients who had PNH, 79 (38%) had an antecedent history of aplastic anemia.[16]

On the other hand, the proportion of patients who have aplastic anemia who have PNH cells at diagnosis or who subsequently develop PNH varies widely among studies, in part, because the criteria for diagnosis of PNH are not uniform. In some cases, a positive Ham's test or sucrose lysis test was required for diagnosis; in other cases, identification by flow cytometry of a population of peripheral blood cells with GPI-AP deficiency was used to classify patients. Using a flow cytometric assay with the capacity to detect 0.004% or more GPI-AP–deficient erythrocytes, Mukhina and colleagues[30] reported that 61% of patients who had aplastic anemia had detectable PNH cells in the peripheral blood before therapy. Similar results were obtained in a more recent study using high-resolution flow cytometry with the capacity to detect 0.003% or more GPI-AP–deficient cells.[31] In most of these cases, the GPI-AP–deficient cells would be undetected by conventional flow cytometry, where the sensitivity threshold for detecting cells with the PNH phenotype is 1% to 3%. For example, using a flow cytometric technique in which more than 1% GPI-AP–deficient granulocytes was considered abnormal, Dunn and colleagues[32] reported that 25 of 115 patients (22%) who had aplastic anemia and who were studied before initiation of therapy had a detectable PNH population. Two older studies reported 38% of patients (11/29)[33] and 32% of patients (12/37)[34] who had aplastic anemia treated with immunosuppression developed laboratory evidence of PNH during the course of their disease. In the latter study, 23% of patients had clinical signs and symptoms of PNH. Together, these studies suggest that PNH is subclinical in most patients who have aplastic anemia (**Table 1**). The time between the diagnosis of aplastic anemia and the development of PNH has been reported to vary from a few months to several years and depends on the method and criteria used to diagnose PNH. For example, in the initial French study,[19] the median time between diagnosis of aplastic anemia and laboratory evidence of PNH was 3.1 years (range, 0.17–15 years), but high-resolution flow cytometry was not used for diagnosis in that study, and patients who had aplastic anemia were not analyzed systematically at diagnosis or prospectively for development of PNH. Therefore, it is likely that most of the patients who had aplastic anemia in whom PNH subsequently was diagnosed in the initial French study developed signs or symptoms of disease that led directly to a diagnostic study. In contrast, PNH cells are detected in a much higher percentage of patients who have aplastic anemia who are analyzed at diagnosis using high-resolution flow cytometry.

In summary, although at diagnosis 50% to 60% of patients who have aplastic anemia have a population of GPI-AP⁻ hematopoietic cells detectable by high-resolution flow cytometry,[30–32] only 10% to 15% subsequently develop clinically apparent PNH,[35] and the development of clinical disease, when it occurs, typically follows the diagnosis of aplastic anemia by several years. In the remainder, GPI-AP⁻ cells persist subclinically or disappear; suggesting that mutant *PIGA* (and the consequent deficiency of GPI-APs) is necessary for clonal selection but is insufficient to account for the clonal expansion required for clinical manifestations of PNH to become apparent. One interpretation of these observations is that factors in addition to mutant *PIGA* determine the clinical phenotype of the disease by affecting the extent to which the *PIGA*-mutant stem cells expand. Conceivably, a second genetic event that works additively or synergistically with mutant *PIGA* is required for clonal expansion.[25] That the extent of clonal expansion varies markedly among patients, however, suggests that the second event may have diverse etiologies and could involve somatic mutations, epigenetic phenomena, or stochastic processes.

Because expansion of the mutant clones occurs later in the course of aplastic anemia, the process could be influenced directly or indirectly by therapy.[35] Although many patients who have aplastic anemia and who develop PNH are treated with immunosuppressive therapy (eg, anti-thymocyte globulin and cyclosporin), there is no evidence that immunosuppression causes PNH. Patients who have aplastic anemia who respond to androgens seem equally likely to develop PNH.[19]

The basis of the relationship between PNH and aplastic anemia is speculative. Most patients who have PNH have some evidence of bone marrow failure (eg, thrombocytopenia, leukopenia, or both) during the course of their disease.[16–19] Therefore, bone marrow injury may play a central role in the development of PNH by providing the conditions that favor the growth/survival of *PIGA*-mutant, GPI-AP–deficient stem cells. Alternatively, *PIGA*-mutant stem cells may have a direct role in the pathophysiologic process that mediates marrow hypoplasia. There is no evidence that the types of *PIGA* mutations that occur in PNH/aplastic anemia are different from those observed in classic PNH.[36] Further, a distinction between classic PNH and PNH/aplastic anemia (**Table 1**) may be artificial, because the underlying pathophysiologic process could be the same. According to this hypothesis, in classic PNH, the aplastic or hypoplastic component is subclinical and short-lived with disease noted only after the *PIGA*-mutant clone has expanded sufficiently to dominate hematopoiesis. A two-step model that incorporates the concepts of immune-mediated clonal selection with a second genetic event that leads to clonal expansion is depicted in **Fig. 2**.

Paroxysmal Nocturnal Hemoglobinuria and Myelodysplastic Syndrome

The presence of PNH cells also has been observed in patients who have myelodysplastic syndrome (MDS).[32,37–39] Of note, the association between PNH and MDS seems to be confined to low-risk categories of MDS, particularly the refractory anemia (RA) variant.[37–39] Using high-sensitivity flow cytometry in which 0.003% or more GPI-AP–deficient RBCs or PMNs was classified as abnormal, Wang and colleagues[38] reported that 21 of 119 patients (18%) who had RA MDS had a population of PNH cells, whereas GPI-AP–deficient cells were not detected in patients who had refractory anemia with ringed sideroblasts (RARS), refractory anemia with excess of blasts (RAEB), or refractory anemia with excess of blasts in transformation. Compared with patients who had RA without a population of PNH cells (RA-PNH⁻), patients who had RA with at population of PNH cells (RA-PNH⁺) had a distinct clinical profile characterized by less pronounced morphologic abnormalities of the blood cells, more severe thrombocytopenia, lower rates of karyotypic abnormalities, lower rates of progression to acute leukemia, higher probability of response to cyclosporine therapy, and higher incidence of HLA-DR15. More recently, the findings of Wang and colleagues[39] that a population of PNH cells is associated only with low-risk MDS variants in Japanese patients were confirmed in a North American study of 137 patients classified by World Health Organization criteria.[40] That study found a population of PNH cells in one of five patients (20%) who had 5q- syndrome, in 6 of 17 patients (35%) who had RA, and in 2 of 37 patients (5%) who had refractory cytopenias with multilineage dysplasia (RCMD). No patients who had RARS (0/9), RCMD-ringed sideroblasts (0/6), RAEB (0/26), MDS-unspecified (0/10), myelodysplastic/myeloproliferative disease (0/10), chronic idiopathic myelofibrosis (0/5), chronic myelomonocytic leukemia (0/5), or acute myeloid leukemia (0/6) had a detectable population of GPI-AP–deficient blood cells.

When combined with evidence of polyclonal hematopoiesis (based on the pattern of X-chromosome inactivation in female patients), the presence of a population of PNH cells in a patient who has MDS predicts a relatively benign clinical course and a high probability of response to immunosuppressive therapy.[37] A relatively good response to immunosuppressive therapy for patients who have MDS and aplastic anemia also is predicted by expression of HLA-DR15 in studies of both North American and Japanese patients.[41,42] Together, these observations provide compelling indirect evidence that aplastic anemia and a subcategory of low-risk MDS are immune-mediated

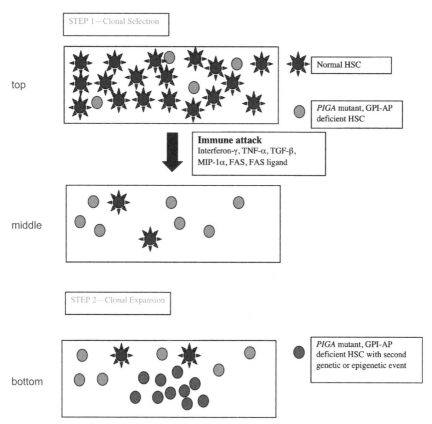

Fig. 2. Model of the two-step hypothesis of PNH pathophysiology. (*Top panel*) Hematopoietic stem cells and primitive progenitors with mutant *PIGA* are present in normal marrow, but they are not apparent because no selection pressure has been applied, and they have no intrinsic growth/survival advantage. (*Middle panel*) In the setting of immune-mediated bone marrow injury, *PIGA*-mutant cells are selected because they have a growth/survival advantage based on their GPI-AP–deficient phenotype. Additional *PIGA*-mutant HSC may be produced as a consequence of this process because the mutational frequency of the gene may be enhanced by stress erythropoiesis. (*Bottom panel*) Clonal expansion is the result of genetic, epigenetic, or stochastic events affecting genes that work in concert with mutant *PIGA* (and the consequent deficiency of GPI-APs) to enhance further the proliferative/survival advantage of the mutant cells. Under these conditions, PNH has the characteristics of a benign clonal myeloproliferative process. (*Modified from* Parker CJ. The pathophysiology of paroxysmal nocturnal hemoglobinuria. Exp Hematol 2007;35:523–33; with permission.)

diseases and that the immune pathophysiologic process provides the selection pressure that favors the outgrowth of *PIGA*-mutant, GPI-AP–deficient stem cells (see **Fig. 2**).

Management of Patients Who Have Bone Marrow Failure and Paroxysmal Nocturnal Hemoglobinuria

The complement-mediated intravascular hemolysis of PNH can be inhibited by blocking the formation of the membrane attack complex (MAC), the cytolytic component of the complement system. The MAC consists of complement components C5b, C6, C7,

C8, and C9. Eculizumab is a humanized monoclonal antibody that binds to complement C5, preventing its activation to C5b and thereby inhibiting MAC formation. In 2007, eculizumab was approved for treatment of the hemolysis of PNH by both the Food and Drug Administration in the United States and the European Union Commission. Treatment with eculizumab reduces transfusion requirements, ameliorates the anemia of PNH, and markedly improves quality of life by resolving the debilitating constitutional symptoms associated with chronic complement-mediated intravascular hemolysis.[43] Following treatment, serum lactate dehydrogenase concentration (a surrogate marker for intravascular hemolysis) returns to normal, but mild to moderate anemia and reticulocytosis usually persist, probably because of ongoing extravascular hemolysis mediated by opsonization of PNH erythrocytes by activated complement C3, because eculizumab does not block the downstream effects of complement activation. Thromboembolic events are the major cause of morbidity and mortality in PNH,[20] and eculizumab seems to ameliorate the thrombophilia of PNH, although the studies that support that conclusion were flawed by suboptimal design.[44]

Eculizumab is expensive ($400,000/year in the United States), and it has no effect on either the underlying stem cell abnormality or on the associated bone marrow failure. Consequently, treatment must continue indefinitely, and leukopenia, thrombocytopenia, and reticulocytopenia, if present, persist despite treatment with eculizumab.

Before eculizumab was available, the primary indications for bone marrow transplantation in patients who had PNH were bone marrow failure, recurrent, life-threatening thrombosis, and uncontrollable hemolysis (**Table 2**).[20] The last process can be eliminated by treatment with eculizumab, and the thrombophilia of PNH also

Table 2
Clinical activity of eculizumab

What It Does	What It Does Not Do	What It May Do
Blocks complement-mediated intravascular hemolysis	Eliminate anemia and reticulocytosis[e]	Reduce the risk of thromboembolism[f]
Reduces transfusion requirement[a]	Affect the underlying marrow dysfunction	—
Improves quality of life (particularly fatigue)	Affect the PIGA-mutant stem cell clones	—
Increases the proportion of circulating type III PNH erythrocytes[d]	Increase the risk for a catastrophic hemolytic crisis if the drug is discontinued[c]	—
Increases the risk of infection with Neisseria meningitides[b]	—	—

[a] Eliminates transfusion requirement in some patients.
[b] Vaccination against N. meningitides is required before initiation of eculizumab therapy.
[c] Of 195 patients in the clinical trials, 16 have discontinued therapy with no catastrophic hemolysis reported.[44]
[d] PNH III cells are completely deficient in GPI-APs.
[e] Following treatment with eculizumab, serum lactate dehydrogenase concentration returns to normal, but mild to moderate anemia and reticulocytosis usually persist, probably as the result of ongoing extravascular hemolysis mediated by opsonization of PNH RBCs by activated complement C3. (Eculizumab does not block the formation of the alternative pathway C3 convertase).
[f] A clinical study[44] that used non-uniform documentation of thromboembolic events and compared retrospective data with observational data suggested that eculizumab ameliorates the risk of thromboembolic complication. Interpretation of these findings is debatable because of the suboptimal experimental design.

may respond to complement inhibition by eculizuab.[44] Nonetheless, transplantation is the only curative therapy for PNH, and the availability of molecularly defined matched unrelated donors, less toxic conditioning regimens, reductions in transplantation-related morbidity and mortality, and improvements in posttransplantation supportive care make this option increasingly attractive. The decision to transplant is complex, however, and requires an understanding of the unique pathobiology of PNH.

For patients who are receiving transplantation for bone marrow failure, the focus of management is on the etiology of the bone marrow failure (**Box 1**). For patients who have aplastic anemia and a small PNH clone who undergo matched sibling donor allotransplantation, the conditioning regimen of anti-thymocyte globulin and cyclophosphamide coupled with graft-versus-host effects seem sufficient to eradicate the PNH clone.[20] In the unusual situation in which the patient has a syngeneic twin, a more intense conditioning regimen seems to be required, because the graft-versus-host effect does not contribute to clonal eradication in this circumstance (**Fig. 3**).[45] If a patient who has low-risk MDS requires allotransplantation, the conditioning regimen (marrow ablative or reduced intensity) in combination with graft-versus-host effects is sufficient to eradicate the PNH clone.

Patients who have classic PNH have clinical signs and symptoms of intravascular hemolysis but have no evidence of another defined bone marrow abnormality. A cellular marrow with erythroid hyperplasia and normal or nearly normal morphology but without nonrandom karyotypic abnormalities is consistent with classic PNH.[20] Transplantation

---

Box 1
Hematopoietic stem cell transplantation for PNH

Indications for transplantation

Bone marrow failure: approach to management depends primarily on the underlying marrow abnormality (eg, aplastic anemia), but the treatment regimen must be sufficient to eradicate the PNH clone

Major complications of PNH

Refractory transfusion dependent hemolytic anemia[a]

Recurrent life-threatening thromboembolic complications[b]

Conditioning regimens and donors

Ablative and reduced-intensity conditioning regimens have been successful.

For transplantations involving syngeneic twins, an ablative regimen is recommended.[c]

Matched unrelated donor transplantations have been successful, but experience is limited.

Outcomes

There are no PNH-specific adverse events. Severe, acute graft-versus-host disease occurs in approximately 33% of patients, and the incidence of chronic graft-versus-host disease is roughly 35%.

Overall survival for unselected patients who have PNH and who undergo transplantation using an HLA-matched sibling donor is in the range of 50% to 60%.

[a] Treatment with eculizumab controls the intravascular hemolysis of PNH. Mild to moderate extravascular hemolytic anemia persists in most patients who have PNH treated with eculizumab, probably because of the opsonization of erythrocytes by activation and degradation products of complement C3.
[b] Eculizumab may ameliorate the thrombophilia of PNH.
[c] Absence of graft-versus-host effect may render nonablative approaches inadequate.

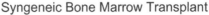

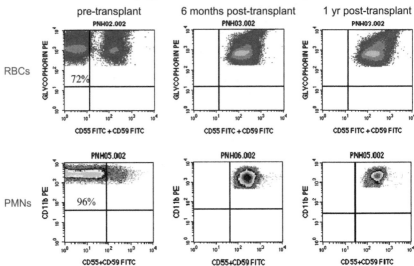

Fig. 3. Outcome of syngeneic transplantation for PNH. A patient who had classic PNH underwent marrow ablative conditioning with busulfan (1mg/kg × 16 doses) and cyclophosphamide (50 mg/kg × 4 doses) followed by stem cell rescue from a syngeneic donor. The presence of PNH cells in the peripheral blood RBCs and PMNs was detected using high-sensitivity flow cytometry (see **Fig. 1**). (*Left column*) Before transplantation, 72% of the patients' peripheral blood RBCs had the PNH phenotype, and 96% of the PMNs were GPI-AP deficient. (*Middle column*) Six months and (*Right column*) 12 months after transplantation, no PNH cells were detected in the patient's peripheral blood.

for classic PNH is aimed at eradicating the PNH clone, and both marrow-ablative[46–48] and reduced-intensity[49,50] conditioning regimens seem to be effective, although experience with the latter is more limited. Successful outcomes have been reported using matched unrelated donors as well as matched sibling donors.[49,51]

There are no PNH-specific adverse events associated with transplantation; severe, acute graft-versus-host disease occurs in more than a third of the patients, and the incidence of chronic graft-versus-host disease is roughly 35%. Overall 5-year survival rates for unselected PNH patients who undergo transplantation using an HLA-matched sibling donor are in the range of 50% to 60%.[20]

PNH can occur in the young (about 10% of patients are younger than 21 years at the time of diagnosis).[20] A retrospective analysis of 26 cases underscored the many similarities between childhood and adult PNH.[52] Signs and symptoms of hemolysis, bone marrow failure, and thrombosis dominate the clinical picture, although gross hemoglobinuria as a presenting symptom may be less common in young patients. A generally good response to immunosuppressive therapy was observed,[52] but, based on poor long-term survival, hematopoietic cell transplantation is the recommended treatment for childhood PNH. A more recent study confirmed the common presentation of bone marrow failure in 11 children who had PNH and reported that five patients eventually underwent hematopoietic cell transplantation (three had matched unrelated donors, and two had matched family donors); four of these children were long-term survivors.[53] Although eculizumab currently is not approved for PNH in patients younger than 18 years old, approval probably will be sought once the pharmacodynamic and pharmacokinetic characteristics of the drug are defined for the pediatric population. The availability of eculizumab for pediatric PNH may be particularly advantageous as a bridge before implementation of more definitive therapy such as hematopoietic stem cell transplantation.

SUMMARY AND FUTURE DIRECTIONS

The defining clinical pathology of PNH (ie, complement-mediated intravascular hemolysis) seems to be an epiphenomenon that is a consequence of an orchestrated response (ie, natural selection of *PIGA*-mutant stem cells) to a specific type of bone marrow injury (ie, immune mediated). Without the hemolytic anemia (and thrombophilia), benign clonal expansion of *PIGA*-mutant hematopoietic stem cells might be the ideal treatment for immune-mediated bone marrow failure, because treatment with the complement inhibitor eculizumab suggests that PNH is relatively benign when hemolysis is inhibited.[43] Studying the unique properties of PNH provides an opportunity to understand the molecular basis of benign clonal hematopoiesis, and identifying and characterizing the mechanisms that underlie the clonal selection, clonal expansion, and clonal dominance of PNH may suggest novel therapeutic strategies for enhancing hematopoietic stem function in patients who have bone marrow failure and for augmenting the function of normal hematopoietic stem cells for use in gene therapy and transplantation.

REFERENCES

1. Dacie JV. Paroxsymal nocturnal haemoglobinuria. Proc R Soc Med 1963;56: 587–96.
2. Kinoshita T, Inoue N, Takeda J. Defective glycosyl phosphatidylinositol anchor synthesis and paroxysmal nocturnal hemoglobinuria. Adv Immunol 1995;60:57–103.
3. Parker CJ. The pathophysiology of paroxysmal nocturnal hemoglobinuria. Exp Hematol 2007;35:523–33.
4. Parker CJ. Hemolysis in PNH. In: Young NS, Moss J, editors. Paroxysmal nocturnal hemoglobinuria and the glycosylphosphatidylinositol-linked proteins. San Diego (CA): Academic Press; 2000. p. 49–100.
5. Aster RH, Enright SE. A platelet and granulocyte membrane defect in paroxysmal nocturnal hemoglobinuria: usefulness for the detection of platelet antibodies. J Clin Invest 1969;48:1199–210.
6. Miyata T, Yamada N, Iida Y, et al. Abnormalities of PIG-A transcripts in granulocytes from patients with paroxysmal nocturnal hemoglobinuria. N Engl J Med 1994;330:249–55.
7. Takeda J, Miyata T, Kawagoe K, et al. Deficiency of the GPI anchor caused by a somatic mutation of the PIG-A gene in paroxysmal nocturnal hemoglobinuria. Cell 1993;73:703–11.
8. Sloand EM, Young NS. Thrombotic complications in PNH. In: Young NS, Moss J, editors. Paroxysmal nocturnal hemoglobinuria and the glycosylphosphatidylinositol-linked proteins. San Diego (CA): Academic Press; 2000. p. 101–12.
9. Endo M, Ware RE, Vreeke TM, et al. Molecular basis of the heterogeneity of expression of glycosyl phosphatidylinositol anchored proteins in paroxysmal nocturnal hemoglobinuria. Blood 1996;87:2546–57.
10. Miyata T, Takeda J, Iida Y, et al. The cloning of PIG-A, a component in the early step of GPI-anchor biosynthesis. Science 1993;259:1318–20.
11. Davitz MA, Low MG, Nussenzweig V. Release of decay-accelerating factor (DAF) from the cell membrane by phosphatidylinositol-specific phospholipase

C (PIPLC). Selective modification of a complement regulatory protein. J Exp Med 1986;163:1150–61.

12. Nicholson-Weller A, March JP, Rosenfeld SI, et al. Affected erythrocytes of patients with paroxysmal nocturnal hemoglobinuria are deficient in the complement regulatory protein, decay accelerating factor. Proc Natl Acad Sci U S A 1983;80:5066–70.

13. Pangburn MK, Schreiber RD, Muller-Eberhard HJ. Deficiency of an erythrocyte membrane protein with complement regulatory activity in paroxysmal nocturnal hemoglobinuria. Proc Natl Acad Sci U S A 1983;80:5430–4.

14. Holguin MH, Fredrick LR, Bernshaw NJ, et al. Isolation and characterization of a membrane protein from normal human erythrocytes that inhibits reactive lysis of the erythrocytes of paroxysmal nocturnal hemoglobinuria. J Clin Invest 1989; 84:7–17.

15. Holguin MH, Wilcox LA, Bernshaw NJ, et al. Relationship between the membrane inhibitor of reactive lysis and the erythrocyte phenotypes of paroxysmal nocturnal hemoglobinuria. J Clin Invest 1989;84:1387–94.

16. Nishimura JI, Kanakura Y, Ware RE, et al. Clinical course and flow cytometric analysis of paroxysmal nocturnal hemoglobinuria in the United States and Japan. Medicine (Baltimore) 2004;83:193–207.

17. de Latour RP, Mary JY, Salanoubat C, et al. Paroxysmal nocturnal hemoglobinuria: natural history of disease subcategories. Blood 2008;112:3099–106.

18. Hillmen P, Lewis SM, Bessler M, et al. Natural history of paroxysmal nocturnal hemoglobinuria. N Engl J Med 1995;333:1253–8.

19. Socie G, Mary JY, de Gramont A, et al. Paroxysmal nocturnal haemoglobinuria: long-term follow-up and prognostic factors. French Society of Haematology. Lancet 1996;348:573–7.

20. Parker C, Omine M, Richards S, et al. Diagnosis and management of paroxysmal nocturnal hemoglobinuria. Blood 2005;106:3699–709.

21. Dausset J, Paraf A, Maupin B. [Immunological study in nine cases of Marchiafava-Micheli syndrome.] Sem Hop 1956;32:366–71 [in French].

22. Dacie JV, Lewis SM. Paroxysmal nocturnal haemoglobinuria: variation in clinical severity and association with bone-marrow hypoplasia. Br J Haematol 1961;7: 442–57.

23. Lewis SM, Dacie JV. The aplastic anaemia–paroxysmal nocturnal haemoglobinuria syndrome. Br J Haematol 1967;13:236–51.

24. Dunn DE, Liu JM, Young NS. Bone marrow failure in PNH. In: Young NS, Moss J, editors. Paroxysmal nocturnal hemoglobinuria and the glycosylphosphatidylinositol-linked proteins. San Diego (CA): Academic Press; 2000. p. 113–38.

25. Inoue N, Izui-Sarumaru T, Murakami Y, et al. Molecular basis of clonal expansion of hematopoiesis in two patients with paroxysmal nocturnal hemoglobinuria (PNH). Blood 2006;108:4232–6.

26. Murakami Y, Kinoshita T, Maeda Y, et al. Different roles of glycosylphosphatidylinositol in various hematopoietic cells as revealed by a mouse model of paroxysmal nocturnal hemoglobinuria. Blood 1999;94:2963–70.

27. Maciejewski JP, Sloand EM, Sato T, et al. Impaired hematopoiesis in paroxysmal nocturnal hemoglobinuria/aplastic anemia is not associated with a selective proliferative defect in the glycosylphosphatidylinositol-anchored protein-deficient clone. Blood 1997;89:1173–81.

28. Chen G, Kirby M, Zeng W, et al. Superior growth of glycophosphatidylinositol-anchored protein-deficient progenitor cells in vitro is due to the higher apoptotic rate of progenitors with normal phenotype in vivo. Exp Hematol 2002;30:774–82.

29. Chen R, Nagarajan S, Prince GM, et al. Impaired growth and elevated fas receptor expression in PIGA (+) stem cells in primary paroxysmal nocturnal hemoglobinuria. J Clin Invest 2000;106:689–96.
30. Mukhina GL, Buckley JT, Barber JP, et al. Multilineage glycosylphosphatidylinositol anchor-deficient haematopoiesis in untreated aplastic anaemia. Br J Haematol 2001;115:476–82.
31. Sugimori C, Chuhjo T, Feng X, et al. Minor population of CD55-CD59- blood cells predicts response to immunosuppressive therapy and prognosis in patients with aplastic anemia. Blood 2005;107:1308–14.
32. Dunn DE, Tanawattanacharoen P, Boccuni P, et al. Paroxysmal nocturnal hemoglobinuria cells in patients with bone marrow failure syndromes. Ann Intern Med 1999;131:401–8.
33. Schubert J, Vogt HG, Zielinska-Skowronek M, et al. Development of the glycosylphosphatidylinositol-anchoring defect characteristic for paroxysmal nocturnal hemoglobinuria in patients with aplastic anemia. Blood 1994;83:2323–8.
34. Griscelli-Bennaceur A, Gluckman E, Scrobohaci ML, et al. Aplastic anemia and paroxysmal nocturnal hemoglobinuria: search for a pathogenetic link. Blood 1995;85:1354–63.
35. Frickhofen N, Heimpel H, Kaltwasser JP, et al. Antithymocyte globulin with or without cyclosporin A: 11-year follow-up of a randomized trial comparing treatments of aplastic anemia. Blood 2003;101:1236–42.
36. Nagarajan S, Brodsky RA, Young NS, et al. Genetic defects underlying paroxysmal nocturnal hemoglobinuria that arises out of aplastic anemia. Blood 1995;86:4656–61.
37. Ishiyama K, Chuhjo T, Wang H, et al. Polyclonal hematopoiesis maintained in patients with bone marrow failure harboring a minor population of paroxysmal nocturnal hemoglobinuria-type cells. Blood 2003;102:1211–6.
38. Wang H, Chuhjo T, Yasue S, et al. Clinical significance of a minor population of paroxysmal nocturnal hemoglobinuria-type cells in bone marrow failure syndrome. Blood 2002;100:3897–902.
39. Wang SA, Pozdnyakova O, Jorgensen JL, et al. Detection of paroxysmal nocturnal hemoglobinuria clones in patients with myelodysplastic syndromes and related bone marrow diseases, with emphasis on diagnostic pitfalls and caveats. Haematologica 2008;94:29–37.
40. Harris NL, Jaffe ES, Diebold J, et al. The World Health Organization classification of neoplastic diseases of the hematopoietic and lymphoid tissues. Report of the Clinical Advisory Committee meeting, Airlie House, Virginia, November, 1997. Ann Oncol 1999;10:1419–32.
41. Saunthararajah Y, Nakamura R, Nam JM, et al. HLA-DR15 (DR2) is overrepresented in myelodysplastic syndrome and aplastic anemia and predicts a response to immunosuppression in myelodysplastic syndrome. Blood 2002;100:1570–4.
42. Sugimori C, Yamazaki H, Feng X, et al. Roles of DRB1 *1501 and DRB1 *1502 in the pathogenesis of aplastic anemia. Exp Hematol 2007;35:13–20.
43. Hillmen P, Young NS, Schubert J, et al. The complement inhibitor eculizumab in paroxysmal nocturnal hemoglobinuria. N Engl J Med 2006;355:1233–43.
44. Hillmen P, Muus P, Duhrsen U, et al. Effect of the complement inhibitor eculizumab on thromboembolism in patients with paroxysmal nocturnal hemoglobinuria. Blood 2007;110:4123–8.
45. Endo M, Beatty PG, Vreeke TM, et al. Syngeneic bone marrow transplantation without conditioning in a patient with paroxysmal nocturnal hemoglobinuria: in

vivo evidence that the mutant stem cells have a survival advantage. Blood 1996; 88:742–50.

46. Bemba M, Guardiola P, Garderet L, et al. Bone marrow transplantation for paroxysmal nocturnal haemoglobinuria. Br J Haematol 1999;105:366–8.

47. Raiola AM, Van Lint MT, Lamparelli T, et al. Bone marrow transplantation for paroxysmal nocturnal hemoglobinuria. Haematologica 2000;85:59–62.

48. Saso R, Marsh J, Cevreska L, et al. Bone marrow transplants for paroxysmal nocturnal haemoglobinuria. Br J Haematol 1999;104:392–6.

49. Hegenbart U, Niederwieser D, Forman S, et al. Hematopoietic cell transplantation from related and unrelated donors after minimal conditioning as a curative treatment modality for severe paroxysmal nocturnal hemoglobinuria. Biol Blood Marrow Transplant 2003;9:689–97.

50. Takahashi Y, McCoy JP Jr, Carvallo C, et al. In vitro and in vivo evidence of PNH cell sensitivity to immune attack after nonmyeloablative allogeneic hematopoietic cell transplantation. Blood 2004;103:1383–90.

51. Woodard P, Wang W, Pitts N, et al. Successful unrelated donor bone marrow transplantation for paroxysmal nocturnal hemoglobinuria. Bone Marrow Transplant 2001;27:589–92.

52. Ware RE, Hall SE, Rosse WF. Paroxysmal nocturnal hemoglobinuria with onset in childhood and adolescence. N Engl J Med 1991;325:991–6.

53. van den Heuvel-Eibrink MM, Bredius RG, te Winkel ML, et al. Childhood paroxysmal nocturnal haemoglobinuria (PNH), a report of 11 cases in the Netherlands. Br J Haematol 2005;128:571–7.

Hypocellular Myelodysplasia

Elaine M. Sloand, MD

KEYWORDS

• Myelodysplasia • Cellularity • Hypoplastic • Immune-mediated

The term "myelodysplasia syndrome" (MDS) refers to a group of diverse diseases characterized by ineffective hematopoiesis, cytopenias, and a proclivity to develop leukemia. Although some cases of MDS, particularly those in which the marrow is hypocellular, show evidence of evidence of immune activation and respond to immunosuppressive therapy (IST), other groups of patients, primarily the elderly, do not share these characteristics. Several fundamental questions affecting the current understanding of MDS remain unanswered. Do patients who have hypocellular bone marrows differ from patients who have MDS whose cellularity is normal or increased? Can patients who have MDS who respond to IST be distinguished from patients who have aplastic anemia (AA)? Clearly, some patients who have hypercellular marrows respond to IST, and these responsive patients seem to differ from patients who have AA in many ways. This article evaluates the clinical and molecular data examining these issues and discusses areas of future investigation.

DIFFERENTIATING APLASTIC ANEMIA FROM HYPOPLASTIC MYELODYSPLASIA SYNDROME

Although it generally is accepted that hypoplastic patients who have bone marrow cytogenetic defects or classic morphologic abnormalities on bone marrow smears have MDS, the diagnosis may be somewhat difficult in hypocellular MDS if the aspirate is so sparsely cellular as to preclude such studies. Significant clonal cytogenetic abnormalities are present in only half of all MDS cases, and full karyotypic analysis, which requires cells in metaphase, may not be possible because cells may be scarce or senescent. Other diagnostic difficulties arise when the dysplastic changes are mild and/or when only one lineage is involved. Mild dysplasia, particularly that involving only the erythroid lineage, may be observed in other bone marrow failure states. For example, erythroid dysplasia is present in some cases of AA.

Distinguishing hypoplastic MDS from AA may be even more difficult as technology advances. Now that fluorescent in situ hybridization (FISH) is more readily available, small clones of aneuploid cells may be detected in patients who apparently have AA at diagnosis[1,2] and may not necessarily influence response to IST.[3] Additional

Hematology Branch, National Heart Lung and Blood Institute, 10 Center Drive, Bldg10, CRC Rm 4E5230, Bethesda, MD 20892, USA
E-mail address: sloande@nih.gov

Hematol Oncol Clin N Am 23 (2009) 347–360
doi:10.1016/j.hoc.2009.01.015
0889-8588/09/$ – see front matter © 2009 Published by Elsevier Inc.

hemonc.theclinics.com

clonal changes may be appreciated when single-nucleotide polymorphism (SNP) analysis is used to examine patients who have bone marrow failure.[4]

ARE THERE DIFFERENCES BETWEEN HYPOCELLULAR MYELODYSPLASIA AND NORMO- OR HYPERCELLULAR MYELODYSPLASIA?

Unfortunately no data were collected by the International MDS Research Analysis Workshop on the bone marrow cellularity of their cohort[5] to determine if patients who had hypocellular bone marrows had a better prognosis than patients who had normocellular or hypercellular marrows. Examination of this issue would be difficult, because many patients have variable cellularity depending on the site of biopsy. One retrospective study examined 163 patients who had hypocellular MDS from a pool of 1049 consecutive MDS adult patients seen over an 11-year period (1995–2006). Compared with patients who had normal/hypercellular MDS, the patients who had hypocellular MDS were younger, less anemic, but more neutropenic and thrombocytopenic, and had a comparable cytogenetic risk group distribution and International Prognostic Scoring System (IPSS) scores. Patients who had hypocellular MDS showed a favorable overall survival (56 months versus 28 months, log-rank $P <$ .0001) compared with patients who had normal/hypocellular MDS in all IPSS groups and cytogenetic risk groups.[6] These patients received divergent treatments, but the treatment-algorithm applied to each group was independent of cellularity. In another study karyotypic abnormalities were present in 12.5% of hypocellular cases, in contrast to 44.6% of normo/hypercellular cases ($P = $ .0025). These changes may be attributed to the adequacy of the sample for cytogenetic analysis, however.[7] Basic laboratory studies to define the pathogenesis of the disease do not seem to vary with the cellularity. Apoptosis seems to be excessive in both hypo- and hypercellular MDS.[8] The number of colony-forming units is decreased in MDS, but this number is not significantly different when patients who had hypocellular MDS are compared with patients who had hyper/normocellular MDS.[9]

SOME MYELODYSPLASIA IS IMMUNOLOGICALLY MEDIATED

Laboratory and clinical evidence suggests that some cases of MDS are immune mediated. Bone marrow cells from patients who have low-risk MDS express apoptotic markers and show evidence of programmed cell death. Simultaneously, there are signs of immune activation with expansion of specific Vβ subfamilies consistent with an antigen-mediated CD8 response. Cytotoxic T-lymphocyte expansions can be detected in as many as 81% of patients who have MDS.[10] The fact that lymphocytes within these Vβ subfamilies obtained before successful IST diminish hematopoietic colony formation in vitro, whereas lymphocytes obtained after IST do not, suggests that these cytotoxic T cells may play a role in the pathophysiology of these disorders.[11]

Multiple studies have demonstrated cytokine dysregulation in patients who have MDS.[12,13,14,15] Peripheral blood lymphocytes from patients who have MDS overexpress tumor necrosis factor-α (TNF-α), TNF-related apoptosis-inducing ligand (TRAIL),[16] and interferon-γ (IFN-γ).[17,18] Flice (caspase-8) inhibitory protein (FLIP), an adaptor molecule that modulates TNF-α–, Fas-, and TRAIL-initiated signals, also is abnormally expressed in MDS.[19] TNF-α and IFN-γ suppress hematopoiesis and promote apoptosis and programmed cell death in otherwise normal CD34 cells[11,20,21] as well as in more mature progeny. Levels of TNF-α are highest in patients who have low-risk MDS (ie, refractory anemia [RA] and refractory anemia with ringed sideroblasts). The major sources of TNF-α are bone marrow mononuclear (nonstromal) cells[22] and activated T lymphocytes.[23] Interestingly, TRAIL produced apoptosis selectively in cytogenetically abnormal cells, identified by FISH markers.[16] These findings were attributed to up-regulation of TRAIL receptors 1 and 2 on the aneuploid clone and to differential expression (or function) of intracellular inhibitors of apoptosis such as FLIP.[19]

Immune dysregulation has been described in both hyper- and hypocellular MDS,[11,24] suggesting a similar pathophysiology that is independent of marrow cellularity. Differences in cellularity may be related to the relative resistance of the bone marrow cells to undergoing apoptosis or to the strength of the immune attack. Although in normal cells, early apoptotic changes evidenced by annexin binding and caspase 8 activation are followed inexorably by programmed cell death, this scenario does not always hold true in MDS.[24,25] Annexin-positive, caspase-positive marrow does not always show evidence of DNA degradation in MDS, particularly in trisomy 8.[26] In these circumstances, when annexin-binding bone marrow cells are sorted by flow cytometry and are plated in short-term culture, annexin-positive and -negative cells show comparable growth. The ability to bind annexin results from alterations in membrane phosphatidylserine, which occur early in apoptosis before activation of caspase 8.

The mechanism for immunologically mediated marrow damage in MDS has been defined most clearly in patients presenting with trisomy 8 as a single karyotypic abnormality. The author and colleagues chose to investigate trisomy 8 because patients who have this cytogenetic abnormality are likely to respond to IST,[27] and the dysplastic clone can be identified easily by FISH. In early studies these investigators showed that early apoptotic changes seemed to be restricted to the trisomy 8 clone; flow cytometric–sorted Fas-positive, annexin-positive cells were enriched in or composed entirely of trisomy 8 cells.[8] Expanded Vβ T cells were capable of killing trisomy 8 cells selectively in vitro, suggesting that trisomy 8 cells were an immunologic target. T-cell–depleted marrow showed preferential improved growth of trisomy 8 colonies. The persistence of trisomy 8 cells could be attributed to trisomy 8 up-regulation of the anti-apoptotic protein, survivin, an apoptotic protein. Compared with diploid cells, trisomy 8 bone marrow showed up-regulation of c-Myc, cyclin D1, and survivin,[26] all of which may facilitate the cell's survival despite an immune attack.

Patients who have trisomy 8 are likely to respond to IST. Moreover, following IST, the trisomy 8 clone, unlike other cytogenetic abnormalities, expands. The presence of a neoantigen or of a normal antigen that is overexpressed on the clone could explain these findings. The author and colleagues investigated this possibility by examining microarray data on CD34 cells obtained from patients who had MDS with trisomy 8 as well as other cytogenetic abnormalities,[28] instead of laboriously testing peptide libraries. Wilms tumor protein 1 (WT1) was immunogenic and overexpressed on trisomy 8 cells. WT1 is a zinc-finger transcription factor located on chromosome 11p13, which was discovered because of its involvement in the pathogenesis of the Wilms' tumor.[29,30] This antigen is expressed normally in a number of tissues, including kidney, ovary, testis, and spleen. Although not detected in normal bone marrow or peripheral blood, WT1 is overexpressed in most cases of myeloid and lymphoid malignancies, including MDS,[31,32,33,34] as well as in acquired hematologic diseases such as paroxysmal nocturnal hemoglobinuria.[35] WT1 transcript levels increase with disease progression and correlate with the IPSS stage.[32] In studies conducted by the author and colleagues, both WT1 mRNA and protein were increased in many patients who had IPSS intermediate 1 MDS but were most prominent in patients who had trisomy 8. WT1-evoked TNF-α and IL-2 CD8 responses could be elicited in pretreatment specimens from patients who ultimately responded to IST.[36] CD8 cytotoxic T cells, which recognized WT1$_{126-134}$ peptides, also could be detected by tetramer analysis in the same patient population (**Fig. 1** examines a possible scenario in which trisomy 8 cells are targeted by the immune system). There probably are other antigens recognized by the immune system on the trisomy 8 cell and in MDS in general, but their identification may require careful testing of peptide libraries. In this regard, PR1, a myeloid restricted azurophil granule protein, seems capable of provoking an immune response in patients who have MDS. Proteinase 3 is threefold to sixfold overexpressed in cytotoxic lymphocytes, acute myelogenous leukemia, and MDS cells and has been shown to be a target epitope of cytotoxic lymphocytes that preferentially lyse myeloid leukemia cells.[37,38]

HYPOPLASTIC MYELODYSPLASIA SYNDROME ARISING FROM APLASTIC ANEMIA

MDS may develop de novo in patients without a pre-existing history of bone marrow failure or may arise in patients who have AA.[39,40] The two most frequent cytogenetic abnormalities appearing in patients who have a prior history of AA are monosomy 7 and trisomy 8. Patients who have AA who develop monosomy 7 generally are refractory to immunosuppression, whereas those who have trisomy 8 continue to respond to IST, becoming dependent on its continuation for normal hematopoiesis.[41] In many patients who have normal cytogenetics at disease presentation, chromosomal abnormalities can be detected by FISH.[26,42] Likewise SNP studies demonstrate mutations in apparently straightforward cases of AA that are negative for FISH.[10] One could hypothesize that these abnormalities give rise to antigenic change that elicits an immune response.

Autoimmune bone marrow also may foster the development of chromosomal abnormalities. Inflammatory states such as Barrett's esophagitis, hepatitis, graft-versus-host disease of the skin, and ulcerative colitis result in aneuploidy and tetraploidy that may precede malignant transformation.[43,44,45,46] In ulcerative colitis,[47] nitric

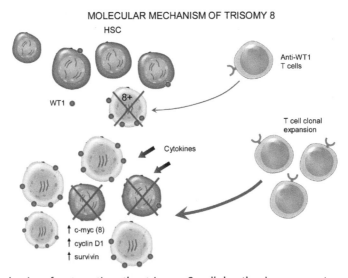

Fig. 1. Mechanism for targeting the trisomy 8 cell by the immune system. Innocent bystanders (diploid cells) are killed after exposure to cytokines secreted by activated T cells. Trisomy 8 cells survive because of up-regulation of c-Myc, cyclin D1, and the anti-apoptotic protein survivin HSC, human stem cells.

oxide–induced cell cycle arrest may lead to tetraploidy and DNA repair, but repeated oxidative stress may lead to mutation or loss of the tumor suppressor gene, *p53* muta-tion.[43,48] *p53* responds to aneuploidy by blocking progression through the cell cycle and triggering apoptosis. In colitis, loss of heterozygosity of *p53* increases with increasing dysplasia. Colon cancers resulting from chronic colitis and inflammatory bowel disease demonstrate almost 85% loss of *p53* heterozygosity.[43] Both *p53* muta-tion and deletion have been described in MDS.[49,50,51] An alternative and not mutually exclusive possibility is that continued inflammation necessitates an increased turnover of cells coupled with an increased possibility of non-disjunction during metaphase and shortening of telomere length. Shortening of telomere length results in aneuploidy in a mouse model, possibly because shortened telomeres tend to fuse end-to-end, pre-venting disjunction of chromosomes during metaphase.[52] Diminished telomere length has been described in both AA[54] and MDS.[55]

Once present, viable aneuploid cells with comparative growth advantages or resis-tance to apoptosis have a survival advantage over their diploid counterparts; this advantage results in expansion of the clone. Trisomy 8 cells are more resistant to apoptosis than are their diploid counterparts by virtue of increased expression of cyclin D1 and c-Myc and up-regulation of the anti-apoptotic protein survivin.[26] These cells are resistant to radiation and withdrawal of serum from media but die quickly when c-Myc, cyclin D1, or survivin is knocked down in vitro.[26] Monosomy 7 cells over-express the maturation-defective granulocyte colony-stimulating factor receptor (GCSFR) isoform IV, rendering them nonviable at ambient concentrations of GCSF seen in normal individuals but driving their growth at the high concentrations seen in patients who have marrow failure.[42] The isoform IV of GCSFR seems to have decreased affinity for GCSF.[56] It seems likely that this decrease is overcome by high concentrations of GCSF, commonly seen in patients who have bone marrow failure,[57,58] because monosomy 7 cells expand at concentrations greater than 200 ng/mL.[42] The truncated GCSFR IV, like the truncated form of GCSFR seen in severe congenital neutropenia, lacks the dileucine residue required for normal inter-nalization and recycling of the GCSFR-GCSF complex,[59] resulting in constitutive up-regulation of Jak-2 and continued proliferation. Akt, a potent anti-apoptotic protein, is up-regulated in turn by Jak-2 and confers resistance to apoptosis relative to diploid cells.[60] The fact that patients who have monosomy 7 show elimination of or a decline in their monosomy 7 clone following clinical responses to immunosup-pressive therapy[61,62,63] further supports the role of GCSF in allowing the expansion of that clone. Others have reported similar declines in monosomy 7 after withdrawal of GCSF administration.[64]

TREATMENT AND ITS RELATION TO CELLULARITY

Cytopenias account for almost half the deaths attributed to MDS, and leukemia accounts for the remainder.[65] Treatment thus has focused not only on the elimination of the dysplastic clone but also on improving bone marrow function. Following the success of IST in patients who had AA, several investigators in the 1980s also used anti-thymocyte globulin (ATG) to treat the bone marrow failure accompanying hypo-plastic MDS. Some of these patients had sustained recovery of their blood cell counts.[66,67] This treatment subsequently was applied also to patients who had hyper-cellular disease.[68] Cyclosporin was used subsequently to treat MDS and generally has yielded equal results in patients, regardless of cellularity.[69,70,71]

Now more treatments are available for patients who have MDS, some of which target genes that are overexpressed in these patients. Patients who have hypocellular

MDS are a diverse group, and the choice of therapy should be based on age, the availability of a suitable matched sibling donor, cytogenetics, and the presence of blasts in the bone marrow. Young patients who have a sibling donor and unfavorable cytogenetics or IPSS score[5] should consider bone marrow transplantation, which is the only curative option for the patient. Supportive care or treatment with lenalidomide, immunosuppressive therapy, or azacitidine may benefit older patients who have comorbidities or those without a suitable bone marrow donor. Choice of therapy should be individualized for each patient. Lenalidomide benefits patients who have MDS regardless of cytogenetic abnormality but seems to produce the best responses in patients who have the chromosomal abnormality, 5q-. About 43% of patients without 5q- respond,[72] whereas 76% of patients with 5q- benefit regardless of the complexity of the karyotype.[73] Interestingly, cytopenias were not worse in patients who had hypocellular bone marrows but seemed to be greatest in patients who had 5q-; this finding was attributed to specific toxicity of the drug for cells with this cytogenetic abnormality.[74] 5-azacytidine preferentially benefits patients who have blasts, patients who have high-risk MDS, and patients who have monosomy 7. Significant cytopenias may complicate treatment, however, and it would seem likely that patients who have hypocellular MDS would be preferentially affected. The prognosis following bone marrow transplantation seems to be related most closely to factors such as disease burden, age,[75,76] and performance status rather than cellularity. The presence of excess blasts in the marrow is the factor that affects the outcome most negatively.[77,78]

ROLE OF IMMUNOSUPPRESSIVE THERAPY IN HYPOCELLULAR VERSUS HYPERCELLULAR MYELODYSPLASIA SYNDROME: DOES CELLULARITY AFFECT RESPONSE TO IMMUNOSUPPRESSIVE THERAPY?

Many physicians believe that hypocellular MDS is best treated with IST. Although some studies show better responses in this patient population, improvements in hematopoiesis certainly are not limited to this population, and in some studies other factors seem more important for predicting response. The initial prospective trials using ATG or cyclosporine A (CsA) were published in the late 1900s, and now there are data from more than 10 centers worldwide on a large number of patients treated with IST in clinical protocols.[68,70,71,79,80,81,82] What seems evident from these studies is that successes generally were reported in younger patients who had low-risk MDS. Older patients were more likely not to respond and also were more susceptible to the vasomotor instability associated with ATG and the renal failure associated with long-term use of CsA.

Cyclosporine

CsA is effective for some patients who have low-risk MDS, regardless of cellularity.[69] One group reported prolonged responses in as many as 82% of patients, all of whom achieved transfusion independence: responses occurred in eight of nine patients who had hypocellular MDS and in six of eight patients who had normo/hypercellular MDS. In a larger multicenter study in Japan,[83] 50 patients who had "low-risk" (blasts < 10%) MDS with variable marrow cellularity were treated. Of these, 30 patients (60%) showed hematologic improvement and responses independent of marrow cellularity. CsA was well tolerated generally, but serious toxicities, primarily renal failure, made termination of therapy necessary in a minority of patients, most of whom then sustained hematologic relapse. Another study reported no substantial responses to CsA but unacceptable toxicity.[84] One explanation for the poor responses and high toxicity in this cohort may be their older age, which puts them at greater risk for CsA-related renal toxicity (**Table 1**).

Anti-Thymocyte Globulin–Based Regimens

Horse and more recently rabbit ATG have proven utility in treatment of both AA and MDS. Although ATG rapidly depletes peripheral and lymphoid T cells, its effect is transient, and repopulation greatly precedes hematologic response. In vitro data suggest that ATG may interfere with the function of dendritic cells and inhibit the interaction between the T cell and the antigen-presenting cell.[85] Other in vitro data support a role for ATG in facilitating expansion of T-regulatory cells.[86]

In the National Institutes of Health (NIH) trials using ATG-based treatment, 129 patients were treated with ATG (40 mg/kg of body weight) daily for 4 days and CsA, or both ATG and CsA. Thirty-nine patients (30%) receiving a single course of immunosuppression responded with significant improvement in cytopenia and transfusion independence.[27] Thirty-one percent of the responses (12/39) were complete, resulting in transfusion independence and nearly normal blood counts. Factors affecting responses included younger age, low IPSS score, and the presence of HLA DR15. Although responses were equal in patients regardless of MDS cellularity, complete responses were more common in patients who had hypocellular MDS. The addition of CsA seemed to increase the response rate ($P = .048$), but a controlled, randomized trial comparing the two regimens is required to verify these results. Age was a continuous variable: the younger the patient, the better the response to treatment. Median survival of responders was superior to that of nonresponders. The survival of patients 60 years of age or younger who had IPSS intermediate 1 MDS treated with IST was superior to that of the historical sample of similar patients treated with supportive care.[27] Multifactorial analysis showed that cellularity did not affect survival. In contrast Lim and colleagues[81] in the United Kingdom studied a group of 96 patients who had MDS, 40 (42%) of whom achieved a hematologic response. This group reported that patients who had hypocellular bone marrow were most likely to respond and that age did not influence response. Differences in patient recruitment, data analysis, and criteria for diagnosis of MDS may have been responsible for these differences in results.

Trials with younger patients tend to show improved response rates as well as decreased morbidity associated with the ATG.[87] Geary and colleagues[62] from

Table 1							
Clinical trials of ATG to treat cytopenia in MDS							
Center	N	Median Age	% RA	Response n (%)	Response RA (%)	% Hypocellular	Response Hypocellular
National Institutes of Health[53]	129	60	87 (67)	39 (30)	36 (40)	41 (34)	18 (44)
London	96	56	74 (77)	40 (42)	34 (46)	53 (55)	27 (51)
MD Anderson[11,71]	31	59	18 (58)	5 (27)	2(11)	—	2
Hanover[90]	35	63	24 (68)	12 (34)	10 (42)	4 (11)	2 (50)
Mayo Clinic[82]	8	71	2 (25)	0	0	—	0
Karolinska[87]	20	85	—	6 (30)	5 (29)	4 (20)	2 (50)
Total	253	—	—	71 (28)	61 (41)	—	—

Manchester, United Kingdom, reported the use of ATG with CsA or oxymetholone in 13 patients who had hypoplastic MDS with cytogenetic abnormalities (average age, 40 years). All patients ultimately responded to immunosuppression (with or without androgens), but three eventually relapsed into aplasia. In contrast, Steensma and colleagues[82] from the Mayo clinic studied a group of older patients (median age, 69 years) and found no responses and considerable toxicity in eight patients who had MDS (two had RA, and six had refractory anemia with excess of blasts) treated with ATG, 40 mg/kg/d for 4 days. At the M.D. Anderson Cancer Center, a group of 32 patients who had MDS were treated with ATG (40 mg/kg/d) intravenously (iv) for 4 days plus CsA daily orally for 6 months and methylprednisone, 1 mg/kg/d, iv before each dose of ATG. Of the 31 evaluable patients, 4 had a complete remission, and 1 had a partial remission (16% response rate); three of these responses were durable remissions (12–60+ months). The inclusion of older patients with excess blasts may account for the results that are relatively poorer than those in other studies.

IST seems to improve non-clonal hematopoiesis. Aivado and colleagues[88] from Dusseldorf studied this phenomenon in 10 female patients who had low-risk MDS treated with antilymphocyte globulin or ATG. The four responders demonstrated a "non-clonal" marrow defined by X chromosome inactivation patterns, suggesting improved normal progenitor function.

The use of rabbit ATG has not been studied thoroughly in MDS, although it is used commonly to treat AA.[89] Stadler and colleagues[90] compared the efficacy of horse ATG (15 mg/kg/d) with rabbit ATG (3.75 mg/kg/d) in a cohort of 35 patients who had MDS treated for 5 days. There were no significant differences between the two treatment arms with regard to clinically relevant responses or adverse effects. Although only small numbers of patients were enrolled, this study suggested that results were comparable in the two arms. The overall response rate was 34% and 42% in RA patients receiving horse and rabbit ATG respectively.

Although patients who have MDS relapse following treatment with ATG, they frequently respond to reinstitution of immunosuppression, often with CsA. In the NIH study, there were 13 relapses among the 39 responders. Among the 12 patients who had complete responses, four relapsed within the first year, but all responded to re-initiation of immunosuppression; of these patients, two only required re-initiation of CsA. Three of these patients remain in remission without further treatment at a median follow-up of 6.2 years. Median relapse-free survival was greater than 10.5 years. Of the 40 responders in the European study, 30 (75%) had a durable hematologic response with a median duration of 31.5 months at the time of reporting (range, 6–92 months).[81] Ten patients had a transient response to ATG with a median duration of 22 months (range, 2–46 months). Of the 10 patients who had a transient response to initial ATG therapy, 3 patients subsequently received a second course of ATG, with 2 patients achieving a hematologic response. The duration of response among trials varied considerably (see **Table 1**); the variation may be related to differences in the definition of relapse and to differences in immunosuppressive regimen. A randomized study comparing ATG and ATG plus CsA has not been performed to determine if the addition of CsA has positive effects on the duration of remission. Despite concerns regarding the potential for escape of a malignant clone, IST has not been associated with an increased progression to leukemia.[27] FISH and cytogenetic analysis of a patient's bone marrow before and following immunosuppression have demonstrated no consistent increase in chromosomal abnormalities indicative of clonal expansion other than in patients who have trisomy 8.[24] Trisomy 8 cells increase in IPSS intermediate 1 patients following ATG treatment when the cytotoxic T cell specific for this clone is eliminated. The trisomy 8 clone expands but, interestingly, is capable of sustaining normal hematopoiesis for protracted periods of time.[24]

SUMMARY

Cellularity may not affect either response to therapy or prognosis substantially. Whether the pathophysiology differs is unclear. Cellularity does not seem to affect response to IST significantly and does not seem to be the major factor affecting improvements in response to lenalidomide, stem cell transplantation, or hematopoietic growth factors. Difficulties encountered when comparing patients who have hypocellularity and those who have hypercellularity include variability in cellularity and difficulties in distinguishing between AA and hypoplastic MDS.

REFERENCES

1. Kojima S, Ohara A, Tsuchida M, et al. Risk factors for evolution of acquired aplastic anemia into myelodysplastic syndrome and acute myeloid leukemia after immunosuppressive therapy in children. Blood 2002;100(3):786–90.
2. Sloand EM, Scheinberg P, Fenlon E, et al. Monosomy 7 detected by FISH at disease presentation is a marker for non-response to immunosuppression. Blood 2007;110:1697 [abstract].
3. Gupta V, Brooker C, Tooze JA, et al. Clinical relevance of cytogenetic abnormalities at diagnosis of acquired aplastic anaemia in adults. Br J Haematol 2006; 134(1):95–9.
4. Tiu R, Gondek L, O'Keefe C, et al. Clonality of the stem cell compartment during evolution of myelodysplastic syndromes and other bone marrow failure syndromes. Leukemia 2007;21(8):1648–57.
5. Greenberg P, Cox C, LeBeau MM, et al. International scoring system for evaluating prognosis in myelodysplastic syndromes. Blood 1997;89(6):2079–88.
6. Yue G, Hao S, Fadare O, et al. Hypocellularity in myelodysplastic syndrome is an independent factor which predicts a favorable outcome. Leuk Res 2008;32(4): 553–8.
7. Marisavljevi-ç D, -îemeriki-ç V, Rolovi-ç Z, et al. Hypocellular myelodysplastic syndromes. Med Oncol 2005;22(2):169–75.
8. Sloand EM, Kim S, Fuhrer M, et al. Fas-mediated apoptosis is important in regulating cell replication and death in trisomy 8 hematopoietic cells but not in cells with other cytogenetic abnormalities. Blood 2002;100(13):4427–32.
9. Sato T, Kim S, Selleri C, et al. Measurement of secondary colony formation after 5 weeks in long-term cultures in patients with myelodysplastic syndrome. Leukemia 1998;12(8):1187–94.
10. Wlodarski MW, Gondek LP, Nearman ZP, et al. Molecular strategies for detection and quantitation of clonal cytotoxic T-cell responses in aplastic anemia and myelodysplastic syndrome. Blood 2006;108(8):2632–41.
11. Kochenderfer JN, Kobayashi S, Wieder ED, et al. Loss of T-lymphocyte clonal dominance in patients with myelodysplastic syndrome responsive to immunosuppression. Blood 2002;100(10):3639–45.
12. Allampallam K, Shetty V, Mundle S, et al. Biological significance of proliferation, apoptosis, cytokines, and monocyte/macrophage cells in bone marrow biopsies of 145 patients with myelodysplastic syndrome. Int J Hematol 2002;75(3):289–97.
13. Allampallam K, Shetty VT, Raza A. Cytokines and MDS. Cancer Treat Res 2001; 108:93–100.

14. Kitagawa M, Saito I, Kuwata T, et al. Overexpression of tumor necrosis factor (TNF)-alpha and interferon (IFN)-gamma by bone marrow cells from patients with myelodysplastic syndromes. Leukemia 1997;11(12):2049–54.

15. Koike M, Ishiyama T, Tomoyasu S, et al. Spontaneous cytokine overproduction by peripheral blood mononuclear cells from patients with myelodysplastic syndromes and aplastic anemia. Leuk Res 1995;19(9):639–44.

16. Zang DY, Goodwin RG, Loken MR, et al. Expression of tumor necrosis factor-related apoptosis-inducing ligand, Apo2L, and its receptors in myelodysplastic syndrome: effects on in vitro hemopoiesis. Blood 2001;98(10):3058–65.

17. Kitagawa M, Takahashi M, Yamaguchi S, et al. Expression of inducible nitric oxide synthase (NOS) in bone marrow cells of myelodysplastic syndromes. Leukemia 1999;13(5):699–703.

18. Verhoef GE, Schouwer P, Ceuppens JL, et al. Measurement of serum cytokine levels in patients with myelodysplastic syndrome. Leukemia 1992;6:1268–72.

19. Benesch M, Platzbecker U, Ward J, et al. Expression of FLIP(long) and FLIP(short) in bone marrow mononuclear and CD34+ cells in patients with myelodysplastic syndrome: correlation with apoptosis. Leukemia 2003;17(12):2460–6.

20. Maciejewski JP, Selleri C, Anderson S, et al. Fas antigen expression on CD34+ human marrow cells is induced by interferon-gamma and tumor necrosis factor-alpha and potentiates cytokine-mediated hematopoietic suppression in vitro. Blood 1995;85:3183–90.

21. Sato T, Selleri C, Anderson S, et al. Expression and modulation of cellular receptors for interferon-t, tumor necrosis factor, and Fas on human bone marrow CD34+ cells. Br J Haematol 1997;97:356–65.

22. Deeg HJ, Beckham C, Loken MR, et al. Negative regulators of hemopoiesis and stroma function in patients with myelodysplastic syndrome. Leuk Lymphoma 2000;37(3–4):405–14.

23. Stifter G, Heiss S, Gastl G, et al. Over-expression of tumor necrosis factor-alpha in bone marrow biopsies from patients with myelodysplastic syndromes: relationship to anemia and prognosis. Eur J Haematol 2005;75(6):485–91.

24. Sloand EM, Mainwaring L, Fuhrer M, et al. Preferential suppression of trisomy 8 compared with normal hematopoietic cell growth by autologous lymphocytes in patients with trisomy 8 myelodysplastic syndrome. Blood 2005;106(3):841–51.

25. Michalopoulou S, Micheva I, Kouraklis-Symeonidis A, et al. Impaired clonogenic growth of myelodysplastic bone marrow progenitors in vitro is irrelevant to their apoptotic state. Leuk Res 2004;28(8):805–12.

26. Sloand EM, Pfannes L, Chen G, et al. CD34 cells from patients with trisomy 8 myelodysplastic syndrome (MDS) express early apoptotic markers but avoid programmed cell death by up-regulation of antiapoptotic proteins. Blood 2007;109(6):2399–405.

27. Sloand EM, Wu CO, Greenberg P, et al. Factors affecting response and survival in patients with myelodysplasia treated with immunosuppressive therapy. J Clin Oncol 2008;26(15):2505–11.

28. Chen G, Zeng W, Miyazato A, et al. Distinctive gene expression profiles of CD34 cells from patients with myelodysplastic syndrome characterized by specific chromosomal abnormalities. Blood 2004;104(13):4210–8.

29. Call KM, Ito CY, Lindberg C, et al. Mapping and characterization of 129 cosmids on human chromosome 11 p. Somat Cell Mol Genet 1992;18(5):463–75.

30. Haber DA, Housman DE. Role of the WT1 gene in Wilms' tumour. Cancer Surv 1992;12:105–17.

31. Cilloni D, Gottardi E, Fava M, et al. Usefulness of quantitative assessment of the WT1 gene transcript as a marker for minimal residual disease detection. Blood 2003;102(2):773–4.
32. Cilloni D, Gottardi E, Messa F, et al. Significant correlation between the degree of WT1 expression and the International Prognostic Scoring System Score in patients with myelodysplastic syndromes. J Clin Oncol 2003;21(10):1988–95.
33. Cilloni D, Saglio G. WT1 as a universal marker for minimal residual disease detection and quantification in myeloid leukemias and in myelodysplastic syndrome. Acta Haematol 2004;112(1–2):79–84.
34. Ellisen LW, Carlesso N, Cheng T, et al. The Wilms tumor suppressor WT1 directs stage-specific quiescence and differentiation of human hematopoietic progenitor cells. EMBO J 2001;20(8):1897–909.
35. Shichishima T, Okamoto M, Ikeda K, et al. HLA class II haplotype and quantitation of WT1 RNA in Japanese patients with paroxysmal nocturnal hemoglobinuria. Blood 2002;100(1):22–8.
36. Sloand EM, Rezvani K, Yong A, et al. Cytotoxic CD8 T cell immune responses to Wilms tumor protein (WT-1) characterizes immunosuppression-responsive myelodysplasia (MDS) [abstract]. Abstracts of the ASH Annual Meeting 108, 255a. 2006.
37. Molldrem J, Dermime S, Parker K, et al. Targeted T-cell therapy for human leukemia: cytotoxic T lymphocytes specific for a peptide derived from proteinase 3 preferentially lyse human myeloid leukemia cells. Blood 1996;88(7):2450–7.
38. Molldrem JJ, Clave E, Jiang YZ, et al. Cytotoxic T lymphocytes specific for a nonpolymorphic proteinase 3 peptide preferentially inhibit chronic myeloid leukemia colony-forming units. Blood 1997;90(7):2529–34.
39. Rosenfeld S, Follmann D, Nunez O, et al. Antithymocyte globulin and cyclosporine for severe aplastic anemia: association between hematologic response and long-term outcome. JAMA 2003;289(9):1130–5.
40. Socie G, Rosenfeld S, Frickhofen N, et al. Late clonal diseases of treated aplastic anemia. Semin Hematol 2000;37(1):91–101.
41. Maciejewski JP, Risitano A, Sloand EM, et al. Distinct clinical outcomes for cytogenetic abnormalities evolving from aplastic anemia. Blood 2002;99(9):3129–35.
42. Sloand E, Yong S, Barrett J, et al. Granulocyte colony stimulating factor preferentially stimulates proliferation of monosomy 7 cells bearing the isoform IV receptor. Proc Natl Acad Sci USA 2006;103(39):14483–8.
43. Goodman JE, Hofseth LJ, Hussain SP, et al. Nitric oxide and p53 in cancer-prone chronic inflammation and oxyradical overload disease. Environ Mol Mutagen 2004;44(1):3–9.
44. O'Sullivan M, Bronner MP, Brentnall TA, et al. Chromosomal instability in ulcerative colitis is related to telomere shortening. Nat Genet 2002;32:280–4.
45. Svendsen LB, Sondergaard JO, Hegnhoj J, et al. In vitro tetraploidy in patients with ulcerative colitis. Scand J Gastroenterol 1987;22(5):601–5.
46. Ying L, Marino J, Hussain SP, et al. Chronic inflammation promotes retinoblastoma protein hyperphosphorylation and E2F1 activation. Cancer Res 2005;65(20):9132–6.
47. Hofseth LJ, Saito S, Hussain SP, et al. Nitric oxide-induced cellular stress and p53 activation in chronic inflammation. Proc Natl Acad Sci U S A 2003;100(1):143–8.
48. Perwez HS, Harris CC. Inflammation and cancer: an ancient link with novel potentials. Int J Cancer 2007;121(11):2373–80.

49. Misawa S, Horiike S, Kaneko H, et al. Genetic aberrations in the development and subsequent progression of myelodysplastic syndrome. Leukemia 1997;11(Suppl 3):533–5.
50. Nakamura K, Inokuchi K, Dan K. [Abnormalities of the p53, N-ras, DCC and FLT-3 genes in myelodysplastic syndromes.] J Nippon Med Sch 2001;68(2):143–8.
51. Sugimoto K, Hirano N, Toyoshima H, et al. Mutations of the p53 gene in myelodysplastic syndrome (MDS) and MDS-derived leukemia. Blood 1993;81(11):3022–6.
52. Blasco MA. Mice with bad ends: mouse models for the study of telomeres and telomerase in cancer and aging. EMBO J 2005;24:1095–103.
53. Molldrem JJ, Leifer E, Bahceci E, et al. Antithymocyte globulin for treatment of the bone marrow failure associated with myelodysplastic syndromes. Ann Intern Med 2002;137(3):156–63.
54. Brummendorf TH, Maciejewski JP, Mak J, et al. Telomere length in leukocyte subpopulations of patients with aplastic anemia. Blood 2001;97(4):895–900.
55. Sieglova Z, Cermak J, Zilovcova S, et al. Measurement of telomere length in patients with early MDS may serve as a prognostic factor. Leuk Res 2005;29:S3 [abstract].
56. Dong F, van BC, Pouwels K, et al. Distinct cytoplasmic regions of the human granulocyte colony-stimulating factor receptor involved in induction of proliferation and maturation. Mol Cell Biol 1993;13(12):7774–81.
57. Kavgaci H, Ozdemir F, Aydin F, et al. Endogenous granulocyte colony-stimulating factor (G-CSF) levels in chemotherapy-induced neutropenia and in neutropenia related with primary diseases. J Exp Clin Cancer Res 2002;21(4):475–9.
58. Watari K, Asano S, Shirafuji N, et al. Serum granulocyte colony-stimulating factor levels in healthy volunteers and patients with various disorders as estimated by enzyme immunoassay. Blood 1989;73(1):117–22.
59. Ward AC, van Aesch YM, Schelen AM, et al. Defective internalization and sustained activation of truncated granulocyte colony-stimulating factor receptor found in severe congenital neutropenia/acute myeloid leukemia. Blood 1999;93(2):447–58.
60. Hunter MG, Avalos BR. Granulocyte colony-stimulating factor receptor mutations in severe congenital neutropenia transforming to acute myelogenous leukemia confer resistance to apoptosis and enhance cell survival. Blood 2000;95(6):2132–7.
61. Delforge M, Demuynck H, Verhoef G, et al. Patients with high-risk myelodysplastic syndrome can have polyclonal or clonal haemopoiesis in complete haematological remission. Br J Haematol 1998;102:486–94.
62. Geary CG, Harrison CJ, Philpott NJ, et al. Abnormal cytogenetic clones in patients with aplastic anaemia: response to immunosuppressive therapy. Br J Haematol 1999;104(2):271–4.
63. Smith DA, Green SW, Epstein ND, et al. Reversion to polyclonal hematopoiesis after successful treatment of aplastic anemia [abstract]. Blood 1992;80(Suppl 1):283a.
64. Nishimura M, Yamada T, Andoh T, et al. Granulocyte colony-stimulating factor (G-CSF) dependent hematopoiesis with monosomy 7 in a patient with severe aplastic anemia after ATG/CsA/G-CSF combined therapy. Int J Hematol 1998;68(2):203–11.
65. Barrett J, Saunthararajah Y, Molldrem J. Myelodysplastic syndrome and aplastic anemia: distinct entities or diseases linked by a common pathophysiology? Semin Hematol 2000;37(1):15–29.

66. Biesma DH, van den Tweel JG, Verdonck LF. Immunosuppressive therapy for hypoplastic myelodysplastic syndrome. Cancer 1997;79(8):1548–51.
67. Tichelli A, Gratwohl A, Wuersch A, et al. Antilymphocyte globulin for myelodysplastic syndrome. Br J Haematol 1988;68(1):139–40.
68. Molldrem J, Caples M, Mavroudis D, et al. Antithymocyte globulin (ATG) abrogates cytopenias in patients with myelodysplastic syndrome. Br J Haematol 1997;99:699–705.
69. Jonasova A, Neuwirtova R, Cermak J, et al. Cyclosporin A therapy in hypoplastic MDS patients and certain refractory anaemias without hypoplastic bone marrow. Br J Haematol 1998;100(2):304–9.
70. Killick SB, Mufti G, Cavenagh JD, et al. A pilot study of antithymocyte globulin (ATG) in the treatment of patients with 'low-risk' myelodysplasia. Br J Haematol 2003;120(4):679–84.
71. Yazji S, Giles FJ, Tsimberidou AM, et al. Antithymocyte globulin (ATG)-based therapy in patients with myelodysplastic syndromes. Leukemia 2003;17(11):2101–6.
72. Raza A, Reeves JA, Feldman EJ, et al. Phase 2 study of lenalidomide in transfusion-dependent, low-risk, and intermediate-1 risk myelodysplastic syndromes with karyotypes other than deletion 5q. Blood 2008;111(1):86–93.
73. List A, Kurtin S, Roe DJ, et al. Efficacy of lenalidomide in myelodysplastic syndromes. N Engl J Med 2005;352(6):549–57.
74. Sekeres MA, Maciejewski JP, Giagounidis AAN, et al. Relationship of treatment-related cytopenias and response to lenalidomide in patients with lower-risk myelodysplastic syndromes. J Clin Oncol 2008;26(36):5943–9.
75. Deeg HJ, Shulman HM, Anderson JE, et al. Allogeneic and syngeneic marrow transplantation for myelodysplastic syndrome in patients 55 to 66 years of age. Blood 2000;95(4):1188–94.
76. Deschler B, de Witte T, Mertelsmann R, et al. Treatment decision-making for older patients with high-risk myelodysplastic syndrome or acute myeloid leukemia: problems and approaches. Haematologica 2006; 91(11):1513–22.
77. de WT, Hermans J, Vossen J, et al. Haematopoietic stem cell transplantation for patients with myelo-dysplastic syndromes and secondary acute myeloid leukaemias: a report on behalf of the Chronic Leukaemia Working Party of the European Group for Blood and Marrow Transplantation (EBMT). Br J Haematol 2000;110(3):620–30.
78. Venditti A, Maurillo L, Buccisano F, et al. Pretransplant minimal residual disease level predicts clinical outcome in patients with acute myeloid leukemia receiving high-dose chemotherapy and autologous stem cell transplantation. Leukemia 2003;17(11):2178–82.
79. Asano Y, Maeda M, Uchida N, et al. Immunosuppressive therapy for patients with refractory anemia. Ann Hematol 2001;80(11):634–8.
80. Joachim Deeg H, Jiang PYZ, Holmberg LA, et al. Hematologic responses of patients with MDS to antithymocyte globulin plus etanercept correlate with improved flow scores of marrow cells. Leuk Res 2004;28(11):1177–80.
81. Lim ZY, Killick S, Germing U, et al. Low IPSS score and bone marrow hypocellularity in MDS patients predict hematological responses to antithymocyte globulin. Leukemia 2007;21(7):1436–41.
82. Steensma DP, Dispenzieri A, Moore SB, et al. Antithymocyte globulin has limited efficacy and substantial toxicity in unselected anemic patients with myelodysplastic syndrome. Blood 2003;101(6):2156–8.

83. Shimamoto T, Tohyama K, Okamoto T, et al. Cyclosporin A therapy for patients with myelodysplastic syndrome: multicenter pilot studies in Japan. Leuk Res 2003;27(9):783–8.

84. Atoyebi W, Bywater L, Rawlings L, et al. Treatment of myelodysplasia with oral cyclosporin. Clin Lab Haematol 2002;24(4):211–4.

85. Haidinger M, Geyeregger R, Poglitsch M, et al. Antithymocyte globulin impairs T-cell/antigen-presenting cell interaction: disruption of immunological synapse and conjugate formation. Transplantation 2007;84(1):117–21.

86. Lopez M, Clarkson MR, Albin M, et al. A novel mechanism of action for anti-thymocyte globulin: induction of CD4 + CD25 + Foxp3 + regulatory T cells. J Am Soc Nephrol 2006;17(10):2844–53.

87. Broliden PA, Dahl IM, Hast R, et al. Antithymocyte globulin and cyclosporine A as combination therapy for low-risk non-sideroblastic myelodysplastic syndromes. Haematologica 2006;91(5):667–70.

88. Aivado M, Rong A, Germing U, et al. Long-term remission after intensive chemo-therapy in advanced myelodysplastic syndromes is generally associated with restoration of polyclonal haemopoiesis. Br J Haematol 2000;110(4):884–6.

89. Di Bona E, Rodeghiero FBB, Gabbas A, et al. Rabbit antithymocyte globulin (r-ATG) lus cyclosporine and granulocyte colony stimulating factor is an effective treatment for aplastic anaemia patients unresponsive to a first course of intensive immunosuppressive therapy. Gruppo Itlaian Trapianto di Midollo Osseo (GITMO). Br J Haematol 1999;107:330–4.

90. Stadler M, Germing U, Kliche KO, et al. A prospective, randomised, phase II study of horse antithymocyte globulin vs rabbit antithymocyte globulin as immune-modulating therapy in patients with low-risk myelodysplastic syndromes. Leukemia 2004;18(3):460–5.

Myelodysplasia and Acute Leukemia as Late Complications of Marrow Failure: Future Prospects for Leukemia Prevention

Grover C. Bagby, MD[a,b,c,d,]*, Gabrielle Meyers, MD[b,e]

KEYWORDS

- Clonal evolution • Myelodysplasia • Aplastic anemia
- Natural selection • Fanconi's anemia
- Apoptosis • Leukemogenesis

Patients with bone marrow failure syndromes are at risk for the development of clonal neoplasms including acute myeloid leukemia (AML), myelodysplastic syndrome (MDS), and paroxysmal nocturnal hemoglobinuria (reviewed elsewhere in this issue and in).[1,2] From 10% to 20% of survivors of acquired aplastic anemia develop a clonal disease within the decade following their diagnosis,[3–6] and the relative risk of clonal neoplasms is even more significantly increased in children and adults with inherited bone marrow failure syndromes.[7] Informed by advances in studies on evolutionary adaptation,[8–10] recent studies testing the adaptive nature of clonal evolution in mammalian hematopoietic stem cells are clearly positive.

This work was supported in part by grants from the National Institutes of Health, 1P01 HL48546 (GB), R01 CA138237-01 (GB), and K23 RR 020043 (GM); the Veterans Affairs Merit Review Program (GB); the Aplastic Anemia and MDS International Foundation (GM); and the Children's Leukemia Research Association (GM).
[a] Department of Molecular and Medical Genetics, Oregon Health and Sciences University, Portland, OR, USA
[b] Department of Medicine, Oregon Health and Sciences University, Portland, OR, USA
[c] Knight Cancer Institute at Oregon Health and Sciences University, Portland, OR, USA
[d] NW VA Cancer Research Center, VA Medical Center Portland, R&D2, Building 103, E221B, 3710 SW Veteran's Hospital Road, Portland, OR 97239, USA
[e] Hematologic Malignancies Program, Knight Cancer Institute at Oregon Health and Sciences University, Portland, OR, USA
* Corresponding author. NW VA Cancer Research Center, VA Medical Center Portland, R&D2, Building 103, E221B, 3710 SW Veteran's Hospital Road, Portland, OR 97239.
E-mail address: grover@ohsu.edu (G.C. Bagby).

Hematol Oncol Clin N Am 23 (2009) 361–376
doi:10.1016/j.hoc.2009.01.006
0889-8588/09/$ – see front matter

THE INFLAMMATION AND CANCER CANON

Inflammatory disorders, infectious and noninfectious, are known to predispose patients to neoplastic diseases. Although the type of inflammatory disorder can be variable, one constant is that the tissue at risk is the inflamed tissue itself. For example, inflammatory bowel disease is a risk factor for colon cancer, hepatitis C infection is a risk factor for hepatocellular carcinoma, and so forth. A recent wave of interest in the linkage between inflammation and cancer has resulted in a canonical view that the neoplastic cells grow because they respond to the proliferative, antiapoptotic, and proangiogenic effects of the cytokines released in the inflamed tissue. Given that a large population of stem cells is under the influence of these proproliferative cytokines, if this feed-forward model is sufficient to account for subsequent neoplasia the neoplasms themselves ought to be polyclonal; yet, they are not. Because neoplasms are usually clonal (arising from one mutant stem cell) the model fails to explain a key step in this process: the emergence and domination of the niche by the progeny of a single mutant stem cell. An alternative model, one that applies the rules of natural selection, better reconciles the clinical course of disease in humans and mice. To compare this model with the more canonical one requires a thorough understanding of the concept of "selection coefficients."

SELECTION COEFFICIENTS AND DETERMINANTS OF CLONAL EVOLUTION

Principles of natural selection were developed in reference to studies on species but are legitimately applicable to asexual populations.[9] When these principles are tested in the laboratory using hematopoietic stem cells of mice with marrow failure, they have informed clinicians about the importance of the microenvironment in processes of clonal evolution.[11,12] In selection of species and subspecies, emergence and fixation of adaptive mutations depends first on an environmentally induced stress on a population that makes that population less fit. An apt example is found in studies on selection of dark and light colored rock pocket mice[13] that differ in only one allele that influences coat color. In a neutral environment, both strains survive equally well but in the real world (in this case an environment with owls in it), the dark colored mice are easier for the predators to spot if they are running about on sand. Conversely, the light colored ones are easy pickings sitting on lava-beds. In effect, the environment does its work to select the fit population not by influencing directly that population but by purging its unfit competitors. There is evidence that this is true not only for bacteria in which adaptation to antibiotic challenge results in resistance,[14,15] but also for mammalian cells.[16] This unabashedly Darwinian model is a perfectly applicable model to apply to populations of stressed hematopoietic stem cells.

To develop a clear picture of clonal evolution that occurs in the setting of bone marrow failure requires clarification of the relationships that exist between the target cells and the selective forces in the environment that determine fitness.[17] Some mathematical models have even suggested that selective pressure is a more important determinant in initiation of a tumor than is an increased baseline mutation rate,[18] but it is intuitively more appealing to accept that variations in fitness in stem cell populations increase not only as a function of the relative fitness differences between two competing populations (a notation of which is known as the "coefficient of selection") but in proportion to the population size and mutation rate.[9]

The likelihood of clonal evolution depends on the relative fitness differences between normal stem cells and mutant (potentially adapted) stem cells. This relative difference is expressed as the selection coefficient. A high selection coefficient exists when a somatic mutation accords to cells a uniquely strong advantage. Two models of clonal evolution are presented in **Fig. 1**. Note that each model results in the same coefficient of selection. Studies on clonal evolution using murine stem cells clearly support the model in **Fig. 1**B.[11] The model in **Fig. 1**B. makes the argument that the selectability of a specific mutation is highest when the reference population is disadvantaged at the outset. This model suggests that if one wants to prevent clonal evolution, one must focus on restoring the fitness of the unfit stem cells. This requires that the precise molecular mechanisms that reduce fitness in the stem cell pool are clarified. The focus needs to be both on mechanisms intrinsic to stem cells and pathways that influence the microenvironment.

PATHOGENESIS OF ACQUIRED APLASTIC ANEMIA

In the past two decades experimental evidence from translational studies places acquired aplastic anemia squarely into the category of autoimmune diseases. The evidence from a number of laboratories, recently summarized by Young and colleagues,[1] has revealed that (1) aberrantly activated oligoclonal T-cell populations[19] suppress hematopoiesis by releasing cytokines (importantly interferon [IFN]-γ and tumor necrosis factor [TNF]-α); (2) these cytokines and other factors induced by them cause apoptotic responses in hematopoietic stem cell and progenitor cells; (3) clinical responses to immunosuppressive therapy correlate directly with the capacity of the treatment to suppress T-cell function; and (4) immune-mediated bone marrow failure can now be modeled in mice and in that model monoclonal antibodies to TNF-α and IFN-γ prevent fatal aplasia. Recent gene expression microarray analysis confirms predicted abnormalities in both the attacking T-cell populations[20] and the progenitor cell pool.[21]

CLONAL EVOLUTION IN ACQUIRED APLASTIC ANEMIA

Stem cells assaulted by cytotoxic lymphoid populations[22] represent perfect models of a disadvantaged population (**Fig. 2**). Unless the offending T-cell population is eradicated or inactivated, the selective pressure they exert on the stem cell pool favors the evolution of somatically mutated stem cells that had acquired, by virtue of the mutation, the capacity to resist the attack of T cells. The requirements for clonal evolution are (1) that a sufficiently high coefficient of selection exists (ongoing selection against the nonadapted stem cells as is the case with ongoing immune attack in acquired aplastic anemia); (2) that a stem cell population is of sufficient size (as is the case before the onset of aplasia); and (3) that there is an appreciable mutation rate (as is the case in many of the congenital aplastic states because of the additional feature of genetic instability).

As shown in **Fig. 2**, an identical somatic mutation could occur randomly in an otherwise normal stem cell pool but because there is a low selection coefficient (the mutant cell exists in a large pool of nondisadvantaged stem cells) clonal evolution is less favored (see **Fig. 2**, pathway 1). This situation may explain how covert leukemic clones can be found during normal fetal development yet not raise their heads even later in life (ie, these clones have no advantage).[23] If some degree of bone marrow failure develops in a way that disadvantages the greater pool without influencing the mutant stem cell, the situation changes greatly in favor of clonal evolution (see **Fig. 2**, pathway 2). This paradigm fits very nicely with observations in humans and mice with acquired and inherited aplastic anemia.

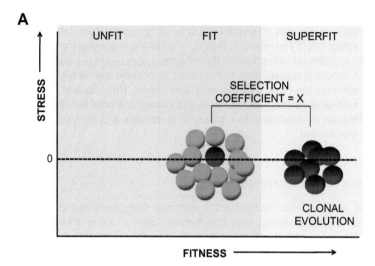

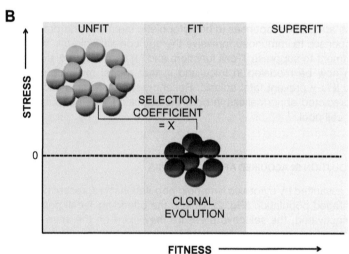

Fig. 1. The fitness landscape for hematopoietic stem cells. (*A*) A popular model of clonal evolution in hematopoietic stem cells proposes that somatic mutations occur stochastically in hematopoietic stem cells and that rare mutations of this kind confer on the mutant stem cell (*red*) an inherent proliferative and survival advantage over the nonmutant (*blue*) stem cells. A key principle of this model is that the nonmutant stem cells are not unfit, at least at the time the new clone initially evolves. The fitness differences between the evolving clone and the normal stem cell pool can be described as a selection coefficient, here given a value of X. (*B*) An alternative model, one more consistent with studies on clonal evolution in the setting of marrow failure, is one in which the entire population of normal hematopoietic stem cells is unfit as a result of environmental stress. A somatic mutant (*red*) stem cell has developed resistance to the specific environmental stressor so remains fit while the remainder of the stem cell pool has become unfit as a result of environmental stress. In this instance the coefficient for selection of the abnormal clone is identical (X) to that of the model described in *A*.

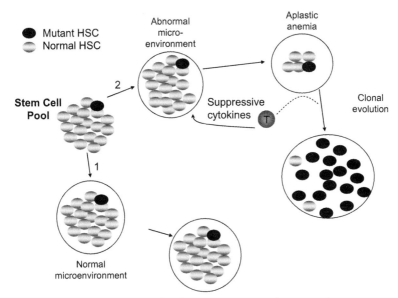

Fig. 2. Clonal evolution in acquired aplastic anemia. In the ground state, somatically mutated stem cells do not expand because the mutation does not confer on that cell a selective advantage. The coefficient of selection for clonal expansion of that cell is low. If the microenvironment remains normal over time (pathway 1), no clonal expansion occurs because the microenvironment is highly supportive of most stem cells in the pool. That is, no clonal evolution occurs in pathway 1 because the relative fitness differences between the normal and mutant cells are trivial. If, however, T lymphocytes arise that inhibit the replication, expansion, or survival of normal hematopoietic stem cells, and if the somatic mutation confers on a stem cell the capacity to resist the effect of the T cells (eg, by resisting the apoptotic effects of suppressive cytokines like TNF-α and IFN-γ), then pathway 2 is most relevant. During the development of aplasia, normal stem cells are suppressed but the mutant one is not and, because the coefficient of selection for that cell is now high (as a result of a decline in fitness of the normal stem cells), it can expand clonally. In some cases the very cytokines that suppress the normal stem cells function to enhance the expansion of the mutant clone. Under continued pressure from the aberrant T-cell population, the neoplastic clone preferentially expands over time while the less fit normal HSC are selected against. Not shown in this figure is a theoretical process by which a mutant stem cell arises in a population only after it is exposed to a hostile environment. This meets strict genetic standards for a truly "adaptive mutation" in which the hostile environment per se induces mutations, some of which permit an adaptive response to the environment. In light of the capacity of TNF-α to induce oxidative DNA damage,[82] this process is not simply a remote possibility. The coefficient of selection idea is still relevant here because relief of the environmental stress (eg, fully effective immunotherapy of aplastic anemia) might lower the coefficient in time to prevent an outgrowth of adapted clonal progeny. Finally, in some cases the new clone is able to subordinate the signals from the suppressive population and convert them to growth and survival signals (represented by the dashed line leading from the T cell in pathway 2). For example, in some cases of MDS arising in the context of bone marrow failure, TNF-α enhances the proliferation of clonal erythroid and myeloid progenitors, a distinctly aberrant response. HSC, hematopoietic stem cells.

INHERITED BONE MARROW FAILURE SYNDROMES: ROLE OF CYTOKINES IN SELECTION

Aberrant interactions of IFN-γ and TNF-α with stem cells are also features of the most well-studied of the inherited aplastic anemias, Fanconi's anemia (FA). Studies on hematopoietic cells from children with FA and later in mice nullizygous for *Fancc* demonstrated not only that FA-C cells release more TNF-α in the ground state,[24,25] but that FA-C progenitor cells are inherently hypersensitive to apoptotic cues, including IFN-γ, TNF-α, macrophage inflammatory protein-1 and tumor necrosis factor ligand superfamily, member 10.[26–28]

Some of the mechanisms by which FA cells are hypersensitive to inflammatory cytokines are being clarified. For example, for TNF-α hypersensitivity in FA cells, two serine-threonine kinases are important because their activity is influenced by FA proteins. The first is the protein kinase PKR, a key molecular effector of the antiviral response, and the second is the apoptosis signal regulating kinase 1 (Ask1).[29,30] Additional work is required to determine whether these pathways might be reasonable therapeutic targets.

OVERPRODUCTION OF CYTOKINES

Not only are FA target cells hypersensitive to apoptosis-inducing cytokines, auxiliary cells that produce them have lower thresholds for cytokine release. Pang and colleagues[31] have reported that Fancc$^{-/-}$ mice treated with endotoxin had higher mortality rates than wild-type mice; had higher serum levels of TNF-α, interleukin-6, and macrophage inflammatory protein-2 and demonstrated hematopoietic suppression that could be directly attributed to TNF-α (anti-TNF antibodies protected FA target cells). They also showed that transplantation of hematopoietic stem cells from wild-type mice protected Fancc$^{-/-}$ mice from endotoxin-induced mortality, clarifying the key role played by auxiliary cells of hematopoietic origin in the microenvironment.[31]

Stem cells in patients with both acquired and certain inherited aplastic anemias are highly apoptotic and the signaling pathways, both within and external to stem cells, which ultimately execute them, are very closely related. In acquired aplastic anemia the stress initially comes from rogue clones of T cells overproducing factors that result in stem cell death. In FA the production of some of the same factors is increased because the normal FA proteins set thresholds for cytokine production responses to cytokine-inducing factors in auxiliary cells (eg, in response to endotoxin).[31] In addition, the stem cell pool is inherently hypersensitive to those factors because the normal FA proteins set their response thresholds for responses to some of the very apoptotic cytokines overexpressed in auxiliary cells.[2] Although the experimental evidence supporting stem cell stress in other inherited marrow failure syndromes is not as robust, evidence is beginning to emerge supporting the idea that the heterogeneous inherited mutations result in higher rates of stem and progenitor cell apoptosis.[32–34] These pools of damaged stem cells are all perfect environments for the selection of somatically mutated stem cell clones that have acquired the capacity to completely ignore those apoptotic cues. These clones have a huge competitive advantage when compared with the highly disadvantaged reference population of stem cells. It is likely that in all aplastic states the coefficient of selection is high in the stem cell pool.

THE NATURE OF THE INSULT AND THE ADAPTIVE TACTIC ARE LINKED

Fortunately, the clonal adaptation-selection model can be best tested directly now that some of the mechanisms that negatively impact stem cells are defined.

Deductively, if the new clone has to be more fit, the type of resistance they exhibit must be precisely to the key factor or factors that put the stem cell pool under pressure in the first place. For example, if an aplastic microenvironment packed with IFN-γ–producing T cells provides the key selective pressure for the emergence of a fit clone of stem cells, the clonal progeny ought to be IFN-resistant. Clinical and laboratory observations have confirmed the accuracy of this notion.

MOSAICISM: THE BEST ADAPTIVE RESPONSE IN INHERITED MARROW FAILURE SYNDROMES

Some patients with FA exhibit a phenomenon (mosaicism) of genetic reversion in which one of the mutant FA alleles has been corrected in a hematopoietic stem cell. This cell and all its progeny have gained fitness in a perfect (not maladaptive) way.[35,36] That is, the growth of clonal progenitors can be inhibited by cytokines but only at high doses (in the way normal progenitors respond). In cases in which the entire hematopoietic organ includes progeny of a stem cell corrected in this way, the occurrence of AML-MDS has not been reported. Indeed, in a patient with incomplete mosaicism (a mixture of unfit and fit [reverted] stem cell pools), clonal evolution has occurred in the uncorrected stem cell pool, not the reverted one.[37] These clinical observations are consistent with the importance of the selection coefficient in stem cells. Even stronger evidence exists from systematic experimental studies.

Paroxysmal Nocturnal Hemoglobinuria

The most common somatic mutation in the context of acquired bone marrow failure is somatic inactivation of the *PIG-A* gene, and although the precise mechanisms involved are not completely known, genome-wide transcriptional surveys of the *PIG-A* mutant progenitor cells indicate that they are less apoptotic than the nonmutant cells (reviewed in).[1]

Myelodysplastic Syndrome and Acute Myeloid Leukemia

MDS or AML clones that evolve in the context of aplastic anemia are characterized by nonrandom chromosomal abnormalities, the most common of which are trisomy 8 and monosomy 7.[38] Cells bearing these abnormalities have a demonstrable advantage over the cells not bearing these rearrangements.[39,40] The authors have observed cytokine hypersensitivity in progenitor cells of patients with FA but have found that progenitor cells from their affected siblings who have clonal evolution[41] are resistant. FA patients in the aplastic phase have hypersensitive progenitors but clonal progenitors from the same patients studied later during the MDS phase are resistant to precisely the same cytokines (TNF-α and IFN-γ). In murine models of FA, although stem cells and progenitors are hypersensitive to a variety of cytokines (reviewed in Bagby and Alter)[2] neoplastic clones are resistant.[11,12,42]

VARIATIONS ON THE SELECTION THEME

The adaptation-selection model of clonal evolution demands that the environmental factor damaging the cells be the one to which the new clone is resistant but it does not mean that the change is sufficient to initiate the entire leukemogenic process. The new clone may also be resistant to other factors,[43] a phenomenon that only makes the neoplastic clone even more capable of competing against the disadvantaged stem cells. In addition, somatic changes that lead to clonal evolution may not always be genetic because epigenetic events have been described as factors in the evolution of hematologic neoplasms. Genetic loss and epigenetic silencing may cooperate in some instances. For example, in myeloid leukemic clones with allelic losses caused by chromosomal deletions, the retained allele can be suppressed epigenetically[44] resulting in a functional loss of heterozygosity.

RELEVANCE OF THE CLONAL SELECTION-ADAPTATION MODEL TO CLINICAL MANAGEMENT
Choosing Proper Therapy

A number of advances in transplantation technology and supportive care have improved the success rates of stem cell transplantation in primary therapy of aplastic anemia.[45–47] In addition, the incidence of clonal evolution after immunosuppressive therapy is high[5,48] but is lower in patients treated only with matched-related donor bone marrow transplantation.[5] In addition, in patients treated only with immunosuppressive therapy, more instances of clonal evolution have been found among those who had incomplete remissions and an ongoing requirement for immunosuppression.[49–52] Although loss of immune surveillance may play a causal role in clonal evolution in such instances, there is to date no direct experimental evidence in support of this. The authors believe that the physiologic basis for the superiority of stem cell transplantation (at least for patients under 41 years of age)[53] over immunosuppressive therapy for acquired aplastic anemia is accounted for by the clonal selection model presented in **Figs. 1B and 2**. Specifically, stem cell transplantation results not only in the replacement of stressed and depleted stem cells, but also replaces the offending auxiliary cells (the stem cell suppressors). In patients treated with immunosuppressive therapy this model is also applicable because the seminal difference between a responder and nonresponder is that the coefficient of selection has been altered in the former but not the latter. Clearly, for patients with a suitable related donor the evidence-based path is bone marrow transplantation and in such cases it is undesirable first to use immunosuppressive therapy.[45]

Therapeutic decisions in older patients are more difficult because complications of transplantation are substantial. Such patients should be treated using clinical trials focusing on improving complete response rates for immunotherapy or improving survival in recipients of bone marrow transplantation. For all severe aplastic anemia patients ineligible for stem cell transplantation the goal must be to terminate the immune attack altogether and thereby normalize hematopoiesis and lower the coefficient of selection for stem cells bearing polymorphisms or mutations that make them much "more fit" than the pressured wild-type stem cell population. The cocktail and doses of immunosuppressive agents should be evidence-based and the therapeutic goals should be aggressive. For example, if a patient treated with antithymocyte globulin and cyclosporine A has an improvement in peripheral blood counts sufficient to reduce their risk of intercurrent infections or bleeding but has not demonstrated normalization of blood counts, ongoing or alternative immunosuppressive therapy should be considered. Although it is also essential to take care in balancing the risks of ongoing immunosuppression, this more aggressive path has the potential advantages of lowering the incidence of relapse[49–52] and reducing the coefficient of selection for new clones. The authors propose that in patients whose remission is incomplete, hematologists should resist temptations to reduce the conventional doses of immunosuppressive agents used or to terminate immunosuppressive therapy early based on strictly theoretical concerns about potential adverse events associated with immunosuppression.

Conducting Surveillance

For some of the inherited aplastic states, general surveillance guidelines are available (eg, at www.fanconi.org) and although they are helpful, the levels of certainty are not particularly high because they are such rare conditions. For some cytogenetic rearrangements, the best action is to do nothing because they are associated with a phenotype that rarely evolves to hematologic neoplasia (eg, isochromosome 7q in patients with Shwachman-Diamond syndrome). Other chromosomal abnormalities, like duplications of chromosome 3q in FA patients, are more ominous and predict leukemic transformations so ought to raise considerations of higher-risk stem cell transplantation options (reviewed in Guinan).[54]

For patients with acquired aplastic anemia, there exist few formal surveillance guidelines. Although transplanted patients and complete responders to immunosuppressive therapy have fewer clonal events,[49] there is no certain way to identify all patients at risk for clonal disease.[48] The authors believe that even stable transfusion-independent patients should be followed at least annually. In the population under surveillance, whether annual bone marrow biopsies provide sufficient information to warrant their use is debatable. Clearly, because of technical considerations, bone marrow hypocellularity alone is not a meaningful data point. Marrow aspirates should be obtained not only as a tool to seek morphologic evidence of trilineage dysplasia, however, but as a source of cells for the application of colony-forming unit or flow cytometric assays that can be used to identify ongoing evidence of hematopoietic inhibitory T-cell activation[22,55] and for cytogenetic analysis using conventional metaphase methods and interphase fluorescence in situ hybridization.

If there are signs that clones of potential significance are evolving (eg, monosomy 7), medical management and the pathways of surveillance must be altered in ways that best fit the medical evidence. For example, if a patient with an evolving monosomy 7 clone is being treated with granulocyte colony–stimulating factor along with immunosuppressive therapy, granulocyte colony–stimulating factor should be discontinued and the clone followed with more frequent surveillance.[40,56] If this approach does not work, a novel transplantation trial should be considered. Patients with trisomy 8 can have a more stable clinical course, however, and high-risk procedures may not be warranted on the grounds of the cytogenetic defect per se.[48]

THE FUTURE OF LEUKEMIA PREVENTION RESEARCH
Basic Research

Much scientific and financial energy today focuses, for good reason, on developing targeted therapies for leukemic disorders. Taking into account the recent evidence, reviewed previously, that new clones arise in the context of an unfit cohort of stem cells, it is a perfect time to apply the same systems, molecular, genetic, and chemical biology approaches to the problem of clonal evolution with the goal of preventing MDS and AML in patients at risk. Novel agents could, by reducing apoptotic stresses on hematopoietic stem cell pool, lower the selection coefficient and thereby lower the risk of clonal evolution. Although this requires matching the screening assay with the particular type of bone marrow failure syndrome, there is sufficient scientific evidence that a stressed stem cell population is a major factor in the evolution of preleukemic clones to warrant such an approach.

Use of New Preclinical Models

Reliable murine models now exist and permit the assessment of new agents. For acquired (autoimmune) aplastic anemia, the infusion of F1 mice with cells from parental lymph nodes results in marrow failure and increases in serum IFN-γ. The F1 mice respond favorably to both immunosuppressive therapy and neutralizing antibodies to IFN-γ and TNF-α.[57] For FA at least two tractable models of clonal evolution now exist. The first is one in which murine Fanconi cells cultured ex vivo and then transplanted into radiated recipients are at risk for clonal evolution,[12] a complication prevented by correcting the FA defect.[42] The second model (**Fig. 3**) is one in which clonal evolution can be forced in vitro by exposing Fancc$^{-/-}$ cells to TNF-α.[11] These models allow identification of small molecules that normalize responses to stress factors, such as TNF-α. Indeed, candidate molecular targets (eg, TNF-α, IFN-γ, reactive oxygen species, p38, and JNK) have already been identified in preclinical models for acquired aplastic anemia[57] and FA.[31] The ultimate goal is to reduce the impact of unusual environmental stress factors on stem cells without reducing the responses of those cells to normal regulatory factors.

Design of clinical prevention trials

Clinical trials designed to increase the number of completely responsive patients are warranted because if the goal is achieved the relative risk of clonal evolution likely declines. It is equally important, however, that long-term interventional trials be developed for patients who have already received immunosuppressive therapy for aplastic anemia. These studies must focus on the goal of reducing late morbidity and mortality including the relative risk of clonal evolution. In light of the limited sensitivity of fluorescence in situ hybridization and Giemsa stain banded cytogenetic analyses, more sensitive methods now available for quantifying genetic losses and gains ought to be exploited.[58] Identification of potential molecular targets for prevention can also be addressed using systems biology approaches. They would necessarily include attempts to define the emergent phenotypes associated with discrete cytogenetic rearrangements on a genome-wide scale (as has been done with 5q$^-$ cells)[44] and to

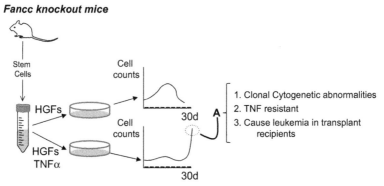

Fig. 3. Clonal evolution is adaptive. Fanconi's anemia group C mutant cells are intrinsically hypersensitive to the apoptotic effects of TNF-α, yet clonally evolved cells are resistant.[41,42] Li and colleagues[11] tested the hypothesis that TNF exposure changes the fitness landscape significantly enough to permit clonal evolution ex vivo. When mutant Fancc stem cells (Kit+, Lin-, Sca1+) were exposed to a combination of hematopoietic growth factors (HGF) in suspension culture they expanded logarithmically. Then, as differentiated cells accumulated cell counts declined. This proliferative capacity of stem cell progeny in vitro was slightly suppressed in Fancc knockout mice, but the slope of the expansion curve did not differ from that of stem cells from wild-type mice. When the Fancc mutant cells were exposed to both growth factors and TNF-α (to which they are intrinsically hypersensitive), however, there was little expansion at all until late in culture. At this late time point (A) cells that began to proliferate in the face of ongoing TNF-α exposure exhibited clonal cytogenetic abnormalities, were TNF resistant, and when injected into sublethally radiated mice gave rise to AML.

establish robust target validation analyses for interventional studies using new targeted agents.

Marrow transplantation

In both acquired and inherited types of aplastic anemia, novel approaches to transplantation ought to be developed because of the clear superiority of that approach in preventing clonal evolution. Key limiting factors for transplantation are lack of perfectly matched donors, age over 40 years, and the high transplant-related mortality for recipients of mismatched marrows, so increasing the safety of transplantation in the mismatch setting is an important objective. To date there has been some improvement in outcomes using alternative donors for aplastic anemia. The improvement has evolved for a variety of reasons including (1) the use of non–total body irradiation or low-dose total body irradiation based conditioning regimens,[59–63] (2) the development of high-resolution histocompatibility typing,[64,65] and (3) improvements in supportive care.[66,67]

In the future, for patients ineligible for transplantation three strategic research paths ought to be considered. First, new immunosuppressive agents and combinations should be developed, ones that induce a higher fraction of complete responses. The second investigative opportunity is to identify or develop agents that suppress discrete apoptotic pathways in stem cells ignited by the immune system (or by inherited mutations that reduce their fitness). The third opportunity is to do both things: combine new immunosuppressive agents with agents that lower the coefficient of selection by raising thresholds of adverse stem cell responses to the activated immune system. This approach is no longer simply theoretically appealing. Robust preclinical models now exist[11] that could facilitate this kind of approach and clearly point the way to agents that first ought to be tested.

Modulating responses to tumor necrosis factor

TNF-α is a key mediator not only in aplastic anemia but in clonal evolution, as described previously. This cytokine also plays a seminal role in the pathogenesis of other autoimmune diseases, and a number of agents targeting the TNF-α pathway have been effective in controlling some of them, including rheumatoid arthritis, psoriatic arthritis, and inflammatory bowel disease.[68–72] The extensive use of these agents in humans to treat multiple disease states and relatively good tolerance of these drugs makes them attractive options for management of the proinflammatory state characteristic of aplastic anemia.

Although there are little preclinical and clinical data for the use of these agents in the treatment of marrow failure, the evidence supports consideration of these or like agents in the treatment of this disease. In their mouse model of aplastic anemia, Bloom and colleagues[57] describe significant improvement in survival in aplastic mice treated with TNF-α blocking antibodies compared with control mice. In addition, Dufour and colleagues[73] have recently reported the successful use of etanercept in a child with refractory aplastic anemia.

More importantly, because TNF is a kind of final common pathway, more work needs to be done to identify the factors that underlie TNF overproduction and, in FA stem cells, the characteristic TNF hypersensitivity of stem cells. Natural modulators of the TNF response are being identified regularly and some of them not only function as nodal points that determine whether the TNF response is cell survival or death,[74] but play key roles in stem cell maintenance.[75] If dysfunction of such molecules underlies the pathogenesis of some marrow failure states, they may prove to be ideal targets. Future approaches need to focus precisely on molecular pathogenesis in individual patients.

Blocking tumor necrosis factor–induced oxidative stress

TNF-α stimulation leads to a rapid increase in intracellular levels of reactive oxygen species, with multiple downstream implications ending in activation of cell death (apoptosis and necrosis) pathways.[76–79] In some instances, antioxidants can protect against TNF-α–induced cytotoxicity,[80] including in hematopoietic cells of FA knockout mice.[31] Some antioxidants, like *N*-acetylcysteine, are safe to use in humans, so use of this and other reactive oxygen species scavengers may find a place in the future management of TNF-α–induced marrow injury and subsequent clonal adaptation.

Other cytokine pathways of potential relevance

Additional biologic agents targeting other inflammatory cytokines, in particular inter-leukin-1, -6, and-15, and TNF superfamily members, in particular LIGHT, BlyS, APRIL, and RANKL, are currently in clinical trials for the treatment of rheumatoid arthritis and other inflammatory diseases.[81] It is fortunate for the bone marrow failure field that the search for additional agents targeting these pathways is brisk.

SUMMARY

From 10% to 20% of acquired aplastic anemia survivors develop a clonal disease within the decade following their diagnosis as do up to 40% of children and young adults with some of the congenital marrow failure syndromes. A good amount of recent evidence from the disparate fields of genetics, adaptation, stem cell biology, and hematopoiesis leads inescapably to the conclusion that clonal evolution in aplastic states arises in the context of ongoing stem cell damage through a process of clonal selection and adaptation. In the past 2 years this theoretical paradigm has been validated in clinical and preclinical models robust enough to inform surveillance strategies and reconsider therapeutic objectives in patients with aplastic states and to support the planning and development of rationally designed leukemia prevention trials in patients with bone marrow failure syndromes.

REFERENCES

1. Young NS, Calado RT, Scheinberg P. Current concepts in the pathophysiology and treatment of aplastic anemia. Blood 2006;108:2509–19.
2. Bagby GC, Alter BP. Fanconi anemia. Semin Hematol 2006;43:147–56.
3. Maciejewski JP, Selleri C. Evolution of clonal cytogenetic abnormalities in aplastic anemia. Leuk Lymphoma 2004;45:433–40.
4. Bacigalupo A, Bruno B, Saracco P, et al. Antilymphocyte globulin, cyclosporine, prednisolone, and granulocyte colony-stimulating factor for severe aplastic anemia: an update of the GITMO/EBMT study on 100 patients. Blood 2000;95:1931–4.
5. Socie G, Henry-Amar M, Bacigalupo A, et al. Malignant tumors occurring after treatment of aplastic anemia. European Bone Marrow Transplantation-Severe Aplastic Anaemia Working Party. N Engl J Med 1993;329:1152–7.
6. Tichelli A, Gratwohl A, Wursch A, et al. Late haematological complications in severe aplastic anaemia. Br J Haematol 1988;69:413–8.
7. Rosenberg PS, Greene MH, Alter BP. Cancer incidence in persons with Fanconi anemia. Blood 2003;101:822–6.
8. Orr HA. Theories of adaptation: what they do and don't say. Genetica 2005;123:3–13.
9. Desai MM, Fisher DS, Murray AW. The speed of evolution and maintenance of variation in asexual populations. Curr Biol 2007;17:385–94.

10. Orr HA. The genetic theory of adaptation: a brief history. Nat Rev Genet 2005;6: 119–27.
11. Li J, Sejas DP, Zhang X, et al. TNF-alpha induces leukemic clonal evolution ex vivo in Fanconi anemia group C murine stem cells. J Clin Invest 2007;117:3283–95.
12. Li XX, Le Beau MM, Ciccone S, et al. Ex vivo culture of Fancc-/- stem/progenitor cells predisposes cells to undergo apoptosis, and surviving stem/progenitor cells display cytogenetic abnormalities and an increased risk of malignancy. Blood 2005;105:3465–71.
13. Nachman MW, Hoekstra HE, D'Agostino SL. The genetic basis of adaptive melanism in pocket mice. Proc Natl Acad Sci U S A 2003;100:5268–73.
14. Bjedov I, Tenaillon O, Gerard B, et al. Stress-induced mutagenesis in bacteria. Science 2003;300:1404–9.
15. Foster PL. Stress responses and genetic variation in bacteria. Mutat Res 2005; 569:3–11.
16. Anderson AR, Weaver AM, Cummings PT, et al. Tumor morphology and phenotypic evolution driven by selective pressure from the microenvironment. Cell 2006;127:905–15.
17. Gatenby RA. Commentary: carcinogenesis as Darwinian evolution? Do the math! Int J Epidemiol 2006;35:1165–7.
18. Tomlinson IP, Novelli MR, Bodmer WF. The mutation rate and cancer. Proc Natl Acad Sci U S A 1996;93:14800–3.
19. Risitano AM, Maciejewski JP, Green S, et al. In-vivo dominant immune responses in aplastic anaemia: molecular tracking of putatively pathogenetic T-cell clones by TCR beta-CDR3 sequencing. Lancet 2004;364:355–64.
20. Zeng W, Kajigaya S, Chen G, et al. Transcript profile of CD4+ and CD8 + T cells from the bone marrow of acquired aplastic anemia patients. Exp Hematol 2004; 32:806–14.
21. Zeng W, Chen G, Kajigaya S, et al. Gene expression profiling in CD34 cells to identify differences between aplastic anemia patients and healthy volunteers. Blood 2004;103:325–32.
22. Sloand E, Kim S, Maciejewski JP, et al. Intracellular interferon-gamma in circulating and marrow T cells detected by flow cytometry and the response to immunosuppressive therapy in patients with aplastic anemia. Blood 2002;100: 1185–91.
23. Mori H, Colman SM, Xiao Z, et al. Chromosome translocations and covert leukemic clones are generated during normal fetal development. Proc Natl Acad Sci U S A 2002;99:8242–7.
24. Dufour C, Corcione A, Svahn J, et al. Interferon gamma and tumour necrosis factor α are overexpressed in bone marrow T lymphocytes from paediatric patients with aplastic anaemia. Br J Haematol 2001;115:1023–31.
25. Dufour C, Corcione A, Svahn J, et al. TNF-{alpha} and IFN-{gamma} are over expressed in the bone marrow of Fanconi anemia patients and TNF-{alpha} suppresses erythropoiesis in vitro. Blood 2003;102:2053–9.
26. Whitney MA, Royle G, Low MJ, et al. Germ cell defects and hematopoietic hypersensitivity to γ-interferon in mice with a targeted disruption of the Fanconi anemia C gene. Blood 1996;88:49–58.
27. Pigullo S, Ferretti E, Lanciotti M, et al. Human Fanconi A cells are susceptible to TRAIL-induced apoptosis. Br J Haematol 2007;136:315–8.
28. Haneline LS, Broxmeyer HE, Cooper S, et al. Multiple inhibitory cytokines induce deregulated progenitor growth and apoptosis in hematopoietic cells from FAC -/- mice. Blood 1998;91:4092–8.

29. Zhang XL, Li J, Sejas DP, et al. The Fanconi anemia proteins functionally interact with the protein kinase regulated by RNA (PKR). J Biol Chem 2004;279:43910–9.

30. Bijangi-Vishehsaraei K, Saadatzadeh MR, Werne A, et al. Enhanced TNF-α-induced apoptosis in Fanconi anemia type C-deficient cells is dependent on apoptosis signal-regulating kinase 1. Blood 2005;106:4124–30.

31. Sejas DP, Rani R, Qiu Y, et al. Inflammatory reactive oxygen species-mediated hemopoietic suppression in Fancc-deficient mice. J Immunol 2007;178:5277–87.

32. Dror Y, Freedman MH. Shwachman-Diamond syndrome marrow cells show abnormally increased apoptosis mediated through the Fas pathway. Blood 2001;97:3011–6.

33. Kollner I, Sodeik B, Schreek S, et al. Mutations in neutrophil elastase causing congenital neutropenia lead to cytoplasmic protein accumulation and induction of the unfolded protein response. Blood 2006;108:493–500.

34. Yoon A, Peng G, Brandenburg Y, et al. Impaired control of IRES-mediated translation in X-linked dyskeratosis congenita. Science 2006;312:902–6.

35. Lo Ten Foe JR, Kwee ML, Rooimans MA, et al. Somatic mosaicism in Fanconi anemia: molecular basis and clinical significance. Eur J Hum Genet 1997;5: 137–48.

36. Mankad A, Taniguchi T, Cox B, et al. Natural gene therapy in monozygotic twins with Fanconi anemia. Blood 2006;107:3084–90.

37. Gregory JJ Jr, Wagner JE, Verlander PC, et al. Somatic mosaicism in Fanconi anemia: evidence of genotypic reversion in lymphohematopoietic stem cells. Proc Natl Acad Sci U S A 2001;98:2532–7.

38. Kearns WG, Sutton JF, Maciejewski JP, et al. Genomic instability in bone marrow failure syndromes. Am J Hematol 2004;76:220–4.

39. Sloand EM, Pfannes L, Chen G, et al. CD34 cells from patients with trisomy 8 myelodysplastic syndrome (MDS) express early apoptotic markers but avoid programmed cell death by up-regulation of antiapoptotic proteins. Blood 2007;109: 2399–405.

40. Sloand EM, Yong AS, Ramkissoon S, et al. Granulocyte colony-stimulating factor preferentially stimulates proliferation of monosomy 7 cells bearing the isoform IV receptor. Proc Natl Acad Sci U S A 2006;103:14483–8.

41. Lensch MW, Rathbun RK, Olson SB, et al. Selective pressure as an essential force in molecular evolution of myeloid leukemic clones: a view from the window of Fanconi anemia. Leukemia 1999;13:1784–9.

42. Haneline LS, Li X, Ciccone SL, et al. Retroviral-mediated expression of recombinant Fancc enhances the repopulating ability of Fancc -/- hematopoietic stem cells and decreases the risk of clonal evolution. Blood 2003;101:1299–307.

43. Kamarajan P, Sun NK, Chao CC. Up-regulation of FLIP in cisplatin-selected HeLa cells causes cross-resistance to CD95/Fas death signalling. Biochem J 2003; 376:253–60.

44. Liu TX, Becker MW, Jelinek J, et al. Chromosome 5q deletion and epigenetic suppression of the gene encoding alpha-catenin (CTNNA1) in myeloid cell transformation. Nat Med 2007;13:78–83.

45. Ades L, Mary JY, Robin M, et al. Long-term outcome after bone marrow transplantation for severe aplastic anemia. Blood 2004;103:2490–7.

46. Kahl C, Leisenring W, Deeg HJ, et al. Cyclophosphamide and antithymocyte globulin as a conditioning regimen for allogeneic marrow transplantation in patients with aplastic anaemia: a long-term follow-up. Br J Haematol 2005;130: 747–51.

47. Kennedy-Nasser AA, Leung KS, Mahajan A, et al. Comparable outcomes of matched-related and alternative donor stem cell transplantation for pediatric severe aplastic anemia. Biol Blood Marrow Transplant 2006;12:1277–84.
48. Maciejewski JP, Risitano A, Sloand EM, et al. Distinct clinical outcomes for cytogenetic abnormalities evolving from aplastic anemia. Blood 2002;99:3129–35.
49. Viollier R, Tichelli A. Predictive factors for cure after immunosuppressive therapy of aplastic anemia. Acta Haematol 2000;103:55–62.
50. Kojima S, Ohara A, Tsuchida M, et al. Risk factors for evolution of acquired aplastic anemia into myelodysplastic syndrome and acute myeloid leukemia after immunosuppressive therapy in children. Blood 2002;100:786–90.
51. Rosenfeld S, Follmann D, Nunez O, et al. Antithymocyte globulin and cyclosporine for severe aplastic anemia: association between hematologic response and long-term outcome. JAMA 2003;289:1130–5.
52. Saracco P, Quarello P, Iori AP, et al. Cyclosporin A response and dependence in children with acquired aplastic anaemia: a multicentre retrospective study with long-term observation follow-up. Br J Haematol 2008;140:197–205.
53. Marsh J. Making therapeutic decisions in adults with aplastic anemia. Hematology Am Soc Hematol Educ Program 2006;78–85.
54. Guinan EC. Aplastic anemia: management of pediatric patients. Hematology 2005;2005:104–9.
55. Maciejewski JP, Selleri C, Sato T, et al. Increased expression of Fas antigen on bone marrow CD34+ cells of patients with aplastic anaemia. Br J Haematol 1995;91:245–52.
56. Yamazaki E, Kanamori H, Taguchi J, et al. The evidence of clonal evolution with monosomy 7 in aplastic anemia following granulocyte colony-stimulating factor using the polymerase chain reaction. Blood Cells Mol Dis 1997;23:213–8.
57. Bloom ML, Wolk AG, Simon-Stoos KL, et al. A mouse model of lymphocyte infusion-induced bone marrow failure. Exp Hematol 2004;32:1163–72.
58. Gondek LP, Tiu R, O'Keefe CL, et al. Chromosomal lesions and uniparental disomy detected by SNP arrays in MDS, MDS/MPD, and MDS-derived AML. Blood 2008;111:1534–42.
59. Bacigalupo A, Locatelli F, Lanino E, et al. Fludarabine, cyclophosphamide and anti-thymocyte globulin for alternative donor transplants in acquired severe aplastic anemia: a report from the EBMT-SAA Working Party. Bone Marrow Transplant 2005;36:947–50.
60. Deeg HJ, Amylon ID, Harris RE, et al. Marrow transplants from unrelated donors for patients with aplastic anemia: minimum effective dose of total body irradiation. Biol Blood Marrow Transplant 2001;7:208–15.
61. Deeg HJ, O'Donnell M, Tolar J, et al. Optimization of conditioning for marrow transplantation from unrelated donors for patients with aplastic anemia after failure of immunosuppressive therapy. Blood 2006;108:1485–91.
62. Gupta V, Ball SE, Sage D, et al. Marrow transplants from matched unrelated donors for aplastic anaemia using alemtuzumab, fludarabine and cyclophosphamide based conditioning. Bone Marrow Transplant 2005;35:467–71.
63. Kang HJ, Shin HY, Choi HS, et al. Fludarabine, cyclophosphamide plus thymoglobulin conditioning regimen for unrelated bone marrow transplantation in severe aplastic anemia. Bone Marrow Transplant 2004;34:939–43.
64. Maury S, Balere-Appert ML, Chir Z, et al. Unrelated stem cell transplantation for severe acquired aplastic anemia: improved outcome in the era of high-resolution HLA matching between donor and recipient. Haematologica 2007;92:589–96.

65. Viollier R, Socie G, Tichelli A, et al. Recent improvement in outcome of unrelated donor transplantation for aplastic anemia. Bone Marrow Transplant 2008;41:45–50.

66. Yagasaki H, Takahashi Y, Kudo K, et al. Feasibility and results of bone marrow transplantation from an HLA-mismatched unrelated donor for children and young adults with acquired severe aplastic anemia. Int J Hematol 2007;85:437–42.

67. Yoshimi A, Kojima S, Taniguchi S, et al. Unrelated cord blood transplantation for severe aplastic anemia. Biol Blood Marrow Transplant 2008;14:1057–63.

68. Elliott MJ, Maini RN, Feldmann M, et al. Randomised double-blind comparison of chimeric monoclonal antibody to tumour necrosis factor alpha (cA2) versus placebo in rheumatoid arthritis. LANCET 1994;344:1105–10.

69. Furst DE, Schiff MH, Fleischmann RM, et al. Adalimumab, a fully human anti tumor necrosis factor-alpha monoclonal antibody, and concomitant standard anti-rheumatic therapy for the treatment of rheumatoid arthritis: results of STAR (Safety Trial of Adalimumab in Rheumatoid Arthritis). J Rheumatol 2003;30:2563–71.

70. Lipsky PE, van der Heijde DM, St Clair EW, et al. Infliximab and methotrexate in the treatment of rheumatoid arthritis. Anti-Tumor Necrosis Factor Trial in Rheumatoid Arthritis with Concomitant Therapy Study Group. N Engl J Med 2000;343:1594–602.

71. Peyrin-Biroulet L, Deltenre P, de SN, Branche J, et al. Efficacy and safety of tumor necrosis factor antagonists in Crohn's disease: meta-analysis of placebo-controlled trials. Clin Gastroenterol Hepatol 2008;6:644–53.

72. Saad AA, Symmons DP, Noyce PR, et al. Risks and benefits of tumor necrosis factor-alpha inhibitors in the management of psoriatic arthritis: systematic review and metaanalysis of randomized controlled trials. J Rheumatol 2008;35:883–90.

73. Dufour C, Giacchino R, Ghezzi P, et al. Etanercept as a salvage treatment for refractory aplastic anemia. Pediatr Blood Cancer 2008;52:522–5.

74. Lee HY, Youn SW, Kim JY, et al. FOXO3a turns the tumor necrosis factor receptor signaling towards apoptosis through reciprocal regulation of c-Jun N-terminal kinase and NF-kappaB. Arterioscler Thromb Vasc Biol 2008;28:112–20.

75. Miyamoto K, Araki KY, Naka K, et al. Foxo3a is essential for maintenance of the hematopoietic stem cell pool. Cell Stem Cell 2007;1:101–12.

76. Larrick JW, Wright SC. Cytotoxic mechanism of tumor necrosis factor-alpha. FASEB J 1990;4:3215–23.

77. Matthews N, Neale ML, Jackson SK, et al. Tumour cell killing by tumour necrosis factor: inhibition by anaerobic conditions, free-radical scavengers and inhibitors of arachidonate metabolism. Immunology 1987;62:153–5.

78. Yamauchi N, Kuriyama H, Watanabe N, et al. Intracellular hydroxyl radical production induced by recombinant human tumor necrosis factor and its implication in the killing of tumor cells in vitro. Cancer Res 1989;49:1671–5.

79. Zimmerman RJ, Chan A, Leadon SA. Oxidative damage in murine tumor cells treated in vitro by recombinant human tumor necrosis factor. Cancer Res 1989;49:1644–8.

80. Delhalle S, Deregowski V, Benoit V, et al. NF-kappaB-dependent MnSOD expression protects adenocarcinoma cells from TNF-alpha-induced apoptosis. Oncogene 2002;21:3917–24.

81. Brennan FM, McInnes IB. Evidence that cytokines play a role in rheumatoid arthritis. J Clin Invest 2008;118:3537–45.

82. Zhang X, Sejas DP, Qiu Y, et al. Inflammatory ROS promote and cooperate with the Fanconi anemia mutation for hematopoietic senescence. J Cell Sci 2007;120:1572–83.

Index

Note: Page numbers of article titles are in **boldface** type.

A

Aase syndrome, 264
Acquired aplastic anemia, antithymocyte globulin in, horse versus rabbit, 162
  bone marrow transplantation in, 164–166
  classification of, by severity, 172
  clinical symptoms of, 159
  clonal evolution of, 163, 363, 365
  cord blood transplants in, 166
  cyclosporin dependence in, 162
  diagnosis of, 159–160
    and treatment of, **159–170**
  differential diagnosis of, 174–175
  differentiation from hypoplastic myelodysplasia syndrome, 347–348
  first-line therapy in, 166–167
  hypoplastic myelodysplasia syndrome arising from, 350–351
  immunosuppressive treatment in, 161–164
    for older patients, 164
    pregnancies after, 164
    response to, 163–164
  in childhood, **171–191**
    hematopoietic stem cell transplantation in, 177–178
      complications of, 178–179
    immunosuppressive therapy of, 179–182
      response after, 172, 173
    management of, 175–182
    supportive care in, 176
  overproduction of cytokines in, 366
  paroxysmal nocturnal hemoglobinuria and, 334, 337–338, 339
  pathogenesis of, 363
  pathophysiology of, 172–174
  presentation of, 171–172
  relapse in, 162
  supportive care in, 160–161
  surveillance guidelines and, 369
  treatment of, 160–164
    designing strategy for, 161
    growth factors in, 162–163
Anemia(s), acquired aplastic. See *Acquired aplastic anemia.*
  Diamond-Blackfan. See *Diamond-Blackfan anemia.*
  dyserythropoietic. See *Dyserythropoietic anemias.*
  Fanconi. See *Fanconi anemia.*

Hematol Oncol Clin N Am 23 (2009) 377–382
doi:10.1016/S0889-8588(09)00054-9
0889-8588/09/$ – see front matter © 2009 Elsevier Inc. All rights reserved.

hemonc.theclinics.com

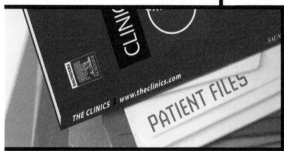

Moving?

Make sure your subscription moves with you!

To notify us of your new address, find your **Clinics Account Number** (located on your mailing label above your name), and contact customer service at:

E-mail: elspcs@elsevier.com

800-654-2452 (subscribers in the U.S. & Canada)
314-453-7041 (subscribers outside of the U.S. & Canada)

Fax number: 314-523-5170

Elsevier Periodicals Customer Service
11830 Westline Industrial Drive
St. Louis, MO 63146

*To ensure uninterrupted delivery of your subscription, please notify us at least 4 weeks in advance of move.